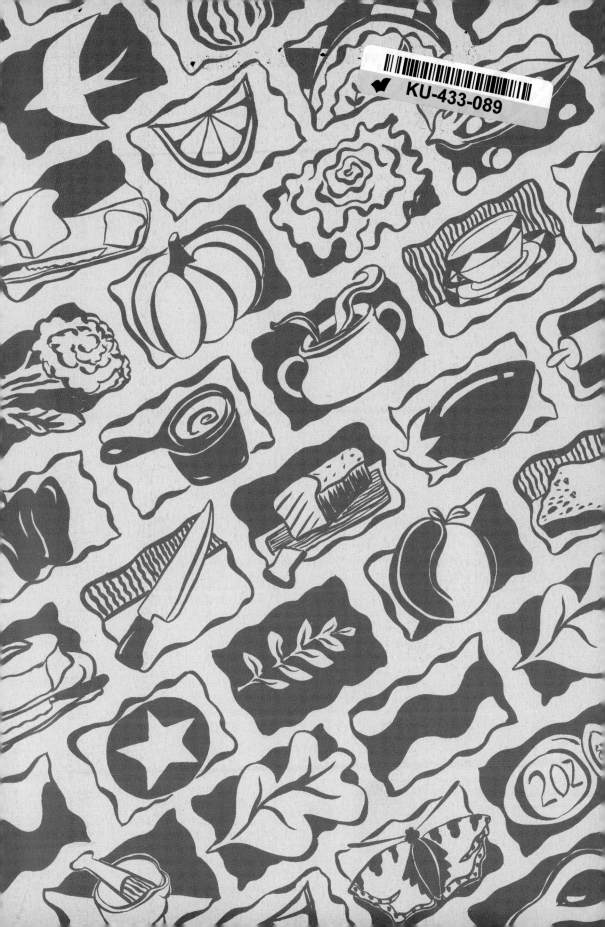

KU-433-089

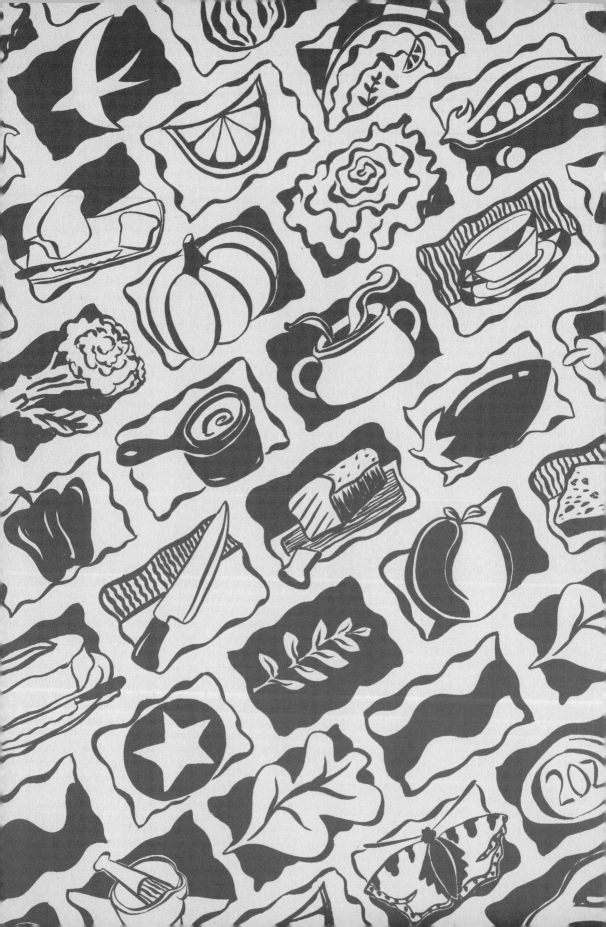

Daverick Leggett

Recipes for Self-Healing

Illustrations and design by
Katheryn Trenshaw

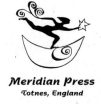

Meridian Press
Totnes, England

Acclaim for *Recipes for Self-Healing:*

A fabulous wealth of wisdom offered with clarity and wit. Daverick Leggett has written in a style that offers real understanding and insight into this fascinating approach to health and wellbeing. The recipes are lovely and make you want to get started right away! *Recipes for Self-Healing* has wonderful accessible information for the intellect, tasty delicious food for the body and wit and levity for the spirit – the complete mind, body, spirit experience.

Jane Sen, author of *The Healing Foods Cookbook*

Daverick Leggett's book is a timely addition to the increasing information in the West about Chinese medicine. In China everyone instinctively knows which foods are appropriate for a healthy life. We have lost this connection in the West. Daverick's book is a reminder of its simplicity.

Building upon solid foundations of Chinese medicine, he comprehensively lists recipes which will nourish our souls as well as our bodies. These recipes are the practical application in the modern world of a 5,000 year old medical tradition. In our increasingly frantic world such wisdoms are greatly needed. This book will be of great benefit to everyone interested in health and developing a healthy way of living.

Dr. Stephen Gascoigne, M.B., Ch.B., C.Ac., Dip. C.H.M., acupuncturist and herbalist

Everyone will love this book because it is about something close to everyone's heart – food! And not just food, nourishment. It is about getting and staying healthy by eating and enjoying delicious foods which suit you the individual; not your doctor, or your spouse, or your mother or the architect of the latest diet fad. It's about self exploration and self understanding and appropriate self nourishment the way Chinese medicine sees it.

Jane Lyttleton, traditional Chinese medicine practitioner and author, Australia

This wonderful book offers words and wisdom – the intelligence and poetry of Chinese medicine reframed for modern life – to cultivate your own capacity to nourish yourself and others in accord with the unique circumstances of TODAY. What a blessing and joy!

Edward Espe Brown, author of the *Tassajara Bread Book* and *Tomato Blessings and Radish Teachings*

A book we've been waiting for! It provides a rich source of information on many aspects of Chinese medicine especially in relation to food and diet. It is a user friendly resource for practitioners, patients and all those interested in Chinese dietary therapy and combines the Chinese principles of diet in relation to foods which are easily available in the west.

Angela Hicks, author of *The Principles of Chinese Medicine* and co-founder of The College of Integrated Chinese Medicine

'Daverick's descriptions of the Chinese medical system are both simple yet profound; his explanation of the crucial balance of our ability to receive and transform as the key to our health are enlightening. But this book is much more than that. *Recipes for Self-Healing* has inspired me to see diet in a totally new way, and has given me the tools necessary to truly use food as medicine. This is a great gift. By following the recipes and engaging actively with our own healing processes, we can begin to take responsibility for our own health. This is the first step towards true healing.'

Sandra Hill, author of *Reclaiming the Wisdom of the Body* and co-author of *A Guide to Acupuncture.*

Acclaim for *Helping Ourselves*, Daverick Leggett, Meridian Press, 1994

'There are other guides to Chinese dietary therapy on the market, but none that I have seen makes the subject so readily accessible.'

Simon Fielding, *European Journal of Oriental Medicine*

'The thing I most like about the presentation of this book is its simplicity. In the introduction the author says that the book is intended both as a learning resource for students and clients of traditional Chinese medicine and as a reference manual for practitioners. In my opinion it succeeds brilliantly in both instances: it explains Chinese energy concepts... in terms that most lay people would understand.'

Altair de Almeida, *Traditional Acupuncture Society News*

'Helping Ourselves takes two important steps towards making Chinese food energetics accessible. Firstly, it is extremely easy to read and explains Chinese energy concepts such as the Spleen, Yin, Yang, Cold, Hot and Damp in terms most lay people would understand. Secondly, it classifies the foods into what they do energetically so you can easily look up which foods help to resolve Dampness and which foods are cooling. To my knowledge this has not been done in English before.'

Bill Palmer, *Shiatsu Society News*

'I particularly like that by using this book we can advise patients to take positive action and enhance their treatment by adding certain foods to their diet, as well as excluding others. It is a useful book to have in practice and I use it regularly.'

Sally Blades, acupuncturist

'Helping Ourselves is a relatively short introduction to the basic principles of Chinese dietary therapy... the foods discussed are easily available and the writing intelligent, clear and concise.'

Peter Deadman, *Journal of Traditional Chinese Medicine*

Disclaimer

Whilst every attempt has been made to present information safely and accurately, this book is only as good as its author. Furthermore, Chinese medicine itself has its limitations and its own internal contradictions and inconsistencies. Readers are therefore encouraged to test the information and ideas of this book against their own experience and to trust their own body knowing. It is profoundly difficult to self-diagnose, especially from a book, and readers are encouraged to actively seek the support and advice of a qualified health professional. This book is not intended as a replacement for such guidance nor may the author or publisher be found responsible for any adverse effects resulting from the use of suggestions in this book.

Acknowledgments and thanks

I would like to acknowledge the help of my partner, Katheryn Trenshaw, who not only produced all the illustrations and conceived the book's design, but also believed passionately in it, and in me, at every stage. My thanks also to Cynthia Trenshaw, my friend and mother-in-law, who generously edited the book with remarkable skill and insight. Thank you to Peter Deadman, Angela Hicks and Sally Blades who read the first manuscript and helped me sharpen the text considerably. Thanks also to Bridget Long for her generous help and advice with the book's design and Jonathan Coleclough for his skilled work on the layout. I am grateful too to all the friends who helped with the testing and shared in the eating of the recipes. Lastly I am thankful for my son, Orion Reed, whose arrival in my life slowed the progress of this book long enough for it to ripen and mature.

Meridian Press PO Box 3, Totnes, Devon TQ9 5WJ; tel/fax: 01803 863552 · e-mail: post@meridianpress.net; website: www.meridianpress.net

First published by Meridian Press 1999. Reprinted 2001.

© 1999 Daverick Leggett

Daverick Leggett asserts the moral right to be identified as the author of this work

A catalogue record for this book is available from the British Library

ISBN 0 9524 640 2 0

Printed and bound in Great Britain by Biddles Limited, Guildford

All rights reserved. No part of this publication may be reproduced, stored in a retrieval system, or transmitted, in any form or by any means, electronic, mechanical, photocopying, recording or otherwise, without the prior permission of the publishers.

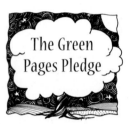

The Green Pages Pledge

Books are made from trees. At all stages of the production of this book care has been taken to minimise the environmental impact: recycled and scrap paper was used for all stages up to publication; printing has been done on recycled paper; packaging has made full use of reclaimed and recycled material; all waste paper has been re-used or recycled. In addition, the author makes a commitment that a percentage of the profits from the sale of this book will be used to plant new trees at least equivalent to the total paper use involved in all aspects of its publication and distribution

Notice how each particle moves,
notice how everyone has arrived here from a journey,
notice how each wants a different food
and how each streams towards the ocean

Rumi

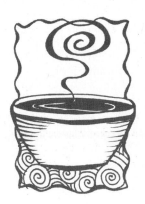

About the author

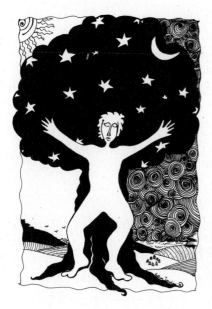

Daverick Leggett BA Hons PGCE MRSS began his working life on a smallholding, growing and producing much of his own food. After five years working as a school teacher he trained in Shiatsu and Qi Gong, which he has practised since the late 1980's. Since then he has become an experienced practitioner and respected teacher. He is committed to self-help and empowering those he works with on their unique path to healing. He teaches Qi Gong, nutrition and traditional Chinese medicine throughout Britain. His first book, *Helping Ourselves*, was published in 1994. Daverick lives with his wife and son in Devon, England.

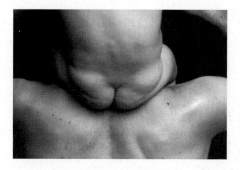

I dedicate this book to my mother and
father who fed and nourished me,

And to my son Orion Reed for whom I
now do the same.

May all be nourished.

Contents

Part Three
Recipes for Self-Healing

Part Four
Leftovers

Foreword

When I opened Daverick Leggett's *Recipes for Self-Healing* for the first time, the book fell open to the section on coffee. In the few words I read, I was amazed at how precisely he had captured the meaning of nutrition and food in Chinese traditional medicine. I knew immediately that I would like this man and his philosophy of healing.

Practitioners of Chinese medicine have debated fiercely whether coffee is 'cold' or 'warming.' Mr. Leggett has resolved it. He presents a unique understanding of the body's complex response to coffee and of the energetic forces at work: coffee, he demonstrates, is both heating and cooling – as a result of its own nature, as well as the nature and condition of the person ingesting it.

Throughout the beautifully written *Recipes for Self-Healing*, Mr. Leggett reminds us that Chinese medicine cannot be described in black or white. Yin and Yang are not fixed entities, and always exist in relationship to one another. *Recipes for Self-Healing* reflects the philosophical strengths of Chinese medicine.

No one could create the perfect diet pill that balances the energetics, flavours, and natures of food needed to achieve wholeness and harmony. Food energetics are not simply the result of chemistry – they are also a result of spiritual forces. The power of food – positive and negative – to influence the mind/body/spirit is affected by how it is prepared, served and eaten. A balanced diet results from the combination of the foods ingested, the way they are prepared and how a person thinks about and eats the food.

Food prepared as a gift, served calmly, eaten with respect and digested in a harmonious atmosphere bestows positive benefits. Food thrown together without regard or with resentment, in a hurry, gobbled down, or eaten while driving, watching TV or even reading cannot be assimilated healthfully.

In our food-obsessed, food-unhealthy culture, it's easy to misinterpret the traditional Chinese medicine perspective on diet. Daverick Leggett helps the reader understand that the traditional Chinese view of diet and nutrition is about creating balance and harmony using a flexible approach to how we eat. There are no 'bad' or 'good' foods. There are only foods that have certain natures, energetics, and flavours. Chinese medicine is traditionally about choosing moderation to maintain wellness and wholeness, and Mr. Leggett reflects this stance throughout the book. He also makes choosing and cooking food clear and readable as well as a fun process.

Recipes for Self-Healing should find a wide audience. It is a useful work which can help anyone who eats food or has an interest in nutrition. I am personally recommending it to my clients, because I believe diet and nutrition are the bottom line for maintaining wellness, wholeness, balance, and harmony.

Thank you, Daverick Leggett, for giving us such an inspiring and useful tool as part of our constant struggle to achieve individual and planetary health.

Misha Ruth Cohen O.M.D.
San Francisco, May 1999

Founder and clinical director of Chicken Soup Chinese Medicine

Author of *The Chinese Way to Healing: Many Paths to Wholeness,
The HIV Wellness An East/West Guide to Living Well with HIV/AIDS,*
and *The Ultimate Hep C Help Book*

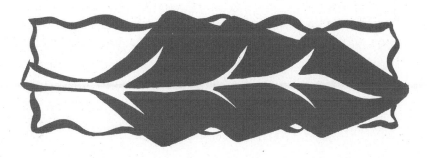

Introduction

The true spirit of traditional Chinese medicine is a living one and it is in this spirit that this book is written. As a westerner I have been drawn to an oriental philosophy and healing system because it offers something I have not found in my own back yard: a coherent, living vision of the world as energy, and a poetic and metaphorical language to express this perception. It suits me, because to perceive the world as energy is natural to me and has been so since childhood; and, besides, I am more inclined towards poetry than science.

I am, however, not Chinese and have no ambition to live anywhere other than the beautiful and sacred landscape of Devon, England. Nor am I interested in living or eating like a Chinese person. So in bringing the profound insights and wisdom of traditional Chinese medicine into my own culture my interest has been to understand how this extraordinary understanding can take root here and become native, how it can enrich rather than supplant my own culture and traditions. For this reason, the suggestions in this book for healing ourselves and eating our way to health are based on primarily western foods and lifestyle practices.

In this book you will find the ideas of eastern medicine explained and interpreted in a western light. I hope that I have sufficiently managed to liberate the ideas of traditional Chinese medicine from their cultural context to make them useful and directly relevant to the western world. I also hope that I have managed to do this without dishonouring their tradition or misrepresenting the ideas through the limitations of my own culture-bound vision.

In presenting these ideas about food I have sought to apply the principles of food energetics to a western cuisine. Most of the ingredients will be familiar and homely and some will reflect the cosmopolitan nature of our eating. Every now and then I have suggested the use of a more unusual ingredient because of its special value. Nevertheless, you should be able to find in your local shops almost any of the ingredients in this book.

The key question in deciding what to eat is not 'What is the best diet?' but 'What is the best diet for me?' or, more precisely, 'What are my constitutional patterns and what are the conditions prevailing in my life and my body today?' What works for one person may not work for another. One man's meat, as the saying goes, is another man's poison. To get the most from this book you will need to understand your own energetic tendencies. Reading the book will take you part way there; but if you are not already familiar with traditional Chinese medicine as a practitioner, or as a student or recipient, it will probably help if you seek out the assistance of a qualified practitioner skilled in traditional diagnosis.

The recipes that form the second part of this book are designed to help you eat according to your own unique needs. If, for example, you are working with a pattern of 'Spleen Qi Deficiency' in your life, you will find several recipes that suit you perfectly. The measure of whether a recipe is right for you is that you can expect to feel good afterwards. Once you have found recipes that work for you, you can apply the principles to recipes of your own making. There is no limit to the number of new recipes you can create.

You can be further helped in this by getting hold of a copy of either the wallchart *The Energetics of Food* and/or the companion volume to this book *Helping Ourselves*. The chart and book list the properties of about three hundred common foods and will enable you to choose ingredients that are well-suited to your individual needs. Both are available from Meridian Press.

Words committed to print tend to become somehow fixed as truth. The recipes in this book are not 'cures' but rather part of a style of eating that, in my judgment, is suited to certain kinds of people and conditions. This book is an adventure and an exploration of how the principles of traditional Chinese medicine and food energetics can be applied in our daily lives. I invite you to test its ideas against your own experience and find your own way of working with the information and principles offered here. I encourage you to be creative in the kitchen and use the recipes as starting points to spin off into your own creations. The principles of a tradition may not change over millennia but the tradition is kept alive only by constant reinterpretation in the light of experience. It is in the creative human spirit that a tradition lives on and its death begins the moment it is 'fixed in stone'.

It must be said that the main ingredient of any recipe never finds its way into a recipe book. Cinema goers may have seen the film 'Like Water for Chocolate'. In this sumptuous film the cook's tears, laughter and desire are at different times infused into the meal, causing hilarious results at the dinner table. It is not mere fancy that the energy with which food is prepared is infused into the meal. From the viewpoint of energy medicine, the Qi of the cook is transmitted to the food and this, in turn, is received through eating.

Cooking is an alchemical process. To liberate the nourishment from food the Qi of the cook must impregnate the food, interacting with the flavours to generate a nourishing message. The energy that goes into creating the ingredients is important too: the grower and the retailer are part of the story. Organically grown food sold by people who know and care about their food carries that caring message to our kitchens. I encourage you to support organic growers and, if you have the opportunity, to grow some of your own food.

Lastly, in using these recipes, I encourage you to relax and have fun in the kitchen. This is your own secret ingredient that no one else can copy. Certainly no one can put it in a recipe book.

Bon appetit

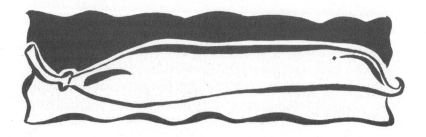

How to use this book

This book may be read from beginning to end, although, like most books, it certainly wasn't written like that. You do not need to read it in that way for it to be useful. You may, for example, simply be trying to understand a particular health pattern such as Kidney Yang Deficiency. If this is the case, first use the contents page to lead you to the section on the Kidney, then the section on Yang Deficiency. If you are looking for suitable recipes, browse through the recipe section to find recipes that match the condition of Kidney Yang Deficiency. Recipes that either strengthen the Kidney or strengthen the Yang will also be helpful.

The recipe index will lead you to recipes that contain a particular food. Alternatively you may simply want to read this as a recipe book or as a stimulus for recipe ideas. In this case, simply browse the recipe index or go directly to the recipe section. The recipes are all tried-and-tested and delicious. They don't taste like medicine! And once you try the recipes, you may want to return to the text to learn more about the principles that underlie them. So feel free to dip in or read it front to back or back to front. However you choose to read it, may it nourish and inspire you.

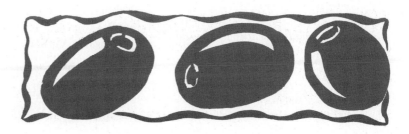

Glossary

Acupoint: a location on the body's surface where pressure, needling or heat is commonly applied to effect change in a person's energy system

Blood: close in meaning to the western concept of blood, a measure of the quality of nourishment available in the body

Bodymind: this term is used to indicate the inseparable nature of body and mind

Cold: a condition of too much cold energy located in the body

Dampness: a condition of too much moisture located in the body

Dan Tian: an energy centre, literally 'field of elixir', one of three centres located in the lower belly, chest or brow

Deficiency: the lack of some substance or function necessary for full health

Essence: (see **Jing**)

Excess: the presence of too much substance or activity which overloads the body

Feng Shui: the art of perceiving the subtle forces of place and their beneficial or negative influence on human life

Heat: a condition of too much hot energy located in the body

Jiao: literally 'burning space', one of the three divisions of the torso into lower, middle and upper sections

Jing (Essence): the fundamental substance from which physical life is created, in part inherited from the blending of man's and woman's energy at conception and in part extracted from air, food and drink

Meridian: part of a network of energy pathways linking all parts of the body

Moxa: the herb mugwort which is burned on or above the body to infuse heat and energy into the system

Organ: a related group of functions and associated structures; clearly different from the western meaning and including expressions at the physical, emotional, mental and spiritual level

Pathogen: an invasive agent such as a virus or bacteria

Phlegm: a congealed form of Dampness, Phlegm may be both substantial and insubstantial manifesting literally as mucus in the lungs but may also manifest as lumps under the skin, blockage in the meridians, stones in the kidney and gallbladder, deformity in the joints, lymphatic congestion and fibroids

Qi: subtle energy, the animating force, similar to 'prana' in Ayurvedic philosophy

Qi Gong: the art of cultivating the subtle energy, Qi, through movement, posture, breath and attention

Shen: consciousness, mind or spirit; the radiance of the spirit shining through the physical body

Shiatsu: Japanese system of applying pressure and stretching to the body to benefit the flow of Qi in the meridians; used both for relaxation and healing

Stagnation: a condition of congestion, impaired flow of Qi or Blood

Syndrome: a collection of related signs and symptoms that indicate a particular pattern of disharmony in the human being

Tai Ji: a branch of Qi Gong consisting of sequences of flowing movements

Traditional Chinese Medicine: a comprehensive system of medicine comprising diet, herbs, acupuncture, bodywork and exercise, used by 25% of the world's population, extensively systematised in the twentieth century

Wind: disturbing symptoms which literally behave like wind in nature, e.g., quick to arise, erratic and affecting the uppermost parts of the body more dramatically

Yin & Yang: complementary natural forces whose dynamic balance is vital for full health

Part One

Nourishment

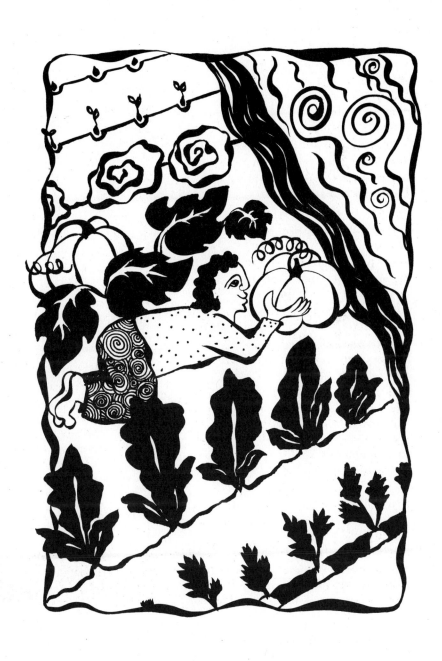

**Food is an
important part
of a balanced diet**

Fran Lebowitz

Chapter One

Perspectives on Nourishment

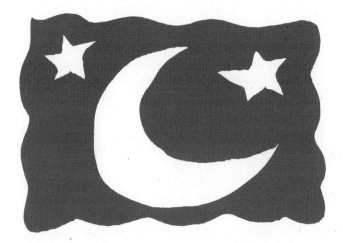

A Cosmic Perspective

In Chinese medicine the human being is seen as a small working model of the universe. The same natural laws that govern the movements of the stars and planets, the weather and the seasons govern the human body and the human journey through life. All things are connected: in every small part or every small event are reflected the workings of a vast cosmos; the microcosm contains the macrocosm. These assumptions underlie everything in this book.

The language of health in traditional Chinese medicine is the language of weather and landscape: we talk of Wind, Heat, Cold or Dampness invading the body, of drought or over-saturation, of problems with the Fire or Water elements. This simple poetic language grows out of centuries of observation of the natural laws of life. Our inner worlds connect with the outer world in both subtle and obvious ways. The sun warms us, the earth feeds us, the breeze feels good on our cheeks and the flowers awaken our delight. We

To see a World in a Grain of Sand

And a Heaven in a Wild Flower

Hold Infinity in the palm of your hand

And Eternity in an hour

William Blake, *Auguries of Innocence*

are connected too by more subtle principles of resonance: our organs resonate with particular planets, our acupoints[1] and meridians vibrate in harmony with stars, and our bodies respond to the subtle essences and vibrations of food in ways that are beyond ordinary perception. These subtle resonances were mapped by the ancient Chinese and continue to be mapped to this day.

In Chinese medicine parts are not just fragments without which the whole is incomplete – parts are also complete in themselves, holographic replicas of the whole. Every event in the life of the body is described not in isolation but in terms of its relatedness to the whole. A hot rash on the face, for example, may be more than a simple event in the local tissues: it is one part of an immensely more complex event in the inner and outer landscapes. All the conditions of the particular time must be considered. Each instance of dysfunction and wellness is felt throughout the whole life web.

Because each part of a person is interconnected with all others, treating any problem in isolation is a mistake. A person whose gall bladder has stopped functioning is not cured by its surgical removal. This is simply 'shooting the messenger'. Modern western medicine lacks a systems model and does not put whatever is happening in the bodymind[2] into a meaningful context. Consequently, when things go wrong, clients of western medicine are too often treated as victims, absolved of any responsibility and denied the opportunity to engage creatively with their own healing.

Although we have come a long way, especially in the realm of surgery and the creation of machinery to see into the body, much of current western orthodox medicine has more in common with warfare than with healing. The illusion that global problems go away if large enough bombs are dropped on them is the same illusion, created from the same mind, that problems of bodily health go away if strong enough drugs are dropped on them. Nowadays the bombs and the drugs are more accurate but the thinking is unchanged.

Just as each part of the body is connected to every other, so is the body connected to the mind. From the perspective of this book, body and mind are inseparable, each influencing and shaping the other. Every thought and feeling has its physical manifestation just as the events of the body generate events in our mental and emotional life.

As body and mind are connected to each other, so too are body and mind in turn connected to the environment. If we fully take on this vision of interconnectedness then we cannot separate our individual health from the health of the planet. 'Whatever befalls the earth befalls the children of the earth' says the American Indian Chief Seattle. Our health is intimately bound up with the health of the planet. Our body is the earth, and we cannot be separate from its sufferings. The poisoning of our lakes and rivers or the erosion of our soils and atmospheric gases is the poisoning and erosion of our own bodies.

> Only when the last tree has died and the last river been poisoned and the last fish has been caught will we realise that we cannot eat money
>
> Cree Indian

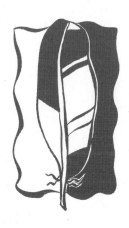

If we accept this principle of interconnectedness we may gain another perspective on some of the more difficult health problems we see today. The erosion of soil and the gases of the upper atmosphere, the deforestation, the over-consumption of resources, all resonate within our bodies. The diseases of any particular time in history reflect the health of the planet itself. The modern phenomena of deficiencies in the immune system have their parallel in the thinning of the earth's protective layer; the increase in lung conditions has its parallel in the destruction of forests; and candida in human intestines has its parallel in the overgrowth of yeast and fungus in much of the earth's soil.

If we are part of Gaia – the planet viewed holistically as a single life form – then our collective health is an expression of the planet's attempts to rebalance life itself. Like our planet and its systems, the body is constantly striving to maintain a state of homeostasis, a balance between hot and cold, activity and rest. We move always towards balance. The further we remain away from balance, the more we are stressed and the more our wholeness is threatened. Our well-being may be seen as our ability to balance the many forces in our lives, our ability to return to and hold the centre.

The ecological message of illness is rarely listened to: we are advised by our doctors to avoid overexposure to sunlight but not advised to behave responsibly towards the planet; genetic manipulation of food is viewed only in terms of its apparent short-term gain with a blind eye turned towards its ecological consequences; asthma is treated by suppressant drugs rather than by facing the need to reduce air pollution. In our individualistic culture we have lost the willingness to connect the personal to the universal.

A Cultural Perspective

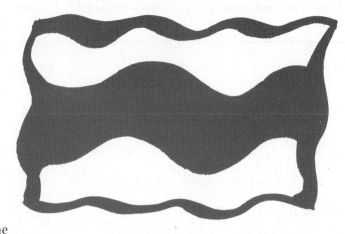

It would be naive to say that every human problem is attributable to the planet's health. We also live in specific cultures with their own lifestyles and belief systems. Many of the diseases we suffer must also be viewed in their cultural context. What is it about the physical and emotional life of the American citizen that makes that person so much more likely to die of heart disease than a Tanzanian or a Sri Lankan? Why is cancer a common cause of death in one culture but rare in another?

When we are born into a culture we take on its evolving story of health and disease. In a less industrial culture most of the threats to health may be from hunger, cold or plague. The mythology of life and death changes with the times. In indigenous society it is common for individual illnesses to be viewed as community and social problems: a person's illness carries some part of the whole community's imbalance and has a social meaning.

In a typically western society which values overwork, continual striving and overachieving, it is not surprising to see diseases of an opposite nature, such as chronic fatigue syndrome. From a cultural point of view, seeing all the people of one culture as one organism, the widespread incidence of chronic fatigue syndrome is an attempt by the organism to rebalance itself, a compensatory mechanism for the madness of over-reaching. An illness can be seen as the culture's attempt to balance its own Excesses, or Deficiencies[3] : diseases of Excess beset the United States, whose five percent of the world's population consumes twenty percent of the world's resources; diseases of Deficiency beset the Third and Fourth World caused largely by the ravenous appetites of developed countries.

The destiny of nations depends upon what and how they eat

Anthelme Brillat-Saverin, *La Physiologie du Gout*

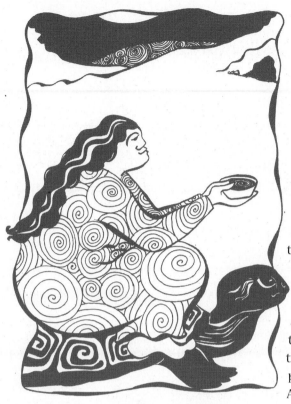

An Ancestral Perspective

Having set human well-being in the context of both planet and culture, let's look at the body familiar: the patterns of health we inherit from our families, and our ability to transform them. We inherit certain health tendencies as a kind of karma passed down from our ancestors. A seventh generation miner is likely to have different tendencies from a farmer or fisherman. Personal health is part of a continuing generational story, a pattern being played out across centuries.

As well as physical tendencies we also inherit psychological patterns from our parents and ancestors, ways of dealing with the world that have become ingrained as the 'family way'. These can be both strengths and limitations. In one family's story an age-old family recipe instructed the cook to cut the end off the ham and discard it before putting the rest in the pot. Finally, many generations on, one woman, puzzled by this apparently meaningless instruction, traced its origin. It turned out that the ancestor who devised the recipe did not have a large enough pot.[4]

In similar ways, habitual behaviours can become outdated. Let us suppose that our great-great-great-great-great-grandparents developed a behaviour of 'putting a lid on' their grief; this strategy served them well in getting through some hard times. And let's suppose that their sons and daughters adopted the same ways without finding reason to challenge them. And so it went, on down the line until it arrived into someone's life who finally said 'Hey, this family way of doing things isn't doing me any good. I'm going to try some other way'. If that person succeeds in transforming this pattern of behaviour, then balance is restored. If they don't, there may come a time in the family lineage when this behaviour has taken such deep root in the body that a generation is born with weak lungs (the organ of grieving in Chinese medicine).

Destructive behaviours, when unchallenged for too long, can become literally embodied. Part of the journey towards well-being may involve the transformation of such family patterns, a refusal to be the lineage-bearers of behaviours or attitudes that we did not choose and that do not serve us.

Biography as Biology

It has been said that 'Our biography becomes our biology'[5]. The formative experiences of our lives do not shape just our character; they also shape our bodies. Physiology, and even physical structure, is shaped in part by life experience. To a skilled health practitioner the body is a book to be read, telling its own unique story. Health is very much a product of beliefs and values, of emotional experiences and patterns of behaviour [see chapter on Qi].

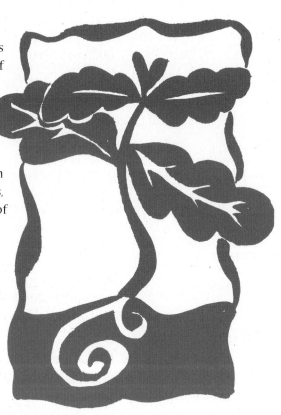

Core feelings are reflected in posture and in physiology. For example, cold hands often reflect the withdrawal of heart energy to the core, or the inability to reach out with heart to another; constant appetite may reflect unfillable needs for emotional nourishment; hunched shoulders may reflect chronic fear. However, tempting though it is to spell out laws for the correspondence of one physical condition with its matching or causative emotion, the reality is that each person's health pattern is unique. For one person a history of back trouble may correlate with her feelings of being unsupported in relationship; for another it may be that he is trying to 'put all his troubles behind him'; for another it may have been the only viable way of getting attention in the family. Each person's story is different, yet we can unlock meaning in an illness by looking at the life story.

As we go through life we process innumerable experiences. Sometimes an experience will be 'indigestible', and we won't know how to process it emotionally. What happens to that experience? Often it will try to resolve through the body. Unshed tears may try to work their way out as chronic sinus congestion; feelings of isolation and loneliness may put strain on the heart; shaming may turn into candidiasis, anger to rheumatoid arthritis, suffocating parenting to asthma. Our stories are many, and unique.

We can come to a partial understanding of biological health through an exploration of personal biography. What messages did we receive about being well or being ill? What messages did we receive about our bodies? How did health or ill-health serve us? Through such questions we may find how much we are creators of our own health; we may also find keys for the transformation of our well-being.

Finding out that they can be responsible for the creation of their health leads some people to feel that they are to blame. There is a kind of compassionless view within the 'new age' that confuses responsibility with blame. We have made the best choices we could at the time; it is useless to be angry or blaming towards ourselves once we see ways that we have helped create our own problems.

Personal responsibility has nothing to do with blame. On the contrary, the realisation of responsibility is the means by which we make the shift from victimhood to self-empowerment.

Cosmos, culture, ancestry: all are part of our health biography. The rest is choice and responsibility – lifestyle, relationship and diet – and these are the subject of this book. One of the most important steps we can take towards self-empowerment is to take responsibility for our own nourishment. This book is essentially written for those people who are taking responsibility for their own lives in this way.

To wait for the illness to develop
Before remedying it,

For the disorder to form
Before taking care of it,

Is to wait until one is thirsty
Before digging the well,

To wait for the battle
Before forging the weapons.

Is this not too late?

Su Wen

Chapter Two

The Sources of Nourishment

Food, although it is the main focus of this book, is only one aspect of human nutrition. We are also nourished by the natural and social environment in ways we may take for granted. In any consideration of nutrition we must look at these things. Air and water combine with food to make energy, blood and substances vital for our well-being. Plants, soil and rock also play their part as do stars and planets; even sound and smell can be said to be an aspect of our nourishment. Touch nourishes us too; so does sleep; so does art. We can also consider relationship as a source of nourishment, relationship both with our fellow beings and with the divine. So how do these factors play their part and what can we do to draw on all the sources of nourishment available to us?

Air

Breathing in we draw nourishment deep into the cells of our bodies; breathing out we expel stale and toxic waste. Through breath we continually revitalise ourselves, from moment to moment. When we restrict our breathing we restrict the flow of our life force. Daring to breathe means daring to experience vitality.

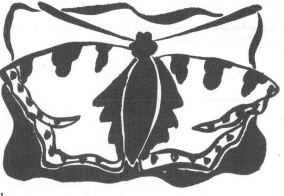

In daily life this means that we need sufficient exercise, open posture and relaxation to fully receive the nourishment of air. We may also need to teach ourselves how to breathe. For some people, reeducation of the breath is the single most potent medicine they ever experience. Its effect is to bring relaxation and deep nourishment into areas of the body previously starved. More powerful than any medicine, air affects nerve, muscle and brain profoundly.

The best teacher for this is a baby. When we watch a young child breathe we can see the soft rising and falling of the belly that shows us that the baby is using the diaphragm to breathe. The diaphragm pushes down on the belly, gently massaging the organs and drawing air deeply into the body. The belly fills first and then the chest. As adults we often restrict our breathing and experience low energy as a result. Over time we get used to this state of underfunctioning and lose access to the feelings of full vitality normally experienced as children.

This 'baby breathing' is the foundation of well-being. Once we have relearned how to breathe like a baby, we can bring mindfulness of our breath into all aspects of daily life. 'Each of us is a flower,' says the Vietnamese monk Tich Nhat Hanh, 'but sometimes our flowerness is tired and needs to be revived. We human flowers need air. If we breathe in and out deeply and consciously, we will bloom right away. We can breathe while sitting, standing, lying down or walking. And, after just a few minutes, we will be fresh enough to share our flowerness with others.'

Breath brings oxygen into the cells. It can also bring awareness to any part of the body. Whenever we need healing at a particular site

When correct breathing is practised, the myriad ailments will not occur. When breathing is depressed or strained, all sorts of diseases will arise. Those who wish to nurture their lives must first learn the correct methods of controlling the breath and balancing energy. These breathing methods can cure all ailments, great and small

Sun Si Miao

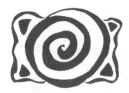

in the body we can direct the breath to that place. If, for example, a knee needs healing we can mentally send the breath there. Breathing in we send healing, breathing out we release pain or illness. This fundamental practice of uniting the breath with an intention can organise the whole being towards self-healing.

The quality of the air we breathe, of course, is important too. The practice of airing the house or going for a walk in the fresh air can revitalise. Even the simple act of bringing green plants into the house or shaking out clothes and bed linen can be helpful. If we live in the city, getting out into a park in the early morning before the traffic fumes have built up can be the best opportunity to renew ourselves through taking in the air.

Even in the city, indoor air quality may be lower than the air on the polluted street[6]. In homes, emissions from the increasing number of synthetic materials commonly used both in construction and furnishing are known to create strain on the immune system. In offices the phenomenon of 'sick building syndrome' is likely to be related to the recycling of stale air combined with an increasingly complex cocktail of chemicals emitted from office machinery and equipment. So staying indoors is not the answer.

Finally it is worth saying that physiologically we obtain most of our energy from air. This simple fact is enough to remind us of the importance of the breath, the dangers of pollution and the necessity of reforestation.

If you have not already reeducated your breath, the following exercise will be helpful. It will help you gain access to higher levels of energy in daily life. Imagine the upper body contains three balloons. One fills the lower abdomen, the second fills the solar plexus and the third fills the chest all the way up to the shoulders. Breathing in, first fill the lower, then the middle and finally the upper balloon. Breathing out, first empty the upper section, then the middle and finally the lower. Be sure to expand the body to the front, the back and the sides as you breathe. Stay as relaxed as you can while you do this.

You can do this exercise standing, sitting or lying down. Placing the hands over the lower belly as you breathe will help draw the breath deeply downwards and encourage good use of the diaphragm. You can even do this exercise in bed. A few minutes every day will bring noticeable benefits.

Water

In William Shakespeare's play, Lady Macbeth compulsively washes her hands after the murder of the king, telling herself repeatedly how a little water washes away the deed. There is a similar blind spot in the modern 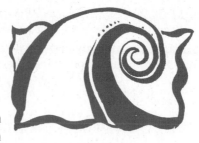 psyche which believes that water will cleanse the polluting lifestyle that we lead. Consequently our rivers and seas are a dumping ground for extraordinary quantities of industrial pollution, and otherwise intelligent people flush toxic chemicals down their drains.

Water, furthermore, is perceived as something which can be owned rather than stewarded by a responsible community. It is a disturbing fact of western life that water is a commodity owned by multinational companies whose raison d'etre is to make profit. As a result our water quality diminishes, short term policies create shortages of supply, and polluters escape public accountability.

Water is the blood of the earth. Its activity and its importance are more subtle than is commonly understood. When water's complex irrigation of our soil is disturbed, ill health follows in the land. Deforestation, building and road-making, damming, mining – all these practices disturb the capillary network of water's pathway through the earth. Stagnation and deficiency of the soil follow. When we add to this the enormous burden of pollution we come face-to-face with an ecological crisis which touches every being on this planet.

Water's needs are subtle. If water is to fully vitalise us it needs to ripen, to spend time underground at cool temperatures, to collect microscopic nutrients, to be filtered through rock, to be aerated as it moves above ground. Those who have tasted fresh water from a mountain spring will know how sweet it tastes and how refreshing it feels. The most vibrant water looks glossy and bluish. It is very high in dissolved carbons and minerals and these fine deposits are part of its aliveness. This water has had the longest maturity cycle. Our domestic water is normally surface water which also contains some mineral deposits but through exposure to the sun and lack of underground filtration, this water is still relatively immature.

From an energetic point of view, the vitality of water is also linked to its movement and aeration. Water naturally moves in a spiral serpentine pattern with a centripetal motion that concentrates its energy; it is purified through filtration and movement. In nature, water carries the memory of its movement and ripening. The memory of water is an aspect of its Qi. What message does today's drinking water carry into the body?

Water has always been recognised as a healer. The landscape of the earth is crowded with sites of holy wells and healing springs. Within energy medicine, water is seen as a message carrier (a principle used by homeopaths). In homeopathy, water is infused with the properties of various plants or substances in such a way that the subtle message of the original substance is impregnated into the water's memory. In many religions blessed water is similarly given a healing message by the community's healer.

The optimistic position is that if water is a message carrier, it can take on a new message. So how can we make tap water more potent, make it glisten with energy once again? Some answers may lie in storing the water for a short while in a clay or glass pitcher, reintroducing movement by stirring, singing to it, pouring it through a spiral funnel, exposing it to magnetic fields or even blessing it ourselves in our own homemade rituals. These proposals may sound outrageous or simply comical but they are in keeping with a view of the world that focuses on the energetic dimension of reality.

The energetic weakness of tap water is not the only problem. Tap water, though far safer than water in many third and fourth world countries, is increasingly polluted by nitrates and other chemicals. In the short term it is advisable to install domestic under-sink water filters. The situation in the western world is that most people use the domestic tap, and I do not want to encourage an

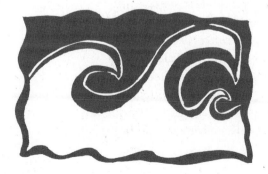

aversion to tap water and the short-sighted and expensive habit of reliance on spring water transported hundreds of miles and packaged in throw-away plastic. In the long term, the real answer lies in reforestation which gives our planet both its oxygen and its water; the reconversion to organic farming practices; and the vigorous regulation of water-polluting industries.

It is easy to overlook the body's simple need for water. Many health problems are actually due in part to local dehydration of the body. We mistakenly believe that we are drinking adequate fluids when a simple glass of water hardly passes our lips. Caffeinated drinks, sugared drinks and concentrated juices, though mostly water in composition, will not properly irrigate our bodies. In fact the diuretic properties of caffeinated drinks and colas disturbs the body's water balance and sets up patterns of dehydration. The result of overuse of these drinks at the expense of simple water is constriction of the vascular system, tiring of the heart muscle and lowered physical and mental energy. This means that nourishment will be restricted and blood pressure will increase.

As with all aspects of diet, individual water consumption will vary according to constitution and condition, to season and to climate. Thirst is generally the best indicator of how much each person should drink, although when we are out of touch with our bodies we may not be able to read its signs very clearly; sometimes water cravings are misread as the desire for sugar, stimulants or foods. So the following guideline may be helpful: more water for excessive and toxic conditions, less for deficient and cold conditions. More water when consuming rich food and meat, less for diets high in vegetable and fruit.

Western doctors commonly recommend drinking large volumes of water daily. Water helps to purify the body; given that many western health problems are caused by toxicity, this approach makes sense. However, a more effective approach is to stop the dietary habits which cause accumulation of toxins, i.e., eating rich, acidic, processed or adulterated food and overeating generally. In the long term, excessive consumption of water will disrupt the harmony between the Stomach and the Spleen, causing digestive weakness. The Kidney will also become exhausted.

As for when it is best to drink, it is generally good to drink something on rising in the morning to rehydrate the body before eating. Most fluid consumption is best kept away from meal times so as not to over-dilute the digestive juices. Generally a small glass of water is sufficient with a meal. A practice that some people find useful is to fill a bottle of water in the morning and have it with them during the day, taking sips as and when desired. This is a good way to keep track of how much water is being consumed.

In 1987 the soda (liquid phosphoric acid) consumption in the US was 45 gallons for every man, woman and child, exceeding the consumption of water for the first time in history

Karen and Jim Ehmke
Food for Life

Trees and Plants

Trees and plants are often a source of food. They are also living beings and when we interact with them there is an exchange of energy; a relationship is established. Generally the movement of energy is a discharge of negativity from human to plant and the giving of positive energy from plant to human. In Qi Gong[7] practice we exchange energy with trees and plants, allowing the tree/plant to transform our chaotic or negative energy, to reorder our energy patterns.

It does not take a special ability in order to experience the transformative power of the natural world upon the human spirit. We need only go for a walk in the woods or sit and contemplate a flower to feel our energy shift. It is important to recognise that we are nourished constantly by the green world. When our perception becomes more subtle we may notice that different species of tree affect us in different ways and that different colours affect us differently too. An apple tree, for example, will tend to uplift the energy of the Heart, a plane tree will tend to remove excess energy and an oak tree will tend to restore at all levels.

We can take this principle of resonance into our lives, finding the trees and plants that resonate with our energetic needs most strongly, and opening to receive help from them. The helpers that we need are often within a few hundred yards of our homes. As a general principle it is better to work with trees when they are awake, i.e., in spring and summer, to work with evergreens in winter and to work with native or well established plants. A window box or a small garden can be a valuable and handy source of energetic nourishment if there is no easy access to land and trees.

It is not possible to teach Qi Gong methods of natural resonance within the limitations of this book, but gathering nourishment from the plant kingdom need not be complicated. Simply giving time and attention is enough: sitting against a tree to rest or standing beside it and opening to sense the exchange of energy. Or we can take time simply to receive the visual nourishment of flowers, the sounds of wind and water, the song of birds and so on.

Rocks can help ground energy; they are related to the Earth element in Chinese medicine. Some rocks are especially powerful and can recharge us or speed our healing from illness. Many of the granite stones of southwest England have reputations as healing stones. In the ceremonial stone rows and circles the carefully positioned stones act as amplifiers of the earth's energy currents and create a ritual space where human Qi can work with the earth's Qi. Most of this energy technology is lost to us now but a visit to an ancient site of power may stir rememberings in the psyche.

A simple practice for tuning into the regenerative power of the natural world is to find a place in the land where we feel an affinity. We can make this our special place which we can grow to know intimately and return to whenever we need. Over time our visits to this personal power place can become a significant part of our lives, connecting us to nature and to ourselves, allowing us to absorb the healing power of earth, rock, plant and tree.

Reverence for trees and rocks is no longer at the heart of our culture. To the Druids, forest glades were temples. Now the British countryside has only ten percent tree cover and worldwide deforestation threatens both the planet's air and its water. Such visionaries as the hero of Jean Giono's *The Man Who Planted Trees*[8] are needed now. Reforestation is probably the single most constructive step towards planetary healing in the twenty-first century.

Cosmic Energy

It is obvious that we receive energy from the sun. At a more subtle level we also receive energy from the moon, stars and planets. This subtle energy is received through the body's meridians and acupoints, discussed in a later chapter. Each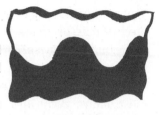
point on the body is an opening for the cosmic energy to pour through. This vibrational energy carries information and nourishment to every cell in the body, connecting the body to the cosmos.

From the viewpoint of Qi Gong, which forms the root of Chinese medicine, the apparent separation of the body from the cosmos is an illusion. As we turn our perception inward and explore deeper and deeper levels of our being, we reach a point where the distinction disappears. When we enter the molecular structure of the human body we find that our 'solidity' is composed mostly of emptiness, of space. If seen from this perspective, the human body would appear like a thick cluster of stars in the vastness of space. The mind too, in deep states of meditation, may dissolve its sense of separateness.

Trapped in the illusion of separateness it is easy to lose connection with and to be closed to the nourishment constantly entering us from the cosmos. Within Chinese medicine, cosmic energy is seen as the source of life and within Qi Gong many meditation practices are intended to help us reconnect with the source and so remember our own true nature. A follower of Lao Tsu, the revered Chinese philosopher, once said 'Make love with the invisible subtle origin of the universe, and you will give yourself everything you need'[9] . This 'origin' is the ultimate source of nourishment.

The body cannot live on denatured nutrients of any sort. Light devoid of its natural 'ultraviolet' nutrients is as 'dead' as food without its living enzymes and air without its negative ions. In all these cases, the missing ingredient is a form of Qi

Daniel Reid, *The Tao of Health, Sex and Longevity*

We are constantly affected by vibrational waves of energy, such as light, reaching our planet from space. We depend on light for the synthesis of certain vitamins and minerals and the regulation of our biological clock. Daylight entering the eyes is conveyed by the retina to the pineal and pituitary glands. These glands are important parts of the hormonal system and their functioning strongly influences our mood and vitality. It is ultraviolet light which is vital; and this is the portion of the spectrum not present in artificial light. It is also the portion of the light spectrum which is filtered out by glass and by air pollution.

It may be surprising to learn that many of the mystical practices of meditation which focus on developing the inner circulation of light in the body may have some basis in modern science. It has recently been discovered that photons (particles of light) circulate in the human body, specifically in the spine where they circulate in the cerebrospinal fluid[10] . The subtle perceptions of Qi Gong also have their parallel in modern physics which understands how the most minute event inside an atom has an effect on every other atom in the universe.

Whereas it may be desirable to open ourselves to the subtle vibrational waves of the universe, there are also waves of energy which it would be better to shield ourselves from, if we could. The spread of telecommunications has brought with it the increasing saturation of airspace with all sorts of wave frequencies, some of which are harmful to life; the nuclear industry has also increased our exposure to low level radiation which undermines human health; and electricity brings with it electromagnetic fields which can also be damaging.

An understanding of the energetic influence of the stars and planets also underlies modern day astrology. The subtle energetic forces of the planetary positions at the time of our birth, and the forces within the landscape, are influences on the quality of our Qi vibration. When we choose to see the world as energy, these are not difficult concepts to grasp.

Consciously choosing to spend time absorbing sunlight and directly connecting to the vibrations of the moon, stars and planets may be considered part of our subtle nourishment. Qi Gong methods can also help us to amplify and circulate the light within the body.

Sensual Nourishment

It is through the senses that we make relationship with the world. A full consideration of nourishment needs to include the colours, sounds, tastes, touch and fragrances which are as much a part of human nourishment as food and drink. This is the realm of pleasure, not the overstimulation of the brain that often passes for pleasure, but a deeply engaged sensual relationship with our own bodies and the world around us.

Of all the senses, human touch is perhaps the most significant. Many people live lives afraid to touch, suspicious of their own sensuality and hostile to their own bodies. An untouched baby will not thrive; and older people, often isolated and deprived of touch, will shrink. In infancy the functions of all the internal organs, especially the digestive organs, are stimulated by touch. A well-touched child usually develops good muscle tone, lively responses and a sense of inner security.

Many patterns of insatiable hunger for food stem from an unsatisfied need for touch. For this reason, bodywork is always nourishing to the functions of the Spleen, the Organ governing digestion in Chinese medicine. There is a direct relationship between the amount and quality of touch we receive and our appetite for food, as well as our ability to digest it.

There is huge benefit to be gained by establishing a sensual tactile relationship with ourselves and with our physical environment. Our touch-taboo culture and the increasingly cerebral nature of many people's lives often means a loss of relationship with the physical body. For some people reestablishing this relationship is transformative.

From an energetic perspective, the sensual impressions received from a plant or a creature or a place are an aspect of its Qi. A sensual experience which gives pleasure is nourishing. To pay attention and let pleasure in increases aliveness and strengthens health.

Here in this body are the sacred rivers: here are the sun and the moon as well as the pilgrimage places... I have not encountered another temple as blissful as my own body

Saraha

Relationship

According to the revered Chinese doctor Sun Simiao who wrote fifteen hundred years ago, people become ill 'because they do not have love in their life and are not cherished'. When the heart is open and we are connected to our fellow beings, when we have intimate relationships, when we feel that we belong to a community where we have a valued place and a context in which to give of ourselves, we are more likely to thrive. This is in many ways just common sense but it is interesting to see that many scientific studies are now confirming this.

Statistically it seems that loneliness, isolation and depression make us several times more vulnerable to premature death or disease. In fact, an analysis of a person's social relationships, how well-connected they are to partners, friends, family, community and tribe is a more powerful predictor of well-being and longevity than any of the more commonly studied factors such as gender, race, socioeconomic status or alcohol and tobacco consumption. One study exposed healthy adults to the common cold virus and found that those with healthy social relationships were four times less likely to catch cold[11].

It may be useful to see relationship as an energy field generated by the two or more people involved. Commitment, clear intention, compassion, generosity and humour will generate a strong healthy field which carries individuals through difficulty. In other situations the energy field may drain and limit the people within it. This can be seen in oppressive regimes or in destructive personal relationships.

In other words, the more we are connected to our community, the more our health is supported. To give to our community can be seen as a mutually nourishing act. Through our contribution the community's energy field is strengthened and this in turn strengthens us. The healthier and more functional a community is, the healthier its members are likely to be. When a community is well-integrated, sharing some common values and recognising the value of its own diversity, its energy field becomes well-developed and increasingly able to support its members.

Nourishment from Food

From the viewpoint of traditional Chinese medicine, our nourishment depends on two powers, two essential abilities of the bodymind. The first is an ability to receive, the second a power to transform.

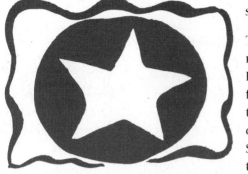

To be nourished by food, both mind and body need to be open to receiving its nourishment. Eating the 'perfect' diet is no guarantee of being fully nourished, as beliefs and feelings, physical tension and underfunctioning Organs can obstruct the receiving of nourishment. Similarly, a weak digestive system may mean that good quality food is poorly absorbed.

Beliefs about food condition the body to receive it. Two people can eat the same meal but receive it differently. One person sitting happily with a cream tea, clear in the belief that 'a little of what you fancy does you good', is predisposed to digest it well and be nourished. Another person sitting with the belief that cream tea is fattening, bad for the arteries and an indulgence, is predisposed to digest it badly. In the second case, the digestive system is programmed to react against the food.

Feelings about essential self-worth, feelings that personal needs can never be met, feelings of wanting nothing to do with the world: any number of feelings can block the ability to receive, and set up the psyche so that nourishment cannot enter. And just as the mind needs to be disposed towards receiving, so does the body. It is important to relax when eating and to give attention to enjoying food. Giving attention to how we eat and the environment we choose to eat in is an important part of receiving the nourishment. If our attention is elsewhere when we eat, perhaps on doing business or watching television, then our energy is diverted from the process of digestion. Similarly, eating on the run or literally while walking along the street, causes a conflict in the demands on our energy: the energy needed for digestion is being called on for movement. The more quiet, calm and relaxed our attitude and environment when eating, the better our digestion is likely to be.

The power to transform food is the other half of the equation. Once received into the body, food must be transformed into energy

> **The greatest force in the human body is the natural drive of the body to heal itself - but that force is not independent of the belief system, which can translate expectations into psychological change. Nothing is more wondrous about the fifteen billion neurons in the human brain than their ability to convert thoughts, hopes, ideas, and attitudes into chemical substances. Everything begins, therefore, with belief**
>
> Norman Cousins

and nutrients which the body can use. This depends on the strength of the digestive system, governed by the Spleen, and the fiery power of the Yang. These two concepts are discussed later in this book. The power to transform is derived from the Fire (Yang) of the body and can be strengthened by exercise and the use of supportive foods.

A relationship with food is central to our lives. It is one of the major ways that we relate to our environment: by eating it, by converting it into us, by the process of transformation. How we eat is a measure of our relationship to nature and in that relationship is mirrored the patterns of all our relating. If, for example, scarcity rules our eating, then scarcity probably also rules our relationships with other beings. If greed rules, or disrespect, then this too is likely to be mirrored in all relationships. Ultimately, in a relationship with food, there is mirrored a relationship with self. An exploration of this relationship can be an uncomfortable but growthful journey.

In the West our relationship with food generally is not based on nutritional needs. Rather, it is based on emotional needs. We eat to feel good, to fill a hole, to distract ourselves, to fulfil craving and addiction. Choice of food is often dictated by the stimulation of the shopping environment and by the manipulation of advertising, and of course by budget. And in a world of overwhelming information, and misinformation, it is easy to be pulled away from our own body wisdom.

But it is in our own bodies that the information about our nutritional needs can be found. The deeper we can listen to ourselves the more appropriate and health-generating our diet will be. To get to that place of listening we sometimes need guidance. This book seeks to offer information as a way in to such deeper knowing and I strongly suggest that, once a clear relationship with inner knowing is established, as many rules as possible be discarded (including any rules presented in this book). I also encourage you to test the information presented here against your own experience.

We move through the world by eating it. We swallow it, taking bits and pieces for ourselves, and push the rest out. One of the principal organising processes of a living organism is its eating behaviour. Food is the means by which we recreate the world as ourselves

Effrem Korngold and Harriet Beinfeld, *Between Heaven and Earth*

Part Two

Working with Chinese Medicine

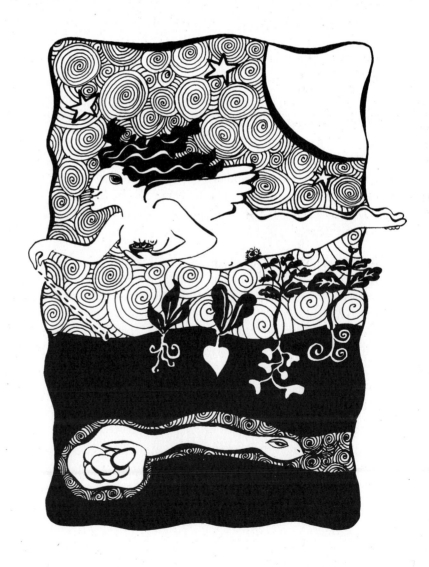

**The doctor of the
future will give
no medicines, but
will interest his
patients in the
care of the human
frame, in diet, and
in the causes of
disease**

Thomas Edison

Chapter Three

Meridians and Organs

What is a Human Being Made Of?

What is a human being made of? In western thought we might answer this question with a list of physical substances such as water, minerals and chemicals; from a Chinese viewpoint the body is a scene of dynamic interplay between energy and matter. The basic Substances of Chinese medicine are Qi, Blood, Jing (Essence), Fluids and Shen (consciousness). These Substances, which comprise the human form, express the interplay of Yin and Yang: they range from the moist and material (Jing, Blood and Fluids) through to immaterial vapour and energy (Qi and Shen).

The Substances are created, processed, renewed or stored by the various Organs. Blood, for example, is said to be governed by the Heart, have its origin in the Spleen and be stored in the Liver. The strength and integrity of each Substance is therefore dependent on the proper functioning of the responsible Organs. When all the Organs are working well and the Substances are vital and abundant, then a person is in good health. Ill health is expressed as disruption in the life of the Organs and Substances.

The Substances also mutually nourish one another. Through the theory of the Substances, body and mind are integrated and their inseparable nature is underlined. The more dense Substances are seen as providing an anchor for the mind in the body: their vitality provides the foundation for mental, emotional and spiritual health. Typically, in Chinese thought the reverse is also true: the immaterial life of spirit, thought and emotion also influences the physical body.

Disharmony in a human being is described either in terms of a weakness within the Organs and Substances, as congestion in the system's flow or as the presence of adverse 'climates' such as Heat or Cold. These are known respectively as conditions of Deficiency,

Stagnation and Excess. Disharmony is also described according to its location (internal or external) and its temperature (hot or cold).

The causes of disharmony are generally attributed to lifestyle (which includes diet, sleep, sex and work), psychological factors (commonly defined as the seven emotions of anger, joy, sadness, worry, pensiveness, fear and shock), and actual environmental influences such as climate and weather. Although described in a language of climates, such as 'Wind Cold' or 'Dampness', the environmental causes of disharmony may be taken to include bacteria, viruses and suchlike.

A person will be predisposed to certain kinds of condition according to their own internal climate and landscape. The strength of Chinese medicine is in its recognition of each person's uniqueness, and therefore of each person's differing needs. People may suffer from the same health problem, but its treatment will vary from person to person, depending on the nature of the person rather than the nature of the problem. Whereas western medicine labels the disease, Chinese medicine describes the unique manifestation in each person.

Illnesses may be the same but the persons suffering from them are different
Hsu Ta-ch'un

The next section of this book presents an overview of traditional Chinese medicine, with a particular emphasis on lifestyle and diet. As far as possible, terminology has been kept simple and new terms explained when they first occur. When an important term is not immediately explained it is likely that its meaning is explained later in the book. In such instances, please either refer to the glossary or use the index to find the relevant pages.

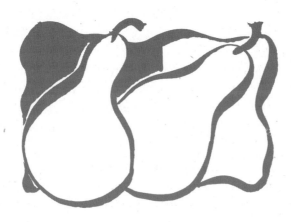

Meridians

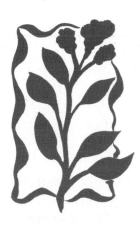

From the viewpoint of oriental Medicine, the body has an energetic structure which is as real as the anatomical structure. The meridians, flowing through the body's soft tissues, integrate body and consciousness the same way that physical anatomy integrates the body's fluid and solid natures. The word for meridian in Chinese is 'Jingluo' which translates roughly as 'threads that connect, like a net'.

The first meridians are formed in the earliest stages of cell division in a developing embryo. The very first cell division, when the first cell becomes two, gives rise to the deepest of all meridians, the Chong Mai or 'Penetrating Vessel'. Later cell divisions give rise to meridians that result in the separation of left and right, front and back, above and below. In the earliest moments of our post-conception life, a deep matrix of energetic pathways is formed which creates a core, around which the complex network of linking energy channels is created.[12]

This deep group of meridians is known as the 'Eight Extraordinary Vessels'. They link us to an undifferentiated experience of self, when we know our connection to the cosmos, our inseparableness from the whole. The awakening of these vessels through bodywork, Qi Gong or acupuncture can put us in touch with a profound experience of this 'original nature'. It may also be that within these vessels lie the inherited patterns of our 'karmic' health.

Around this core energetic structure is the system of energy channels that protect us and distribute nourishment throughout the body. These meridians are not fully formed at birth and take time to develop. They are generally known as the twelve regular meridians (Jing) and their connecting vessels (Luo). The sinew meridians, which are broad superficial pathways largely following the course of their associated meridian, weave together the physical anatomy and are responsible for the strength and suppleness of the physical body. According to some practitioners they also carry the Wei Qi generated by the Lung, the defensive energy that we may call the immune system.

The sinew meridians are closely related to the Liver which regulates them. It is largely within this surface meridian network that patterns of muscle tension can be observed and worked with. The sinew meridians distribute Qi through all the locomotive muscles and irrigate the joints with energy. When Qi is not flowing smoothly, which is normally due to emotional tensions, there will be a direct effect on the physical body.

Most of us are aware of passing tensions in response to life's stresses. If these tensions are chronic and not resolvable, we eventually develop small holdings within the soft tissue that impede flow and create restriction, leading in turn to postural distortions. These constrictions can be felt by the hands and are known as 'kori' to Japanese bodyworkers. They form what has been called the 'emotional anatomy'.

The network of twelve regular meridians travels deeply into the body, linking the inner anatomy to the surface. Each meridian enters the Organ after which it is named and often several others on its journey. These meridians carry nourishment and Qi throughout the body. Their function is partly nutritive and partly communicative.

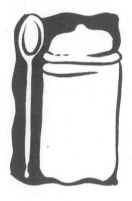

Although the meridians do not have a strictly physical form, they may be detected by modern machinery. A path does not need to be a structure. The pathways of Qi which we call meridians have been shown to have electromagnetic properties. When, for example, an electrical stimulus is applied to a point on a meridian, the electric current follows the meridian pathway rather than any other route. This tells us that a meridian has lower electrical resistance than its surrounding tissue. A meridian is a carrier and receiver of electromagnetic information[13].

In one of the oldest texts of Chinese medicine, known as the Ling Shu, the meridians are described as receiving subtle information from the environment: from stars and planets, from the energy fields of the land and its trees and plants, and from the Qi of other living beings. Each point is seen as a gateway through which the universe pours information into our being and out of which we send information to be received by other beings. Our responses to changes in the weather and to subtler changes in the movements of stars and planets is picked up in the meridian system and relayed around the body. If we work to clear our perception through such practices as Qi Gong[14] we will become more sensitive to the subtle emanations of place, perhaps even able to perceive the subtle movements of Qi which Feng Shui seeks to harmonise.

Many acupoints appear to be directly connected to mast cells[15], cells with a special function within the immune system. This points to a convergence of western and eastern understanding: one of the functions of the meridians in Chinese medicine is the circulation of defensive energy. The pains we often experience at the onset of a cold or flu are, according to oriental medicine, caused by the increased activity within the meridians at the body surface as they fight off the invading forces.

The meridian network has four functions: communicative, defensive, nutritive, integrative. The meridians facilitate communication between the inner and outer realms of the body and among all its parts; they carry the Wei Qi, which circulates beneath the skin and defends the body against attack; they circulate food essences around the body, bringing nourishment to all the cells; and they weave the bodymind together into one integrated unit.

Meridians are named after Organs but do not exclusively belong to that Organ. The meridian of the Spleen, for example, may be stimulated to affect the actions of the Spleen but its pathway also branches into the Stomach and Heart. Organ dysfunction will show at the surface as disturbance to the meridian pathway. Conversely obstruction of or injury to the meridian may eventually lead to some Organ dysfunction.

Individual meridians govern different physical movements according to their route through the musculature. The Bladder meridian, for example, which runs on either side of the spine and along the backs of the legs, governs forward movement and supports erectness. The Liver and Gall Bladder meridians govern sideways and twisting movements and so on. Problems with movement usually develop over time, often starting in early childhood, and these may be observed and treated through the meridian system.

The route of a meridian reflects some of the essential functions of its associated Organ. The Large Intestine meridian, for example, nourishes the muscles responsible for throwing (away) and the gesture of pointing which we use to emphasise the separation of something from ourselves, the naming of something as other. This parallels the Organ's function of separation and purification.

It is somewhat deceptive to speak of each meridian separately, as in reality the meridians form one seamless network and the Qi flows in a biorhythmic pattern around the meridians in sequence. This subtle network, invisibly regulating our being, may be seen as the subtle system through which consciousness inhabits the body. Its invisible threads weave us into the subtle fabric of the universe.

Nourishing the Meridians

The meridians need to be free of congestion to perform their functions. It is easy for congestion to occur as a result of tension, postural distortion, injury or the invasion of Cold, Dampness or Wind from the environment. To maintain the meridians in a state of health it is important to stretch and move the body.

Although there are many specific exercises for the meridians, any exercise which develops suppleness and helps a person to inhabit the body, such as yoga, dance, swimming or Tai Chi, will be helpful. More focused exercises can be found within Qi Gong or amongst the self-development exercises used by Shiatsu practitioners. Of all the exercise forms, Qi Gong, through its special integration of movement, breath and attention, offers the most direct and effective way of clearing and invigorating the meridians.

Touch is also nourishing to the meridians, in particular the combination of perpendicular pressure and stretching applied by Shiatsu practitioners. Shiatsu helps to stimulate and balance the distribution of Qi through the meridians and is effective in keeping the channels clear. The massage techniques of Tuina are also used to correct meridian dysfunction and there are now a range of meridian-focused therapies available. It should be stressed that all massage will have some beneficial effect on the meridians even if the therapy is not specifically meridian-focused.

Although the meridians can only be manipulated through the surface anatomy, the effect of work on the acupoints or along the length of the meridian will be carried to the core of the body. Keeping the meridians healthy will directly benefit the Organs and deeper systems, enabling the circulation of nourishment and supporting the communication between the inner and outer realms.

Finally, it is worth considering that the electromagnetic nature of meridians makes them sensitive to electrical devices and the emanations from TV and computer screens. It would be sensible to reduce unnecessary exposure to these and to learn some Qi Gong exercises for clearing the energy field after exposure.

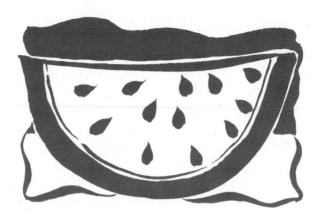

Organs

It may be confusing for a westerner to discover that the names of the organs carry somewhat different meanings when used in the context of Chinese medicine. In the West, an organ is a part of the physical anatomy where various functions are carried out. The liver, for example, is a dense, blood-rich organ that sits at the bottom of the ribcage to the right side. It performs hundreds of different tasks including the secretion of bile and the regulation of iron levels in the blood; it maintains both the fluidity and the coagulating ability of the blood, synthesising proteins, regulating temperature, eliminating toxins and regulating cholesterol.

Western medicine is skilled at detail, at gathering knowledge about structures and substances. In Chinese thought, functions and processes are more significant than structures and the term 'Liver' refers to a wide and interrelated set of functions rather than a fixed object. This set of functions can be observed at work in and around the liver as well as at all other levels of the bodymind: these include physical as well as emotional, mental and spiritual levels. The physical liver organ is simply a site of concentrated energetic activity where many of the physical functions take place. The functions of the physical liver organ are seen as one aspect of a wider picture.

We can summarise this distinction by saying that the Chinese concept of Organ, which throughout this book is indicated by the use of a capital letter, is a description of a wide range of functions and processes which take place in many different aspects and sites of the bodymind. The physical organ, which is indicated by the use of a lower case letter, is a site where many of these functions can be seen happening and the site from which the Organ derives and concentrates its power.

To understand this better, let's take one example of Liver function and see how it manifests at various levels through the bodymind. One of the most important functions ascribed to the Liver in Chinese medicine is the regulation of the smooth flow of Qi: the Liver oversees the processes and movements of the bodymind. At the site of the liver organ itself many of the regulating functions described in the paragraph above are clearly a part of this function. When we widen our view to look at the whole bodymind, then free flow of movement and all physiological processes are seen as an expression of Liver energy: this includes the supple workings of the joints and musculature as well as the opening and closing of valves or the smoothness of peristaltic movement. Psychologically this is reflected in the free flow of emotions. Mentally this is reflected in an ability to think creatively, transform difficulty, and keep in sight the whole picture. The regulating functions of the physical liver are seen as one aspect of the wider function of maintaining the free flow of Qi.

Each Organ has a kind of signature, a resonance, which connects it to other aspects of the cosmos. So the Liver, for example, has a sympathetic resonance with plants such as dandelion or grains such as rye, and these plants will benefit the Liver functions. Various seasons, climates, colours and directions (in this case Spring, wind, green and east) are resonantly linked to the Organ. So too, the Organs vibrate in harmony with certain planets and musical notes. In Qi Gong the Organs are sometimes described as planets within the body's solar system, each emitting a special frequency and possessing its own 'gravitational' field.

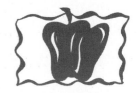

Surface and internal pathways of a meridian circulate from its Organ, linking it to other internal and external sites and structures. The Liver meridian, for example, links its Organ to the foot, the genitals, the throat, the eyes and the top of the head. Internally the meridian pathway connects the Liver to the stomach, lungs, gall bladder and diaphragm. The meridians are the means by which the Organ's physical functions are transmitted through the body.

The following section discusses each Organ in turn and looks at how its health can be supported.

The Spleen

Just as the Earth is the centre of the cosmos from the viewpoint of a human being, 'Earth's Organ', the Spleen, is seen as holding a central place in the human body. Our well-being can be seen as dependent on our ability to absorb and process nourishment. This is the

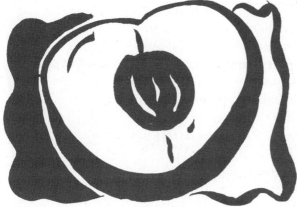

realm of the Spleen in Chinese medicine. The Spleen is responsible for providing the nourishment which supports all aspects of healthy functioning. It is an Organ of transformation and nourishment.

Through the transforming action of the Spleen food becomes nutritional substances, information is digested and transformed into knowledge and sensual experience is received and transformed into a core sense of well-being. It is also through the Spleen that healing energy is received into the body[16]. The Spleen is responsible for nourishment. A strong Spleen ensures that a person is well nourished. A weak Spleen may result in being undernourished. At the physical level it is possible to eat a good diet yet not be strong enough to convert the food into proper nourishment. At the emotional level one may be in an apparently nourishing situation yet still be unable to receive the available nourishment.

In the history of Chinese medicine whole schools have grown up around the idea that in the treatment of all illness we must first address the Spleen and its paired Organ, the Stomach. Without this central ability to transform food and experiences into nourishment, life lacks its central support. So let us look a little more closely at the realm of the Spleen and how we can support and strengthen Spleen energy.

The Spleen's Physical Realm

The Spleen's transformative action is best embodied in the digestive process and the Spleen may be taken to refer to the whole digestive tract from mouth to anus and all the various juices and transformative agents released along the way. This includes the pancreas which secretes enzymes into the small intestine to assist in the assimilation of nutrients. One measure of the Spleen's strength is the vigour of the digestive system. Its transformative action converts food into Blood and Qi.

The strength of Blood and Qi are, therefore, significantly dependent on the Spleen. The nourishment generated by the Spleen is transported along the meridians, through the soft tissues of the body. The Blood and Qi, derived from the original transformation within the digestive system, invigorate the soft tissues and give them tone. Soft tissues support the structure of the physical body, keeping things in place, holding up the body and giving it shape. With poor tone in the soft tissues a body feels and looks saggy and in extreme cases may suffer from prolapse. When the Spleen is strong, physical vitality is also strong and the soft tissues provide the body with good support. The Spleen may therefore be seen as the provider of the body's physical tone.

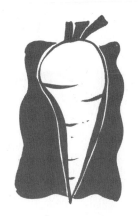

The Spleen's Non-Physical Realm

The Spleen is said to house the power of Thought, the 'Yi' of Chinese medicine, the power to concentrate and apply the mind. This is an odd concept to the western mind, so what does it mean? The digestive process is mirrored at the mental level by the thinking process. Digestion begins with a desire to eat which leads to the intake of food. The food is then sorted into what is usable and sent to where it can be used or stored in the body. What cannot be used is excreted. The thinking process follows a similar path: the desire for knowledge leads to the intake of information which is then sifted and sorted. Whatever can be put to immediate use is applied and the rest is stored for later. Irrelevant or unusable information is rejected and forgotten.

Our everyday language reflects just how similar and related these processes are. We talk of 'food for thought', of being 'unable to digest certain information', of 'verbal diarrhoea', of 'eating our words', of 'chewing over an idea'. Most of us will also recognise more obvious physical connections such as being unable to concentrate after eating too much, or developing food cravings during intense periods of study or not being able to eat when we are worried (a knotted form of thinking). The Latin proverb 'Mens sana in corpore sano', a healthy mind in a healthy body, underlines the relationship between physical vitality and mental alertness.

If the Spleen governs the power of thought at the mental level, at the emotional level it governs feelings of concern both for self and for others. A healthy concern for our own needs leads us to nourish ourselves emotionally and, if we are ourselves emotionally nourished, we can give appropriate nourishment to those we care about. Strong Spleen energy lays the groundwork for a healthy emotional life in which needs are satisfied; we are able to overflow into life with generosity rather than grasp at life from a hungry place of lack.

Turned inward, concern may become self-concern, a self-absorption which leads to Stagnation of energy. Turned outward, concern may become overconcern for the needs of others where, like the naked man who offers another a coat, we project our own need onto others and give from an unbalanced place. This perpetuates a distortion of Spleen energy into the wider community.

Psychologically the Spleen also has to do with issues of nourishment and support. Spleen energy is mature when we are able to nourish ourselves from within, when we feel self-supporting and are not driven so much by need but by an overflowing of our own abundance. This is a tall order! In a culture where traditional systems of support (the sense of community, tribe, family) have largely broken down, most people experience a crying out for support and nourishment. To work with the Spleen we need to work with emotional nourishment as well as physical.

Archetypally the Spleen is related to the mother. In the process of growing up the needs that are initially provided for by the mother are increasingly provided for by the growing child itself. Eventually a person develops an 'internal mother', an ability to find comfort and nourishment from within. At this point in development the Spleen energy can be said to mature.

The Well-Nourished Spleen

Only when you truly inhabit your body can you begin the healing journey

Gabrielle Roth

Abundant Spleen energy will tend to generate a deep inner sense of well-being and a wonderful sense of ease and comfort in the body. We feel content, enjoy the pleasures of life, and have a deep relationship with our own sensuality. We feel abundant at all levels, equally able to give and receive generously. Digestion is relaxed and efficient, the body feels supported and toned, the mind is clear and able to concentrate well. We are grounded, as in touch with the earth as we are with our body, and we rest secure in the knowledge that we are safe and deservedly looked after by the divine Mother, Providence or whatever name we give to the provider of our needs.

When the Spleen is in disharmony there is usually a poor ability to digest food. This will often be mirrored by a decreased ability to receive emotional nourishment. Often weak concentration is linked with difficulty in sifting and sorting nutrients in the physical body. Sometimes, when deeply hungry for love, we turn instead to food to bury our pain. When feeling emotionally unnourished the body may contract and impede the flow of nourishment into the soft tissues; or the posture may collapse, especially the middle section of the torso and at the lumbar-sacral joint, giving up in both an emotional and physical sense.

Nourishing the Spleen

The Spleen loves touch. Anything we can do to feed ourselves at this most fundamental level will strengthen the Spleen. Deprived of touch, the human being shrivels up, behaves crazily and sinks into depression. Touch is as fundamental a need as food, so supporting the Spleen also means entering a deeply sensual relationship with the body. To receive bodywork, to cuddle friends and family, to touch oneself lovingly: all these are ways to strengthen the Spleen. Often we focus on food when in fact this other fundamental need, the need for contact, is the secret cure.

We can maintain the tone and free flow of nourishment in soft tissues by stretching. The Spleen loves to stretch. Stretching eases constriction and opens the flow of nutrients into the muscles. It is a good way to enter into a relaxed relationship with the body. Other ways include learning how to fall, crawl and roll around on the ground. This playful approach reconnects with the earth and helps the body develop trust in the earth's support. When we innately trust the earth to support us, internal resistance to gravity softens, our energy becomes more grounded and the effort used in holding the body upright can be freed to give the body more vitality.

Touch, stretching and physically reconnecting to the earth all direct us to becoming more fully embodied. Being comfortably at

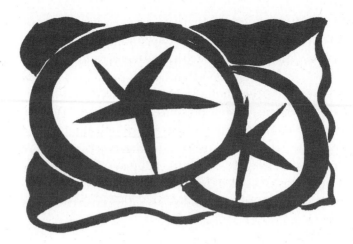

home in the body is the natural expression of Spleen energy. In the touch-deprived, over-sedentary and ungrounded lifestyle typical of modern culture, the Spleen has a hard time. Of all the Organs, the Spleen is the most commonly deficient.

As well as finding groundedness in the body, we can create grounding in our daily lives. We can do this by creating structure and routine in the otherwise chaotic nature of daily life. A structured life is a Spleen-supportive life. This may be as simple as creating a daily space to drink tea, meditate, sit with a book, write in a journal, massage the body, anything which nourishes. It may also mean eating regular meals or keeping regular sleeping and waking times. Routine and structure create a constant, safe and dependable place in our lives, an external support for the Spleen.

> **Regimen is superior to medicine**
>
> Voltaire

We can extend this idea of structure to the physical structure we live in, the home. The home is an external mirror of the internal condition of the Spleen. Creating a comfortable and safe home can also be seen as creating an external support for the Spleen. The Spleen longs for a sense of home and it is no coincidence that people who travel a lot find that their Spleen energy is often put under extra strain. Many illnesses actually have their source in a kind of homesickness, a deep need to feel the security and care that belongs, or should have belonged, to one's childhood home. Creating a sense of home, even when moving from one place to another, will support the Spleen.

A short anecdote illustrates this last point. I once fell into conversation with a man on a train in India. When he found out that I worked within the healing professions he asked me what he could do about his chronic sinus congestion. Our conversation eventually led back to his original home which he had left because of his job. It turned out that, although he had been to several doctors and tried many medicines, the sinus problem was relieved by nothing except his return home. At home his sinus problems would vanish. The deep loss of home was simply too stressful for him. From a Chinese medicine point of view, the Spleen processes the moisture in food and produces mucus which the Lung then stores. In his case, the Spleen was weakened through homesickness and unable to properly process the moisture in food, creating an excess of its by-product (mucus).

The sense of home is vital to the Spleen's health. Ideally, through the childhood experience of secure and nourishing home life, we develop an internal sense of home which enables us to be at home anywhere, independent of place and circumstance. In other words, we become at home in ourselves, accepting of ourselves and comfortably relaxed in our own bodies.

Just as it is helpful to stretch and exercise the body, so it is helpful to train the mind. Learning study skills supports the Spleen's function of sifting and sorting information. Clearing out mental clutter, simplifying involvement with the paperwork of modern life, finding ways of working with the perpetually encroaching chaos: these are all ways of supporting the Spleen.

The Spleen's emotional territory covers the relationship with needs, and inner feelings of trust and safety. The Spleen calls us to honour our needs and attend to them, to enter a nourishing relationship with ourselves, to become self-nourishing. Unattended to, our needs will find their own way to fulfilment and the more they are ignored the more disruptive this way may be. Asking oneself 'What do I truly need to feel nourished, supported and safe in this world?' is a way of engaging with the Spleen at the emotional level.

We can nourish the Spleen in daily life through simple things such as cuddling with someone (even the dog will do!), getting bodywork regularly, making a nesty corner in the home, creating a daily self-nourishing ritual, rolling around on the floor or on the earth, and taking the time to give to ourselves in whatever way we need.

Nourishing the Spleen Through Food

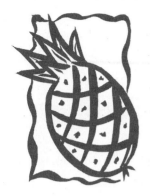

The Spleen likes to feel a satisfied glow of comfort after eating. An eating style that nourishes the Spleen is one that is homely and generous, one that gives attention to the 'feel-good factor', generating a sense of abundance and care.

In Chinese medicine the Spleen is said to be nourished by sweet food. This does not mean sugar but rather the deep sweet taste of grains or root vegetables as in rice pudding or pumpkin soup. Generally speaking the Spleen likes well-cooked food such as thick soups or stews which are easy on the digestion; it has more difficulty with raw and cold food. The weaker the Spleen, the more it benefits from well-cooked meals.

The Spleen also dislikes being flooded with too much fluid so it is helpful to drink only a little fluid with meals and have most fluid intake between meals. It is helpful to separate fruit and sweetened foods from the main meal, eating them instead as between-meal snacks. This assists the Spleen's function of sifting and sorting and helps reduce digestive fermentation.

Chewing well helps the Spleen to digest, and warms chilled or raw food. We can also assist the Spleen by sitting in a relaxed way with an open and untwisted posture. Sitting slumped or twisted will compress the digestive organs and hinder digestion.

Aromatic flavours stimulate the digestion, so the inclusion of aromatic herbs and spices in cooking will encourage the Spleen not to become Stagnant. Sweet-flavoured foods, especially foods rich in complex carbohydrates, are used by the Spleen to release energy steadily into the system; they form the centre of a Spleen-supportive diet.

Finally, according to the system of correspondences in Chinese medicine it is said that yellow/orange foods such as squash, 'red' lentils or carrot are energetically resonant with the Spleen and will support its functions.

Further discussion of the Spleen can be found in this book's sections on Qi, Yang and Dampness.

The Lung

The Lung's task is that of making a boundary between the inner and the outer world. The inner environment needs to be protected by a clear boundary which both defends and defines the person.

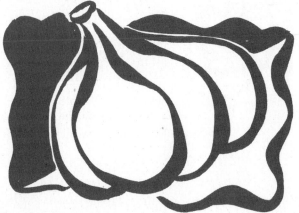

Across this boundary vital materials can be taken in and waste materials excreted. The most vital and obvious material that the Lung takes in is oxygen; but as we shall see, the Lung, in Chinese medicine, is more than the respiratory system. The Lung has to do with boundary, breath and renewal.

The Lung's Physical Realm

At the physical level, boundary, breath and renewal are expressed as the lungs, the skin and the colon. The Lung refers to the whole respiratory system and includes the nose and sinuses. Across the boundary of the lungs oxygen is taken in and carbon dioxide waste is excreted. Since most human energy is derived from air, the Lung is primarily responsible for physical vitality and is said to govern Qi in the body.

The skin is like an outer lung and the pores are seen as the 'doors of Qi'. The skin also breathes and exchanges substances with the outer environment. Its healthy functioning is seen as an aspect of Lung function. Beneath the skin the protective energy known as Wei Qi is said to circulate, defending the body against invasion from pathogenic forces.

The Lung's paired Organ, the Colon, is concerned with release and elimination. The Lung and Colon together are related to immunity, the strength of the protective boundary. Pathogens most easily enter through the respiratory and digestive systems and the Lung and Colon are responsible for maintaining the integrity of these systems so that they are not penetrated by invaders. According to Chinese medicine, the body's defensive energy is directly dependent on the strength of the Lung and Colon[17].

The Lung's Non-Physical Realm

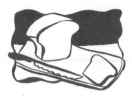

The Lung's physical expression as the boundary between the organism and its environment is expressed at the psychological level as a sense of one's personal boundary. A clear psychological boundary enables us to know who we are, to meet another and to establish clear relationship. When the sense of boundary is strong we can receive experience through the boundary and communicate outwards through it; the boundary is flexible and responsive, opening to receive 'good' influences and closing to screen out 'bad' influences. It enables us to say 'yes' to what we want and 'no' to what we don't want.

Whereas the Spleen is archetypally related to the mother, the Lung is archetypally related to the father. Traditionally it is the father who teaches a sense of self-value and helps us to leave home and find our place in the world. Good fathering teaches boundary, and helps with individuation and separation from the mother. The Lung is therefore concerned with feelings of self-esteem and respect for both ourselves and others. Knowing who we are, believing in our self-worth and taking our place in the world are all part of the realm of the Lung.

The Lung is also said to be the residence of the corporeal soul, or Po. The corporeal soul is the most dense and tangible aspect of the soul which dies with the body at death. The Po gives us awareness of the physical body, of our own aliveness and the physical rhythms of our bodily life. Sometimes translated as the vegetative soul, the Po belongs to the earth, to the material world and to the world of pure sensation. Its counterpart, the Hun, which is housed in the Liver, belongs to the world of spirit and consciousness.

The Well-Nourished Lung

Abundant Lung energy manifests as strong physical vitality. There is a sense of softness and fullness in the chest, strong lungs and a clear powerful voice. Immunity is strong, so recovery from illness is quick and effective, the skin is glossy and the complexion is bright and fresh. The breath is usually clear and pleasant. The body's posture expresses a clear sense of self-worth, presenting the chest openly to the world. Gestures are clear and expansive, a person's gaze is forthright, and their presence is clear and strong. Someone with strong Lung energy usually evokes a response of admiration and respect in another.

In conditions of dysfunction the Lung is either weak or obstructed. Physically weak Lung energy will manifest as low vitality and a poor immune system. The breathing may be shallow, not expanding the lower part of the lungs or the sides, and there may be respiratory problems. The skin may appear unhealthy and circulation of Qi and Blood may be weak. Emotionally there is likely to be constraint and sadness, perhaps a hiding within one's boundary. There may be lack of self-esteem, harsh judgment of both self and others and failure to respect or understand one's own and others' boundaries. Dignity may turn to false pride, leaving a person feeling alone and separate. It may be hard to claim a place in the world.

Nourishing the Lung

The Lung is nourished by breathing. The best way to amplify Lung energy is to take plenty of fresh air, develop the physical capacity of the lungs through exercise such as swimming, and to consciously bring awareness into the breath. A few minutes each day of relaxed breathing, learning to breathe with the diaphragm and relaxing the muscles of the chest and shoulders, can be very effective at building the power of the Lung.

Expansive movements which physically open the chest are also helpful. The intention is to stretch, to bring tone and release contraction in the muscles that surround the rib cage. It is also possible to develop the Lung through voice work such as singing or learning to project the voice. This can be an emotionally charged process for some people, bringing them face-to-face with all the inhibitions which have been allowed to constrain self-expression.

The skin, as part of the Lung system, can be nourished by brushing. Rubbing with a good cotton towel or scrubbing the skin with a brush will maintain the skin's health and support the immune system. Wearing natural fibres will allow the skin to breathe freely; going naked from time to time when weather and circumstances allow will also help the skin to breathe. Moderate sunbathing will nourish the skin, although overexposure may be damaging.

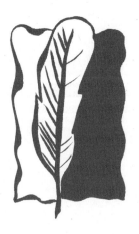

Emotionally the Lung is nourished by respect. Learning to value who we are and what we do will attract respect from those around us. Deeply exploring what we value, and finding ways to express those values in the world, help open us to the energy of the Lung.

In the outer world we can give value to our environment, attend to cleaning out stale corners of our house, or of our life. Clearing up our environment can be a way that we externally support the Lung function and may well bring more clarity into our emotional and mental life. A person's aesthetic life is an outer manifestation of the Lung and attending to beauty and order, making art both of daily environment and of life, will also support and nourish the Lung.

Finally, the Lung's role as boundary-keeper may be metaphorically extended to the boundaries we keep in our own home. Well-maintained fences, sensible security, clean windows and a well-kept exterior are domestic expressions of Lung energy.

Nourishing the Lung Through Food

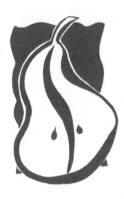

A Lung-supportive style of eating attends to the aesthetics of food and gives food a high value in daily life. A quality of respect for the importance of food and a delight in the simple rituals of eating set the tone for supporting the Lung.

The Lung governs Qi, so a Lung-nourishing approach to food will include many foods known as 'Qi tonics' and fresh foods alive with Qi. A diet high in fresh organic vegetables with some sprouted seeds and grains is helpful. The Lung also needs protein, and a craving for protein often indicates Lung Qi Deficiency. However, the best protein for the Lung is generally low fat such as tofu, beans and white meat.

When tolerated, dairy produce is strengthening for the Lung but in many cases causes congestion and the build-up of Phlegm. If this is the case, use goat or sheep products, or minimise dairy. Some pungent-flavoured foods are helpful to open the lungs and stimulate Lung function. Foods to keep in check are all those which cause congestion, i.e., rich fatty foods and any food which is processed or denatured.

Lastly, white and light-coloured foods are resonant with the Lung, so foods such as radish, white meats and white mushrooms tend to have some benefit.

Further discussion of the Lung can be found in this book's sections on Qi, Yin, Dampness and Wind.

The Kidney

If the Spleen forms the centre of our being and the Lung our boundary, the Kidney gives us our foundation. At the root of all physical functioning lies the activity of the Kidney. The Kidney is the source of both Yin and Yang in the body, or of water and fire. The Kidney stores and activates the watery Jing (the potential for life) giving rise to the physical structure and growth of the body. It also houses the source of fire in the body, the Ming Men, the fire which is said to be produced through the dynamic interaction of the two kidneys, activating the whole metabolism and motivating us to live.

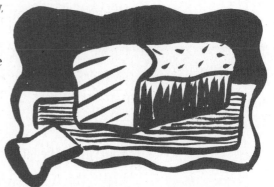

The Kidney is the Organ most closely linked to the source of material life. At both the physical and psychological level the Kidney expresses the most fundamental impulses of survival, reproduction and spontaneous curiosity. The Kidney is responsible for providing the basic impulse towards life and the ability to grow and reproduce.

Being responsible for both the vitality and essential harmony of the Yin and Yang, the strength of the Kidney underpins well-being. Through the Kidney we are most closely connected to the ancestors from whom we inherit our constitutions. A genetic blueprint is stored in the Jing creating a template for growth and development. The task of the Kidney is to make the most of its inherited constitution through the continual renewal and storage of the basic life force and its activation.

The Kidney's Physical Realm

Structurally the Kidney is expressed as the deepest places within our physical structure: the bones and their 'outgrowth' into the teeth. The skeletal structure, the spinal cord and the brain are the realm of the Kidney. Within these structures the Jing is stored, the blood is renewed, and the subtle rhythm of life pulses through the cerebrospinal fluid. The growth of the skeleton and the development of the brain and all its functions are dependent on the power of the Kidney.

The Kidney distributes the activated Jing through the Triple Heater meridian supplying warmth and Qi to all the Organs. This action is most closely expressed through the endocrine system which oversees growth, sexual maturity and fertility through the release of hormones. The pituitary and hypothalamus which regulate the endocrine system may be said to be carrying out the will of the Kidney.

The endocrine system works in conjunction with the autonomic nervous system and it may be useful to see the autonomic nervous system as another part of the Kidney's realm of influence. The autonomic nervous system has two divisions known as the sympathetic and parasympathetic nervous systems. These two branches can be compared to the Yang and Yin aspects of the Kidney.

Broadly speaking, the sympathetic system prepares us for action, mobilising the body's resources and stimulating the brain. It is stimulated by action and may be said to represent the Kidney Yang. The parasympathetic system governs replenishment and renewal, slows us down, and is activated by rest and relaxation. This may be said to represent the Kidney Yin. The balance between these two systems expresses the balance between Yin and Yang.

Chinese medicine divides the torso into three segments known as the three Jiao or burning spaces. This division is part structural, part functional. The upper Jiao contains the Heart and Lungs and is the place of respiration and circulation. The middle Jiao contains the digestive organs governed by the Spleen and is the place of digestion and transformation. The lower Jiao contains the organs of purification and is the place of elimination and sexual function. The lower Jiao is governed by the Kidney.

Structurally this means that the Kidney has a special relationship with the lower back and the pelvic girdle. The knees, which give support to the lower back, are also part of the Kidney's realm. Functionally this means that the Kidney governs the functions of reproduction embodied in the uterus, ovaries, prostate and testes. It also governs the drainage, balancing and purification of fluid through the action of the kidneys, bladder and large intestine.

The Kidney's Non-Physical Realm

It is in the Kidney that we find the deepest impulses of physical life: the impulses towards survival and reproduction. These powerful forces within the psyche are at the root of most behaviour. The Kidney is the source of quite phenomenal power, the will towards life, known as the 'Zhi'. Its natural expression is primal, direct and forceful. How we channel this power into our lives is a measure of how constrained or free the Kidney energy can be.

The will towards life gives rise to sexual energy. It is in relationship with the basic sexual drive that we see the expression of Kidney energy. The more we can maintain contact with the raw fire of sexuality, channelling its abundant energy into our lives, the healthier the Kidney will be. Physically this is expressed as a freely mobile pelvis and good circulation to the sexual and reproductive organs. Psychologically this is expressed as healthy uninhibited sexuality free from shame, guilt and repression.

Sexuality may not express itself directly as sexual behaviour. It may be channelled into art or work. The desire to create has its spark in the Kidney, and so strong is this will to create that to block it is to risk deep levels of emotional, mental and physical disturbance. To liberate it connects us directly to life's desire for itself, to the universal power of creation that unfolds continually throughout the cosmos.

The Kidney can be seen as the source of spontaneity and impulsive curiosity. This natural instinct to explore and express can be seen beautifully in babies. A baby's actions are unrehearsed: meeting life with wonder and acceptance, moving with the natural flow of its curiosity, and unashamedly exploring its own body. The culture into which a baby is born will shape the flow of its Kidney energy, saying yes to some routes of expression and no to others.

In a sexually and emotionally repressive culture such as England's, Kidney energy is over-constrained and it is often difficult for people to fully reclaim this source of their own vitality. The expression of sexual energy in such a culture becomes distorted and either goes underground (into secretive or sometimes abusive practices) or is projected outwards (into the sexualisation of entertainment or consumerism). The more repressive a culture is, the more sexual or creative expression becomes 'deviant'.

Appetite and sex are the great motivators of history…
They preserve and propagate the species, they provoke wars and songs, they influence religions, law and art. All of creation is one long uninterrupted cycle of digestion and fertility

Isabel Allende, *Aphrodite*

The Well-Nourished Kidney

Strong Kidney energy is experienced as a deep reserve of life-force constantly renewed from the source. Though we may naturally tire, the 'batteries' never run flat, and energy soon returns after resting. Reactions are quick, the mind alive and curious, sexual energy abundant and free. The pelvic area is warm and loose, impulses to movement flow unchecked from the hips, and the spine is strong and supple. Abundant Kidney energy overcomes fear and funds will power, the will to live and create. When the Kidney is strong, life is an adventure to be met spontaneously and courageously.

The will towards life gives us both a natural curiosity and a strong survival instinct. The Kidney is highly receptive to signals of danger and can provide huge surges of energy when we are threatened. If we feel threatened all the time, then the Kidney will be drained and so it is important to learn how to manage the stress of life and deal with chronic inner fears. Constant fear will drain the Kidney.

At the psychological level all Kidney disturbances originate from the blocking of spontaneous responses to life. We become out of touch with the instinctual life and the impulses arising from the lower Jiao, from the deep centre in the lower belly known as the Dan Tian. We may be fearful and nervous, easily startled out of this centre. Our sexuality or the fierceness of our instinctive nature may be frightening to us and become disowned. We may be hooked into 'control', unwilling to let life flow freely, and this may lead eventually to depression, exhaustion or disconnected behaviour. Physically, there may be infertility or disturbance in the reproductive system; the waist may feel weak or rigid, the urinary system may be problematic or there may be a range of symptoms in the lower Jiao or in other areas of the Kidney's influence: the knees, ears, teeth or head hair.

Nourishing the Kidney

The Kidney is nourished by balancing activity and rest. Stimulation needs to be balanced by quiet space. Balancing this basic polarity between Yin and Yang means balancing the recipe of 'work, rest and play'. Satisfying activity and stimulation balanced by nourishing rest and sleep is the recipe for balanced Kidney energy.

To nourish the Yang aspect of Kidney we need adventure. Life needs to provide an edge of excitement where there is challenge, and the will towards life is awakened. This may mean finding more motivation in work or daily life or it may mean taking an adventurous holiday every now and again. Physically the Yang aspect of Kidney needs appropriate challenge and stimulus to the body through exercise to fully wake up a sense of aliveness.

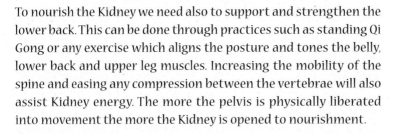

Whereas the Kidney Yang is nourished through movement and action, the Yin of the Kidney is nourished through rest and stillness. Adequate rest is essential to balance activity. At a deeper level we access and nourish the Yin through meditation and quiet contemplation. Turning away from stimulation, including television, and turning the attention quietly inwards, renews the Kidney Yin.

To nourish the Kidney we need also to support and strengthen the lower back. This can be done through practices such as standing Qi Gong or any exercise which aligns the posture and tones the belly, lower back and upper leg muscles. Increasing the mobility of the spine and easing any compression between the vertebrae will also assist Kidney energy. The more the pelvis is physically liberated into movement the more the Kidney is opened to nourishment.

Bodywork practices such as Shiatsu, Zero-balancing or CranioSacral Therapy help to access the deeper rhythms of being (in particular the rhythm of the cerebrospinal fluid) and can free the body into greater spontaneity. We may also be able to reclaim an innate spontaneity through simply playing. Play may be said to be the natural exuberant expression of the Kidney, so finding an adult version of the playfulness often left behind in childhood will nourish the Kidney.

Spontaneous movement practices which release deeply-held constraint can also liberate the Kidney. There are spontaneous practices within Qi Gong, BodyMind Centering and Feldenkrais as well as in many spiritual traditions. One of the earliest Qi Gong practices is to imitate the movement and behaviour of wild animals, one of the animals associated with the Kidney being the Monkey. When we imitate this animal we can tune into its long and free spine, its freedom of movement, its spontaneous curiosity and the demonstrative sexuality of the monkey; this, in turn, helps us to find our own.

Those who act with bravery and courage will overcome diseases, while those who act out of fear will fall ill

Inner Classic

To nourish the Kidney is to become more and more connected to our own spontaneous impulses and the will to live. It is fear which constrains this in us, not a fear that alerts us to real danger, but chronic messages of fear that have worked their way deep into our system. Liberating ourselves from chronic fear, the emotion associated with the Kidney in Chinese medicine, is to open the Kidney to nourishment. Any way that we can explore and release our fearfulness will ultimately nourish the Kidney.

Nourishing the Kidney Through Food

The Kidney is the deepest place in the body and mind where the catalytic processes of creation are happening. To support the Kidney a deep-reaching approach to nutrition is needed. Successful nourishment is dependent on the subtle interaction and balancing of a wide range of essential nutrients. In the world of minerals for example, each mineral is dependent on several other minerals, vitamins and other essential nutrients for its proper transformation and absorption in the body. As the Kidney provides the catalytic power to the transformative action of the Spleen we can support it by ensuring that we have a wide base of essential nutrients. This means that the Kidney likes a wide and varied diet. In particular, foods that come from the water element such as fish and seaweeds are especially nourishing, as are seeds which contain many nutrients to support a plant's growth.

Salty-flavoured foods are directed towards the Kidney, so miso, soya sauce and salted preserves are beneficial (too much salt will have the opposite effect). Dark coloured foods such as red or black beans may also be helpful. Simple water is important as is the avoidance of too many stimulants or dehydrating drinks.

Further discussion of the Kidney can be found in this book's sections on Yin, Yang, and Qi.

The Liver

The complex human system needs regulation. This is the role of the Liver. The Liver has a coordinating role, overseeing the order of the entire system. It is responsible for smoothing the flow of Qi throughout the bodymind, releasing energy and nourishment when they are needed and guiding the Qi into purposeful and graceful manifestation. It is the Organ of the Wood element symbolised by the willow tree: pliant, resilient and powerful in its growth.

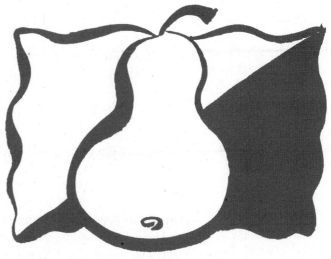

The tough, springy and determined nature of willow is a good metaphorical image for the nature of the Liver. At both the physical and emotional level the Liver gives us willow-like power and flexibility. It may smooth the way, but the Liver is not the peacemaker; it is rather a power for effective action for which a tough kind of pliancy is vital. The Liver gives power to go forward through life; to block this unfolding of purpose is to risk serious disharmony in the Liver's realm.

Going against the flow
Is the catastrophe that destroys life

Su Wen

The Liver houses the aspect of soul known as 'Hun'. The closest expression of this in western terms is the esoteric notion of the astral body. The Hun holds life purpose and guides towards its fulfilment. Unlike its more material counterpart – the Po, housed in the Lung – the Hun survives death and is capable of coming and going in the body. Disharmony in the Liver's realm may be a sign of misalignment with life purpose.

Within the 'five element' system of Chinese medicine, the Liver is associated with the power of spring. Spring is the time of growth and arousal, when the life-force stored and rested in the winter is once again released. The release of this spring-like force is the Liver's realm and this resurgent power, capable of flooding the body with Blood and Qi, is the power we cultivate and draw on from the Liver.

The regulatory and guiding function of the Liver is supported by its other major task of storing the Blood. The Liver oversees the quality of Blood and releases it when needed. When the body is at rest, in particular when lying down, the Liver is said to renew the Blood, giving us the stamina to get through the day and to perform physical work.

The Liver's Physical Realm

Structurally the Liver manifests in those parts of the body which give power, flexibility and grace in movement: the muscles and joints, and their supporting structures: the tendons and ligaments. Strong and flexible joints are essential for coordination and ease of movement. The Liver supplies Blood and, through the action of its Yang partner, the Gall Bladder, supplies Qi to the joints and helps to lubricate all movement.

The Liver's coordinating action is also expressed through the nervous system; the smooth, efficient action of neurons and chemical messengers may be seen as the Liver smoothing the flow of Qi. Awkward physical movement and disrupted internal movement may be seen in part as disharmony in the Liver's realm.

The Liver has a close relationship with the Spleen, and constrained Liver energy easily influences the digestion. The Liver also governs the diaphragm whose action largely determines the smoothness of the digestive process as well as the efficiency of the lungs. Relaxed diaphragmatic breathing is an expression of relaxed Liver energy. Patterns of diaphragmatic tension almost always occur when the Liver Qi is stagnant.

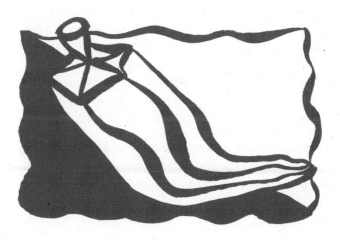

The cyclical movements of life, particularly the menstrual cycle, come under the Liver's sphere of influence. The Liver guides rhythm. In fact a sense of rhythm is an expression of the harmony of Liver, and rhythm itself may be a method for guiding the Liver towards full health.

Likened to an army general in Chinese medicine, the Liver holds the overview of one's life. This is literally expressed through the Liver's relationship with the eyes. The Liver nourishes the eyes and the eyes guide us through life. Also within the Liver's physical realm are the nails, seen as the outgrowth of the tendons; the lustre of the head hair, which reflects the quality of the Blood; and the genitals and breasts, which represent sexual power.

Whereas the Kidney governs fertility and our impulse towards sex, the Liver governs our sexual performance. Sexual arousal, like the awakening of spring, is within the Liver's realm. The Liver releases Blood to the genitals giving the power of erection and sexual opening. The Liver meridian flows through the genitals and breasts and is frequently blocked when sexual energy is obstructed.

The Liver's Non-Physical Realm

Psychologically, the Liver organises us towards the realisation of our potential, helping us to manifest the potential for growth stored in the Kidney. It gives us the desire to assert who we are and express our creative energy in the world. The Liver drives us along the path to self-realisation, determined that we grow. When this force is obstructed, anger is the natural result.

Traditionally, the Liver is associated with anger. Anger pushes through difficulty, giving determination and energy to achieve our goals, defending our right to life. Though often viewed in a negative light in western culture, it is better understood as a necessary companion to growth, the power that drives self-assertion. It can be seen flexing its muscle in very young children going through the 'terrible twos'. Such a powerful force needs a skilful balance of space and boundary provided by the parents.

This natural assertive and creative force becomes damaging when it is chronically obstructed, leading to its pathological state, frustration. Turned inwards, anger frequently attacks the joints and disrupts the body's rhythms or turns to depression or self-

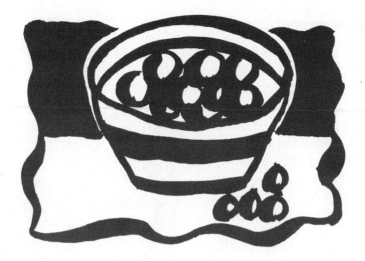

destructive behaviour. When overconstrained and unable to flow freely into life, the Liver Qi is said to be Stagnant, and over time deep disturbance of the bodymind can take root.

The Liver's power may be seen as being in the service of the Hun. According to Dr. Edward Bach, the man who developed the Bach Flower Remedies, all chronic illness is a symptom of the personality's resistance to the soul's purpose in this life[18]. In other words, all chronic illness has a spiritual root and contains information for the spirit. Disturbance in the Liver's realm may also be explored in this light.

The Liver is concerned with planning and organising, deciding the way through. Its decisions are carried out by its Yang partner, the Gall Bladder. We can say that the Liver gives the power of vision, and the Gall Bladder gives the power of courage and decisiveness to carry the vision through. In China and Japan, someone with decisive courage is described as having a big Gall Bladder. We also talk of having gall, usually in a negative sense, but meaning having the audacity to do something.

Assertiveness demands a balance between the qualities of advancing and yielding. The assertive power of the Liver is balanced by flexibility, by suppleness in one's approach to a situation. The Liver gives the ability to yield when appropriate. Just as we need to be physically supple, a psychological suppleness helps us to get what we want and gracefully accept when we cannot. We need to be able to bend without snapping.

The Well-Nourished Liver

Full and vibrant Liver energy manifests as a supple body capable of dynamic movement, like a tiger. Joints flex and extend smoothly and movements are coordinated and graceful. Breathing comes freely with the diaphragm and there is easy access to reserves of energy, plenty of stamina. Eyesight is acute, hair shiny, nails strong. The body rhythms are easy and regular and there is delight in the rhythms of music and dance.

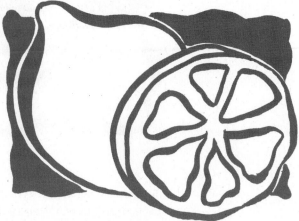

Emotionally there is an ability to express and process what is felt, not tending to store unresolved emotions for too long. There is a strong optimistic yes to life, knowing what is wanted and going for it. With strong Liver energy we can be determined without being a bulldozer, easygoing without being a doormat. We have what is known in Yiddish as 'chutzpah', the skill and courage to risk and progress. We are happy to lead the way, creative in problem-solving, and able to see the big picture. We are essentially aligned with the flow of life.

Nourishing the Liver

Physically the Liver is nourished by attending to the suppleness of the body. This means that exercise and stretching are essential, especially with the Liver's tendency towards Stagnation. Walking is especially helpful, bringing Qi into all the muscles and tendons. More elaborate coordinated movement such as Tai Ji supports and develops the coordinating function of the Liver and is excellent for opening and strengthening the joints.

All sideways bending and twisting movements help keep the Liver free from Stagnation. Martial arts can be useful for channelling unexpressed or disruptive energy into more ordered and purposeful expression and are particularly suited to the Liver, teaching assertiveness and channelling anger. Walking, martial arts and Tai Ji all have a strong element of purposefulness to which the Liver responds well.

All coordinated movement will benefit the Liver. Juggling, for example, develops the power of coordination and activates the Liver. Creative expression can also nourish the Liver. When we create, whether this be a sculpture, a poem, a painting, a garden, a bookshelf or an idea, we are tapping into the Liver's power and giving it expression. Attending to the natural desire to create keeps Liver energy awake and flowing.

There is a flip-side to all this purposeful activity. The Liver also needs good quality rest and relaxation. To balance the drive towards creating and expressing we also need to cultivate the ability to 'kick back' and relax, to take the day off and go to the beach, to have time to simply be or, better still, to develop the quality of beingness within all our doingness.

Giving time to planning and 'seeing the wood for the trees' is helpful for the Liver. Visualising what we want, prioritising a list, creating a business plan, being supervised in our work, doing some assertiveness training – all these activities support the Liver.

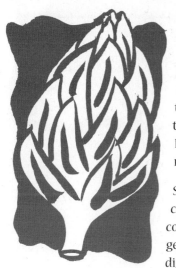

Nourishing the Liver Through Food

The Liver needs to remain clear whilst also maintaining the rich quality of the Blood. The essential principle is therefore to cleanse. Sour foods which stimulate the tissues to contract and release toxins and which stimulate the Gall Bladder to excrete bile to help with the breakdown of fat are helpful. In particular, dark green foods, which combine a mild sourness with vital Blood-nourishing qualities, are essential.

Saturated fats, oversalted and overprocessed foods, chemically adulterated and oversweetened foods will all tend to congest Liver function. Green salads and sprouted foods will generally help the Liver, provided one is not too Cold and the digestion is not too weak. Overeating is especially congesting to the Liver, in particular when the food is rich or fatty.

The other need of the Liver is for food which nourishes the Blood. This and more about the Liver is discussed in this book's sections on Yin, Blood, Heat, Damp and Stagnation.

The Heart

The Heart is the seat of Consciousness. It is the place of saying 'I am', the place from which we radiate our essential presence into the world. The Heart is said to store the 'Shen', usually translated as spirit or mind, whose radiance is known as 'Shen ming'. The radiance of the Heart can be seen in the eye, the complexion and the gestures of the hands. Someone who is vibrant at the core radiates that aliveness outward like a glowing fire.

The calligraphy for Heart shows an empty vessel. This emptiness must remain clear of clouds for the Heart to maintain its clarity and brilliance. The empty vessel of the Heart symbolises open alignment with the will of heaven. When the Heart is clear, an essential divinity shines through, revealing one's true nature. Most pathology of the Heart is described as a misting of this alignment.

Whereas in the West we tend to think of the Heart in a romantic way concerned with human relationships, the Chinese view the Heart as essentially concerned with relationship to the divine. When this is aligned, all other relationships will flow smoothly. The status of the Heart is so important that it is given the title of Emperor. When the Emperor is well and in harmony with the Tao, its radiance shines throughout the whole realm.

The Heart's Physical Realm

More modern Chinese texts stress the importance of the Heart as a physical pump which regulates and powers the flow of Blood through the body. It is in the Heart where the final stage of the manufacture of Blood takes place after the Spleen and the Lung have played their part. The Heart animates the Blood, gives it its vibrancy. When the Blood is strong it can provide a home for the Shen, giving a calm mind and good sleep.

The Heart opens into the tongue which means that the Heart controls the quality of the voice. Whereas the Lung gives the voice power, the Heart gives the voice clarity and brilliance. The tongue is considered to be connected to the heart muscle and the quality of the Blood can be seen in the tongue's redness. Contractions in the tongue causing speech impediments are seen as related to the Heart. More poetically, the truth of our words and the clarity of our songs reflect the condition of the Heart.

The Heart's Non-Physical Realm

The deep nature of the Heart is reflected in its place as the centre of consciousness and spirit. All the Organs of the body are arranged in service to the Heart and the Heart ensures that the 'spirits' are harmonious. A more modern way of describing the Heart's role is to say that the Heart is responsible for psychological integrity. Whatever stresses threaten to fragment the integrity of the psyche, the Heart ensures that we do not disintegrate, do not break our connection with the centre.

To maintain harmony throughout its realm, the Heart must be tranquil and protected. Working closely with the Heart, the Heart Governor mediates between the Heart and the world, acting both as a protector and as a communicator of the Heart's desires. The Heart Governor governs relationships with other beings; it is said that the Heart can never be touched directly.

The Heart is paired elementally with the Small Intestine. The Heart gives, in the sense that it radiates outward, and to do so it must also receive. The Heart receives via the Small Intestine. The Small Intestine filters both physical nourishment in the form of food, and emotional and mental nourishment in the form of experiences. The Small Intestine presents what is nourishing to the Heart; what is not nourishing it passes on to be excreted.

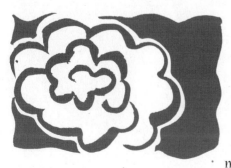

Although the Heart is well-protected, its nature is to connect. Through the Heart we connect to the spiritual source of life, to the deep mystery of the world's turning and to the spirits of our fellow travellers on this earth. The Heart's connection to the 'Great Mystery' of life gives rise to humility, awe and devotion. Prayer and ritual are the natural expressions of the Heart, as are poetry and music and all reverential celebrations of life.

The Well-Nourished Heart

Strong Heart energy manifests as a clear radiance. 'Only with the heart can the eye see clearly' said the fox in Antoine de Saint Exupery's *The Little Prince*: when we look into the eyes of someone with strong Heart energy we may feel that we can see right into their Heart. When Heart energy is strong there is a good capacity to feel emotions and to connect with others. The Heart gives the capacity to truly receive the experiences of life and to integrate those experiences into an increasingly rich wholeness.

Someone with weak Heart energy may be easily troubled, out of touch with the core and unclear what to make of life. It may be hard to make connections with others. There may also be an experience of chest pain, sleeplessness and agitation. The mind may find it difficult to settle; it may become easily overexcited or confused. Circulation may be weak, especially to the hands and there may be sweat for no good reason. In extreme circumstances there may be some level of breakdown in the psyche.

Nourishing The Heart

The Heart is nourished by connecting. Relationships, with all their joys and difficulties, are where the Heart finds its food. To attend to both inner relationship with oneself and outer relationship with others is to nourish the Heart. The key consideration in nourishing the Heart is to maintain its openness, to avoid closing off and becoming isolated.

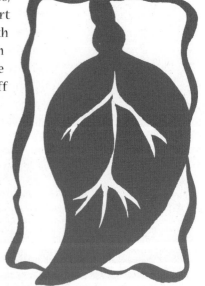

At its deepest level the Heart is nourished by cultivating relationship with the divine, in whatever form. Any way of prayer through which to open to life's mystery keeps the Heart open and able to receive nourishment. Even the simplest gesture of pausing beneath a tree to wonder or stopping to absorb a beautiful view are acts of prayer which open the Heart to its nourishment. We can say simply that any way in which we celebrate life is nourishing to the Heart.

Some people like to keep daily rituals. Creating an altar of personally significant symbols and spending some time each day in prayer, or regularly visiting a favourite place in nature, or giving time to letting go of preoccupations in order to contemplate the big picture – all these are rituals, acts of the Heart. So are the seasonal acknowledgements of the world's turning, the solstices and equinoxes, the harvests and the planting times. Finding our own rituals that have meaning for us helps connect us to and nourish the Heart.

Giving voice, in singing or in speech, may also be Heart-nourishing. The natural state of the Heart is joy, and singing is joy's natural expression. Through singing we can connect to the core. Giving time in our lives to singing, reading poetry aloud or simply playing with the voice will benefit the Heart. In the extraordinary world of the Kogi Indians of South America, certain children are trained as seers and visionaries from birth. Kept in the dark and constantly tended yet kept away from normal human contact, these children spontaneously sing before they learn to talk and spontaneously dance as soon as they can walk.

Meditation is the
mother of nutrition

Unknown

Of all the ways in which we can nourish the life of the Heart, meditation is perhaps the most profound. The Heart's deepest need is to maintain the clarity of the void, to be like an open sky untroubled by clouds. In meditation we learn to calm the distracting chatter of the brain, align with our centre and open the connection to the source. Becoming an empty vessel, we can allow heaven's light to shine through us. To cultivate our essential emptiness is to enter the realm of the Heart.

Nourishing the Heart through Food

A Heart-nourishing approach to eating is a joyful one. There is delight in the tastes, textures and colours of food, enjoyment in sharing food with friends and an impulse to give thanks to the source of our food. We may bring wine and candles or give special attention to the atmosphere in which we eat. We may place flowers at the table or play soft music. We may delight in inviting friends round.

It is not the ingredients that make a meal Heart-nourishing so much as the heartfulness that has gone into its preparation. In the film 'Like Water for Chocolate', whatever was going on in the cook's life was magically transferred to everyone who ate her food, leading sometimes to tears, sometimes to sexual arousal. This alchemical relationship between cook and food affects us more profoundly than we may realise and there is a beautiful mystery in how it is that so-and-so's apple pie is simply the best, no matter what we do to try to imitate it.

Just as in life we need bitter experience in order to fully experience our joy, so it is that the bitter taste nourishes the Heart, although an excess of bitterness will oppress it. A bitter salad, bitter aperitifs or bitter drinks such as dandelion root will stimulate the Heart. The bitter taste is also found in the germ and bran of grains. The habit of drinking bitter elixirs before a meal will prepare the digestive system to most effectively extract nourishment from the food to send up to the Heart. We may have to search hard these days to find bitter foods but only a little is needed and the benefits are worthwhile.

The Heart also responds to the subtle essences of foods and so it is that various flower essences touch the Heart and alter one's mood. I would like to advocate a resurgence of the old tradition of actually eating flowers. Such flowers as English marigolds, borage, sweet violet, nasturtium and rose make wonderful additions to a meal and benefit the Heart. A few petals sprinkled in salad or folded into rice can produce a colourful and vibrant meal. Flowers can also be infused in oil and used in salad dressing.

Foods containing red pigment such as tomato, cherry or red pepper are said to nourish the Heart. Recent research suggests that baked tomatoes strengthen the heart muscle and red wine also has the backing of scientific research in this regard[19]. The moderate use of stimulants such as paprika or black pepper is also helpful. The Heart is nourished by animal heart and blood rich food such as black pudding. Too much red meat can, of course, have the opposite effect. The Heart can be stressed by too much salt, fat and stimulants.

Further discussion of the Heart can be found in the sections on Yin, Yang, Qi and Blood.

Chapter Four

The Substances

Qi

'Just as the world can reveal itself as particles, the Tao can reveal itself as human beings.

Though world and particles aren't the same, neither are they different.

Though the cosmic body and your body aren't the same, neither are they different.'[20]

One translation of Qi is 'breath', the breath of life, the animating principle that has no word in the English language. The visible and tangible world is simply seen as a condensation of Qi. 'When Qi condenses,' says Zhang Zai, 'forms appear'[21] . All matter is a slowed-down vibrational wave, originating from emptiness. Life itself is seen as a condensation of Qi, death as its dispersal. In its broadest sense the concept of Qi is unnameable; the word 'Qi' is an attempt to name the subtle realm of vibration which is the source and true nature of existence.

Through certain Qi Gong and meditation practices, direct perception of Qi is cultivated. As we deepen our connection to Qi, to the subtle vibrational nature of things, we are linked to the universal. To experience Qi is to tap into the unifying principle of all life. In this sense it can be said that Qi belongs to Heaven whilst Blood, which is the subject of the next section, belongs to Earth.

When we start to describe human health and behaviour, the meaning of Qi becomes more specific, and, for the purposes of this book, more useful. Once Qi has manifested in form and function we can more easily name it. We can talk about the Qi of a particular Organ, for example. In this sense we mean the particular vibration and energetic force of the Organ. Kidney Qi, for example, is the vitality of the Kidney Organ and its ability to carry out its associated functions.

And I have felt

A presence that disturbs me with joy

Of elevated thoughts, a sense sublime

Of something far more deeply interfused,

Whose dwelling is the light of setting suns,

And the round ocean, and the living air,

And the blue sky, and the mind of man:

A motion and a spirit, that impels

All thinking things, all objects of all thought

And rolls throughout things

William Wordsworth

Everything has its own characteristic Qi, from rocks to plants, from rivers to landscapes, from jellyfish to human beings; and each Organ of the human body has its own particular quality of Qi. When we talk of the Qi of individual Organs, we are talking about the Organ's vitality and its capacity for work. When an Organ's Qi is weak, we mean that it is underfunctioning. When Qi is strong, everything is working as it should be and the person is fully vibrant, expressive and engaged with life.

Qi Deficiency

It is not really possible to have too much Qi. The pathology of Qi has to do either with its Deficiency or its Stagnation. So what causes the vibrational force of an Organ to become weak? There are, of course, nutritional possibilities, but let's look first at the wider picture.

Trauma. Premature or traumatic birth, or shock in the womb, is sometimes at the root of patterns of Qi Deficiency. Early trauma may leave its imprint so strongly that it chronically suppresses physiological functions. Such an impact can be helped to some extent through nutrition but the trauma is best approached through bodywork. Subtle energy work such as Shiatsu, CranioSacral or Polarity Therapy is known to be helpful. Traumatic events later in life can also set up patterns of Qi Deficiency, whether the shock is physical or emotional.

Lack of oxygenation. Oxygen performs many of the functions in the body which Chinese medicine attributes to Qi. When starved of oxygen, cells underfunction. This is particularly true of the Brain, Heart and Liver. To maintain adequate oxygen intake we simply need to breathe! All physical exercise will increase the intake of oxygen, as will breathing practices. Even sitting still and relaxed whilst focusing on the breath and visualising the nourishing power of oxygen penetrating every part of the body will be helpful. Green plants may also be placed in the home and workplace to keep the atmosphere fresh.

Poor posture. Poor posture, especially compression in the spine, will suppress the Qi of the internal Organs. The more there is space available inside the body for the organs to sit comfortably and the more space there is between the joints, the more easily Qi can flow.

Tao originated from emptiness and emptiness produced the universe. The universe produced Qi... That which was clear and light drifted up to become heaven, and that which was heavy and turbid solidified to form earth

Huai Nan Zi

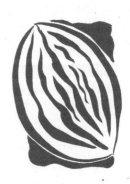

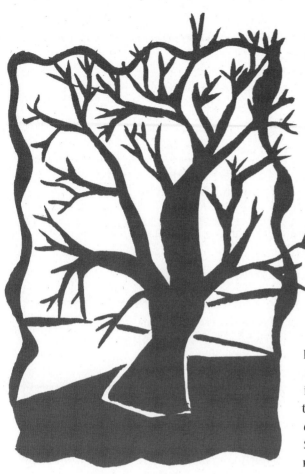

Environmental stress. Some environments are more vital than others. Geopathic or electromagnetic stress may interfere with normal Qi function. It is best not to sleep near electrical equipment, and to minimise exposure where practical. The impact of TV and computer screens can be lessened by placing a cactus or other succulent plant nearby, by shielding with a thick sheet of glass and by drinking extra water when using these electronic devices. Otherwise fresh air and exercise are the best detoxifiers.

Immunisation. The habit of immunising children against an increasing number of illnesses, though well-meant, can often lead to disruption and weakening of the Qi. Some childhood illnesses are in fact necessary for the development of the child. Measles, for example, usually brings on notable changes in a child's emotional growth and is necessary for expelling toxins accumulated in the womb. Chicken pox, mumps and rubella also ultimately have benefits for the child. Chinese medicine and homeopathy both offer ways of overcoming weakness caused by immunisation.

Feng Shui. The arrangement of a room can have surprising effects on our well-being. An understanding of Feng Shui can help keep the Qi flowing clearly around house and support personal Qi in its positive flow. Feng Shui practitioners will cite numerous stories of people's vitality being increased when simple rearrangements are made in the home. Even such simple acts as moving a bed, hanging a mirror or changing the colour of a wall can be effective. We can think of Feng Shui as a way of aligning an environment with our own highest good, or aligning our lives with the Tao.

Overexertion. Certain kinds of physical activity can also deplete the Qi[22] .

- Too much sitting and a lack of physical movement, especially stretching, will tend to deplete the Spleen.

- Lack of full breathing will tend to deplete the Lung.

- Too much standing, especially on hard ground and without awareness of posture, will tend to deplete the Kidney.

- Too much exercise, overstretching or pushing the body to extremes, will tend to deplete the Liver.

- Too much visual and mental stimulation will tend to deplete the Heart.

- The intense energy expenditure of childbirth can also trigger a pattern of Qi Deficiency.

Stress. Sudden stress, whether this be physical exertion, grief, or mental stress, as well as more chronic stress such as long-term worry, overwork or even excessive sex, all can lead to depletion of Qi.

Emotions. Chronic holding of unresolved or unexpressed emotions will impact the physical body and cause underactivity, overactivity or disruptive activity of the Qi. Qi is highly responsive to emotional states. In Chinese medicine the effect of emotional experience on the body has been observantly mapped. The list below is drawn from the ancient writings about Chinese medicine and from the experience of modern-day practitioners[23] . I would like to stress that these are observations rather than 'rules'.

Anger causes energy to rise, joy causes energy to slow down, grief causes energy to descend, fright causes energy to scatter, exhaustion causes energy to wither, worry causes energy to stagnate

Yellow Emperor

- Self-absorption, overconcern with other people or with causes, struggles with dependency, anxiety about the future and any chronic state of insecurity are linked to a pattern of Deficiency in the Spleen.

- Chronic dissatisfaction, disgust, disappointment, greed, compulsive behaviour and chronic hunger are linked to a pattern of Deficiency in the Stomach.

- Grief, a loud self-critic or judgmental attitudes projected outwards, poor self-esteem, and pride are linked to a pattern of Deficiency in the Lung.

- Guilt, shame, depression and an overdeveloped sense of responsibility are linked to a pattern of Deficiency in the Large Intestine.

- Fear, especially of spontaneity and sexual expression, may lead to contraction in the Kidney function.

- Impatience is linked to a pattern of Deficiency in the Bladder.

- Overcontrol of the creative drive, a directionless life, chronic anger and avoidance of personal power are linked to a pattern of Deficiency in the Liver.

- Chronic indecisiveness is linked to a pattern of Deficiency in the Gall Bladder.

- Anger and resentment, lack of forgiveness, restrained love, loneliness, over-stimulation, or life in the 'fast lane' are linked to a pattern of Deficiency in the Heart.

- Feeling full of restrained tears and chronic states of confusion are linked to a pattern of Deficiency in the Small Intestine.

There is a mutual relationship between emotional and physical lives. Physical well-being which we nourish through food, exercise, human contact and rest will influence emotional well-being (e.g., overeating will dull some emotions, jogging may induce feelings of elation, certain minerals or vitamins may help lift depression). Emotional patterns also affect physical bodies. When working with nutrition we need to remember the emotional picture; if food is not helping, our way into healing might be through the emotions.

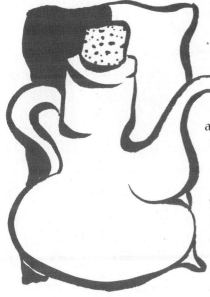

Recognising Qi Deficiency

Qi Deficiency is recognised by a number of general signs and symptoms. These are: low energy, reduced appetite, some shortness of breath, a slight tendency to sweat more than usual in the daytime, loose stools, a pale face, a weak voice and a general sense of functioning 'below par'. Not all of these signs need to be present to confirm the diagnosis. Other signs may also be present, pointing the diagnosis towards particular Organs. The pulse, felt at the wrist, will feel weak, and sensitive practitioners can sometimes sense the weakness of the body's energy field or the weakness of the field generated by certain Organs. Qi Deficiency most commonly involves the Lung and Spleen but all other Organs can also be Deficient in Qi.

Nourishing Qi

Qi can be cultivated by attending to the potential causes of its depletion. Qi is especially nourished by fresh air, exercise and good quality food. We are now discovering how profoundly our beliefs and attitudes affect our body; in the same way Qi is strongly influenced by our mental and emotional life. Strong positive beliefs and a clear emotional life will generate strong Qi.

Opening to the nourishment of the natural world supports strong Qi. Especially, Qi can be nourished through Qi Gong, the art of cultivating the subtle energy through movement, breath and attention. This is the most direct and time-honoured route. It is beyond the scope of this book to suggest Qi Gong practices. However, some guidance towards finding sources of information are included in the Further Reading and Useful Addresses sections at the end of the book.

Dietary Approaches

Qi is made in the body by the interaction of the Spleen, Lung and Kidney. Central to any approach to replenishing the Qi is to strengthen the function of the digestive system and its ability to absorb nourishment. So the first step is to support the Spleen and Stomach as discussed in Chapter Three.

The digestive system begins in the mouth. Well-chewed food will release its nutrients more easily and lessen the burden on the Stomach. Cooked food, especially in the form of soups and stews, also tends to be assimilated more easily. It is not usually necessary to give up raw food but it is made more digestible by fine grating, marinating in vinaigrette and chewing well.

A Qi-nourishing diet features fresh, alive food. The aroma and taste of food is an expression of its Qi. Quite simply, food which tastes and smells good is nourishing. For this reason, fresh foods such as fruit and vegetables should not be over-cooked or allowed to go limp and soggy. Therefore seasonal, locally grown fruit and vegetables are vital, cooked lightly and served up as soon as they are ready.

The Qi of a food or meal is greatly affected by its medium of growth and its preparation. Organically grown food is sig-

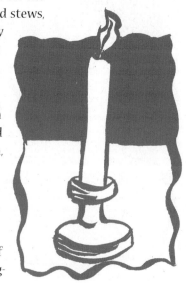

> **The body is the soul. We ignore its aches, its pains, its eruptions, because we fear the truth. The body is God's messenger**
>
> Erica Jong

nificantly more vital than chemically treated foods and traditional varieties are more potent than modern hybrids or genetically manipulated strains. The preparation of food is an energy dance between the cook and the food. All of us have experienced the warm nourishing feeling from food prepared with love and generosity of spirit. The quality of the energy dance between grower and food and between cook and food cannot be listed on the side of a packet but really should be considered an ingredient.

**If you bake bread
with indifference,
you bake a bitter
bread that feeds but
half of man's hunger**

Khalil Gibran

There are many parallels between modern research into the role of oxygen in the body and the functions assigned to Qi in Chinese medicine. Oxygen-rich foods such as fruits and vegetables are needed for full vitality. These oxygen-rich foods balance the oxygen depletion caused by denser foods such as meat and dairy. The key to enhancing the Qi is not so much about avoidance of low-oxygen foods, but about balancing the proportions of oxygen-carrying foods in our diet. A diet high in fruit, vegetables and grains is ideal with seeds, nuts and beans in smaller quantities and meat, dairy and fats in even smaller proportions. In a Qi-enhancing diet proteins are always mixed with a high ratio of vegetables, fruit and grains.

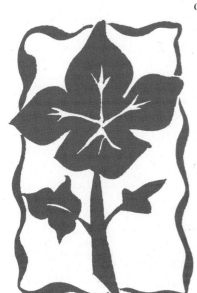

A Qi-enhancing diet, therefore, contains a high level of fresh fruit and vegetables balanced with a small quantity of good quality proteins. A few sprouted seeds are encouraged too. The freshness is important. When used moderately the habit of juicing raw vegetables and fruits can supplement the Qi. Additional principles are the inclusion of complex carbohydrates and the avoidance of refined carbohydrates. Complex carbohydrates release their energy slowly into the body providing a sustained source of nutrition. They are part of the key to strengthening the Qi of the body. This means giving whole grains an important place in the diet.

Grains have been the staple food of all major civilisations. They are the basis of Blood and Qi, essential foods for maintaining strength and vitality. In rural China it is estimated that up to 90% of a person's calories are obtained from grain, as opposed to around 10% in the US. A regular consumption of whole grains will ensure a steady release of energy into the system and support the growth and maintenance of the body. Whole grains also give stability to the system, moderating the influence of more extreme foods or substances.

Foods that nourish the Qi tend to be neutral to warm in temperature and sweet in flavour. Rice, pumpkin or lentils would be considered sweet foods which release their sweetness slowly rather than the quick hit of more 'empty' sugars. Pungent flavours will also stimulate the activity of the Qi and the more aromatic herbs are useful helpers.

When the Qi is weak there are several herbs that can help. Diagnosis needs to be more refined when choosing herbs because their effect is more powerful and a wrong choice could therefore be more damaging. The herbal helpers can stimulate the function of the Organs whereas food nourishes them. For example, hawthorn will stimulate the circulation of Blood and tone the blood vessels, while wheat will nourish the tissues of the heart. This is, of course, a generalisation, but it provides a useful way of thinking about food and herbs. Herbs are often used in cooking to moderate or enhance the effect of food and to direct it towards a particular Organ or function in the body.

There are three other general ways that the Qi can be strengthened. The Qi of each Organ can be helped by eating the corresponding organ from an animal. Kidney Qi Deficiency, for example, is helped by eating kidney. The colour of a food is also an indicator of its action, according to the law of the five elements, i.e., yellow foods tend to nourish the Spleen, white foods the Lung, dark foods the Kidney, green foods the Liver, and red foods the Heart. According to the doctrine of signatures, foods of a similar shape to parts of our anatomy will also be effective, e.g., walnuts are said to nourish the Brain, kidney beans the Kidney, etc.

All grains, legumes, most vegetables, in particular sweet root vegetables and squash, and some fruits are used as basic Qi tonics. Each Organ also has resonant connections to specific foods which reinforce its Qi. These are listed in the next few pages.

Sage is an excellent overall Qi tonic suitable for all Qi Deficient conditions, as is thyme. Pollen and royal jelly are also applicable for all Qi Deficient conditions and ginseng[24] can be used in most cases. More specific recommendations are made according to the nature of the condition.

Qi-strengthening recipes can be found in the main recipe section of this book. The major patterns of Qi Deficiency are discussed below with their appropriate dietary approaches. Deficiency of the Lung and Spleen Qi are seen as the most fundamental. This is because the Lung 'governs' Qi and the Spleen is the 'source' of Qi, which it derives from food. Strengthening the Qi of these two Organs will benefit Qi Deficiency anywhere else in the system.

Spleen Qi Deficiency

The Spleen's sphere of influence is the digestive system, the thinking process, the soft tissue and the limbs. It is also strongly involved in the menstrual cycle and is the key Organ in the production of Blood and Qi. Not surprisingly, a deficiency of Spleen Qi is at the root of many other patterns.

When the Spleen is Deficient we often experience a kind of heaviness. The limbs feel heavy and weak, there is a general tiredness and we easily feel congested. Because the Spleen governs the digestive system, difficulty often focuses there: perhaps a tendency to bloat after eating, problems digesting food, a tendency to ferment inside, tiredness after eating. Stools tend to be loose and appetite low or erratic. There may also be a tendency towards Dampness as the Spleen function of transforming moisture is weak.

The pattern of Spleen Deficiency manifests in many other ways: as poor concentration, as neediness, as collapsed posture, as food intolerances, as prolapse, as menstrual difficulty and so on. It is also at the root of Blood and Qi Deficiency generally. The Spleen could be called the mother of the system, the core supplier of nourishment, the source of well-being and security. The ability to be nourished is dependent on the strength of the Spleen.

In terms of food, all self-help begins with a look at the Spleen to ensure that it is as well nourished as possible. The kind of food that most nourishes the Spleen is often very similar to the food that nourished us as children: thick well-cooked soups and stews, sweet root vegetables and grains, easily-digested food that sits in the belly with a huge sense of satisfaction.

Eating well-cooked food, which is a way of beginning the digestive process outside of the body, and chewing well, assists the Spleen in the breakdown of food. Raw food and complex food combinations are better avoided. Overeating will also worsen conditions of Spleen Qi Deficiency, overwhelming the system and encouraging conditions of Stagnation and Dampness.

Food which nourishes the Spleen Qi is always sweet and often mildly warm in nature. All foods rich in complex carbohydrates such as root vegetables and squash are well-suited. As well as creating a feeling of comfort, Spleen-nourishing food needs to taste and smell good to awaken the digestive system. Aromatic herbs especially stimulate the digestive function and enliven the Spleen. Mild pungent spices such as nutmeg, aniseed, black pepper, fennel and cinnamon are also helpful and the pungent onion family helps reduce any tendency to Stagnation.

Rice, pumpkin, lentil, chicken, carrot, sweet potato/yam, string bean, squash, chestnut, corn, ham, tofu, chickpea, oats, spelt, date, fig, cherry, molasses, herring, mutton, broad bean, mackerel and beef all assist in easing Spleen Qi Deficiency.

Licorice, which is sweet and harmonising in nature, is an excellent Spleen Qi tonic. It can be used as the basis of teas made from such digestive aids as fennel, dill, star anise, cardamom, black pepper, caraway and clove. Jasmine tea is helpful when taken with meals and royal jelly can be used as a supplement.

Stomach Qi Deficiency

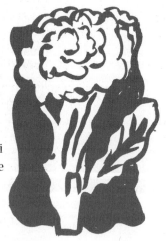

Stomach Qi becomes depleted through poor diet or after a long illness. It is weakened through any patterns of starvation such as excessive dieting or anorexia. It may also become weak through rigorous training, in particular ballet, which tends to damage the Stomach meridian. Stomach Qi Deficiency goes hand in hand with Spleen Qi Deficiency and the general recommendations are the same. However, because the Stomach likes moisture, it is also helpful to include in the diet watery soups and broths. Beef, peas, papaya and shiitake mushrooms have some specific strengthening action

Lung Qi Deficiency

When the Lung Qi is Deficient the voice is often weak, there is a tendency to collect sputum in the lungs and sometimes there is shortness of breath on exertion. The immune system may also be low with a tendency towards coughs and colds. Sometimes there is a tendency to sweat which is an energy loss through the pores of the skin.

Emotionally a pattern of weak Lung Qi will tend to manifest as lack of expressiveness and poorly defined boundaries both in the physical sense of immunity and in the psychic sense of lack of respect for one's own and other people's boundaries. It reflects a poorly defined sense of one's place in the world. Archetypally the Lungs are related to fathering, the way we are taught our value and place in the world outside of home.

Weakness of the Lung Qi is linked to weakness of the Spleen and Kidney. Lung Qi Deficiency is approached in much the same way as Spleen Deficiency because of their close relationship in the manufacture of Qi. Pungent flavours are also used to stimulate the activity of the Lungs so some of the recipes are a little more 'perky'. If the Lung Qi is weak it is sensible to be careful with Dampening foods as these are more likely to cause the accumulation of mucus.

Oats, molasses, carrot, sweet potato, yam, sweet rice, mustard green, ginger, garlic, almond, walnut, squash, potato, date, mutton and grape all nourish the Lung. These strengthening foods can be supported by the use of a few pungent foods, especially those which are also white, such as horseradish and white radish.

The Lungs can be strengthened by a tea of licorice and elecampane in equal parts. Ginger, garlic, cinnamon, black pepper and citrus peels will all stimulate and warm the Lung and expectorants such as coltsfoot and mullein will assist the expulsion of mucus.

Kidney Qi Deficiency

Kidney Qi Deficiency is characterised by weakness or achiness in the lower back and weakness of the urinary and reproductive system. There may also be a general weakness of the skeletal structure especially at the knees or ankles. Poor retention of urine and/or sexual fluids is common so there may be dribbling or frequent urination, wet dreams (usually without dreams) and chronic vaginal dis- 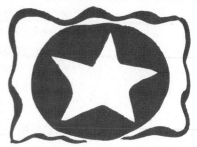 charge. Because of the Kidney's relationship with the Lungs there may also be some shortness of breath and a tendency to feel chilled. The roots of the problem are often in overspending of sexual energy. Loss of energy through childbirth is also common.

Psychologically there may be an over-focus of energy into sexuality, either in a repressive or permissive way. In coming to terms with sexuality, we are learning how to manage the vital force seated in the Kidney, the spontaneous life-affirming energy of creation. Kidney Qi Deficiency is closely linked to Kidney Yang Deficiency.

Weakness of Kidney energy is approached through the inclusion of foods which directly nourish the tissues of the Kidney system (parsley, wheat berry, sweet rice, rosehip, raspberry and blackberry leaf, black sesame seed, string or sword bean, kidney bean, walnut); by eating a wide range of food; by avoiding too much sweetened food, which tends to weaken Kidney function; by including some salted products such as miso or soya sauce and a few astringent herbs; by eating food that is mostly warm; by reducing stimulants.

Millet, kidney, venison, wheat berry, kidney beans, aduki beans, egg, chestnut, walnut, raspberry, string bean, asparagus, parsley, sweet rice, shrimp, lobster, quinoa, oats, sweet potato, blackberry, mussels, nettle and alfalfa sprouts all support Kidney Qi.

Fennel seed makes a delicious tea and is effective in supporting and strengthening the Kidney. Other pungent foods that stimulate the Kidney include fenugreek, star anise and caraway. Astringent herbs such as nettle and blackberry leaf make helpful teas and celery seed can be used in cooking. When the Uterus, which is dependent on the Kidney, needs support, white deadnettle, motherwort and raspberry leaf are helpful remedies and rose oil may be regarded as a general 'cure-all' for virtually all menstrual problems.

Heart Qi Deficiency

Heart Qi Deficiency manifests with many of the classic signs of Qi Deficiency such as tiredness and shortness of breath, with the possibility of heart palpitations. There may also be lethargy and a lack of spiritedness. Heart Qi Deficiency is usually caused by emotional difficulty, especially long-term sadness.

Heart Qi Deficiency is closely linked to Spleen and Lung Qi Deficiency. The dietary approach is as for Lung and Spleen Deficiency, with help given to any accompanying pattern of Liver Qi Stagnation. A few bitter foods can be helpful. Although this pattern may be helped by food, it is primarily helped through calming the mind and dealing with the emotional issues.

From a physiological point of view it is useful to strengthen the nervous system to help with Heart Qi Deficiency. There are some herbs which are good spirit lifters and do not aggravate the nervous system, providing a more helpful kind of stimulation than caffeinated drinks. Some foods are also both calming and tonifying. Don't forget to include the subtle vibration of flowers into Heart cookery.

Raw milk, ghee, reishi mushroom, barley water, corn, chicory, wheat (especially as wheat berry or sprouted wheat), scallion, cherry, date, pomegranate, hawthorn, garlic, apple, flower salads (borage, marigold, nasturtium, rose, violet), oats and quinoa all support Heart Qi. Honey will nourish the Heart and calm the Spirit.

Oat berry and straw, sage, rosemary and skullcap all help lift the spirit and gradually restore Heart function. Cinnamon twig is useful as a general stimulant, especially when the Heart is not strong enough to bring circulation into the fingertips. Arnica restores Heart Qi after a shock and is also an effective general tonic for the Heart, but should only be taken internally under the supervision of a herbalist. Essential oils of lavender and melissa help circulate the Heart Qi and neroli essential oil may be inhaled or used in the bath to relieve anxiety and settle the Heart.

Blood

Blood and Qi have a close interdependent relationship. Both Qi and Blood circulate around the body through the meridians and blood vessels, activating and nourishing the tissues. We could say that Blood is a more dense manifestation of Qi, generated and moved around the body by the power of the Qi and mutually reinforcing the strength of the Qi. Patterns of Qi and Blood Deficiency therefore often occur together.

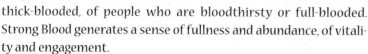

It is through the Blood that we feel embodied. Blood nourishes form and gives us substance. It ties us into the pulse of life and its rhythmic cycles. To be full-bloodedly alive is to be richly and sensuously inhabiting our bodies and emotionally and physically engaged with life. Blood is the carrier of passion in the body. We talk of people who are hot- or cold-blooded, thin- or thick-blooded, of people who are bloodthirsty or full-blooded. Strong Blood generates a sense of fullness and abundance, of vitality and engagement.

Blood is primarily derived from food, which we get from interaction with the physical world. Blood is therefore dependent on the strength of the Spleen which transforms food into nourishment. Renewal of the Blood is dependent on the power of the Liver which is said to store the Blood. The Heart is the place where the Spleen sends the essences of food to be fully transformed into Blood, and the Kidney provides power to the Spleen for the conversion process. The underlying strength of all these Organs will affect the capacity to manufacture good quality Blood.

It is a maxim of Chinese medicine that women rule Blood. Through menstruation and the experience of pregnancy, women are intimately linked to the nature of Blood. It is especially important for women that the Blood is abundant and that the reservoirs do not become depleted. The two vessels known as the Sea of Blood (Penetrating Vessel) and the Sea of Yin (Conception Vessel) need to be kept full to bring abundant nourishing Blood into a woman's reproductive system. Patterns of Blood Deficiency underlie most kinds of menstrual difficulty, infertility and postpartum exhaustion.

In western medicine, blood is known to be the carrier of neuropeptides, chemical messengers that distribute information around the body. In Chinese medicine, Blood is seen as housing the Mind, as the home of consciousness. Consciousness has its anchor in the Blood and weakness of the Blood can also mean that consciousness loses its mooring, that the Mind floats restlessly out of the body giving rise to ungroundedness and feelings of anxiety. In patterns of Deficient Blood this is particularly noticeable before sleeping. Abundant Blood means that the Mind can be fully grounded in the body and can settle down at night, withdrawing inwards and allowing sleep to bring renewal.

When Blood is abundant a person feels well-nourished and has vitality, plenty of stamina and good immunity. He or she is grounded in their body and in their experience, with a strong sense of self. Their complexion is bright and their hair has lustre. When Blood is Deficient such signs appear as low vitality, dull complexion, difficulty going to sleep and anxiety.

How does the Blood become Deficient?

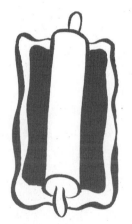

The Blood usually becomes Deficient against a background of Spleen weakness and some toxic accumulation. Like Qi Deficiency, Blood Deficiency may be caused by long-term illness, stress, chronic worry or overwork. Blood is also lost in childbirth, heavy menstrual periods and injury. A period of renewal is always necessary to replenish the loss. It is generally believed to take 120 days to fully renew the Blood, so any programme of Blood renewal needs to be maintained over this long a period.

It is my view that, psychically, Blood Deficiency sometimes expresses the failure of the soul to become fully embodied and the cure has to do with proper incarnation into the physical body. Shock, which sometimes causes dissociation of the soul from the body, may also set up a pattern of Blood Deficiency. (I cannot help thinking of 'vampire' legends when writing this section, those creatures who need human blood to stay incarnate and whose pale lustreless faces are an exaggerated caricature of the classic Blood Deficient complexion.)

Sometimes there are inhibiting factors which interfere with normal digestive processes and prevent the manufacture of good quality Blood. Dampness, for example, inhibits the Spleen's ability to make Blood. Hidden pathogens which have not been successfully resolved by the body's immune system (such as viruses, bacteria, fungi or parasites) can also disrupt the manufacture of Blood, as can a wide range of toxins.

Commonly, however, a prime cause of Blood Deficiency lies in the field of nutrition and diet and this Deficiency is perhaps the easiest to work with. Both the absence of key nutrients and the intake of congesting substances will lead to a pattern of Blood Deficiency.

Blood Deficiency is tied in with the syndromes[25] of Spleen Qi Deficiency, Liver Yin Deficiency, and obstruction through Damp, Cold or Heat, and needs to be treated in this wider context.

Recognising Blood Deficiency

The general manifestations of Blood Deficiency are a pale and dull complexion, dizziness on standing, blurred vision or 'floaters', dry hair and skin, pale lips, scanty or absent menstruation, poor memory, difficulty settling down to sleep, a general sense of anxiety and slight depression. Not all signs need to be present to confirm the diagnosis and other signs and symptoms point towards the involvement of specific Organs. Blood Deficiency usually arises from weakness of the Spleen and mainly affects the Liver and Heart.

Nourishing the Blood

To nourish the Blood all the Organs involved in its creation and maintenance must be supported. These are the Spleen, Kidney, Liver and Heart. Discussion of how to nourish these Organs can be found in the previous chapter.

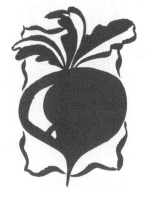

Blood is nourished by fully inhabiting the physical body. Patterns of Blood Deficiency are often seen in people who are not well grounded in their bodies. Movement and physical contact are needed. Whereas the prime physical root of Blood Deficiency is in poor diet or poor assimilation, the mental and emotional root lies in the severance of mind from body. This is more a problem of 'advanced' societies whose life is increasingly detached from the rhythms of the seasons and where survival depends less and less on physical fitness.

Dietary Approaches

The nutritional key lies in adequate protein intake, adequate green leafy vegetables and a wide range of good quality foods. A Blood-building diet of nutritious meals is supported by taking care of the Spleen. The approach is twofold: the diet is aimed at strengthening all the Organs involved in Blood production and at providing nutrients that build the Blood itself.

Blood-nourishing recipes tend to make use of sweet, sour and salty flavours. Almost all foods, when harmoniously prepared, can be said to nourish the Blood; but special consideration is given to the inclusion of green chlorophyll-rich food, good quality protein and grains, and careful combination of foods to enhance the nutritional value. Meat provides one of the easiest sources of Blood enhancement and regular consumption of small amounts of meat can be very helpful.

Some foods are to be avoided or reduced: sugar (the prime Blood imbalancer), alcohol and stimulants in particular must be treated with caution and saturated fats are reduced. Sugar creates sudden imbalance in the composition of the Blood and is highly acidifying. Alcohol creates Heat which in excess can exhaust the Blood. Stimulants overexcite the system and interfere with the timely release of nutrients from the Blood. Many chemical additives can also 'wreck' the Blood, accumulating as toxins which need to be neutralised and expelled. Sea salt, whose mineral profile is very close to that of human blood, is generally beneficial although in excess it becomes weakening. Too much fat will also obstruct the Blood and inhibit its distribution of nutrients.

As a general guideline, the darkness of a food is often an indication of its power to nourish Blood: dark red and black beans, dark fruits such as cherry, date or blackcurrants, black sesame seeds, carrots and beetroot and so forth. However, it is not possible to package the properties of food into neat rules and this guideline has plenty of exceptions. The one thing we can say with regard to colour is that all dark green leafy vegetables are Blood-nourishing.

Highly nutritional foods for the Blood include all dark green leafy vegetables, all grains, meat, eggs, all legumes, fermented soya products (miso, tempeh and tofu), carrots, beetroot, molasses, seaweed, red grapes and dates.

The herbal category which nourishes the Blood is known as 'nutritives'. Nettle tea is a simple, and free, remedy which combines excellent Blood-nourishing qualities with cleansing properties. In China, dangui, the root of Chinese angelica plant, is considered the herb par excellence and can be added to soups and stews, combining very well with chicken. If the Uterus Blood is Deficient, mugwort is a useful herb. Mugwort is combined with sweet rice by the Japanese to make the Blood-strengthening food 'mochi'. Pollen, microalgae, kelp, sage, nutritional yeast and wheatgrass may also be used as tonics. A glass of stout or guinness will also nourish the Blood.

The three Organs most closely involved with Blood are the Spleen, Liver and Heart. Although a pattern of 'Spleen Blood Deficiency' is not listed, Blood Deficiency generally arises from a weakness of the Spleen Qi and the Spleen's failure to effectively extract nourishment from food. Therefore anything which supports the Spleen will improve the quality of Blood.

Liver Blood Deficiency

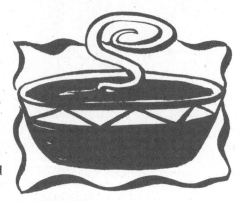

When the Liver is affected by Blood Deficiency there will be signs arising from the Liver's sphere of activity. There may be visual disturbance, numbness or weakness in the muscles and joints, weak nails, dizziness, scanty or even absent menstruation. All Blood tonifying foods will be helpful; liver, alfalfa, nettle, dandelion root and artichoke leaf are additional remedies.

Heart Blood Deficiency

When the Heart is affected there will be signs from the Heart's realm of activity. These may include palpitations, insomnia, anxiety, intense dreaming, memory loss and general nervousness. All Blood tonifying foods will be helpful. Hawthorn berry is particularly recommended and quinoa is an especially nourishing grain. Oats and dates combine well to nourish Heart Blood and beetroot, aduki bean and egg are all supportive foods.

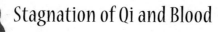

Stagnation of Qi and Blood

Qi Stagnates when the flow of the creative being is stopped. When the Qi is Stagnant, any aspect of harmonious flow can be affected. We may feel frustrated, indecisive or depressed in response to the constraint of our freedom to be ourselves. Physically we may experience uncomfortable digestion, irregular or painful menstruation, headaches, tenderness beneath the ribs or all kinds of pain.

Qi Stagnation underlies all sorts of physical difficulties, from chronic intestinal disorders such as gastritis, cholecystitis and irritable bowel syndrome through to dysmennorhea, premenstrual syndrome and pelvic inflammatory disease. Any problem which involves the Stagnation of natural flow can be said to be a form of Qi Stagnation. Left unattended for too long, Stagnant Qi can transform into Heat in much the same way that a traffic jam can cause tempers to rise.

Stagnant Blood arises from Qi Stagnation or from the influence of Wind, Damp or Cold obstructing the meridians. Sometimes Stagnant Blood is also the result of injury rupturing the blood vessels (bruising is an example of temporary Blood Stagnation). At the external level Blood Stagnation manifests as fixed, stabbing and boring pain in the meridians. More internal conditions of Blood Stagnation manifest as fixed lumps or masses such as ovarian cysts, endometriosis, fibroids and some cancers which are seen as congealed Blood. A milder example of Stagnant Blood is the blood clots often experienced at the beginning of menstruation.

Stagnant Blood in the Heart is a potentially dangerous condition causing heart pain and risking heart attack. Interestingly, some recent research has explored the potential benefits of heart attack for people with blockages around their heart. A heart attack is an attempt by the body to clear obstruction and, if successful, better circulation will follow.

When the Blood is Stagnant, vital nourishment and moisture are prevented from reaching the place where it is congealed. It is important, therefore, not to allow this condition to carry on for too long.

How do we become Stagnant?

It is helpful to consider Stagnation as having two
levels of manifestation. The first is Constraint. This
is the realm of the psyche, the subtle and shifting
ways in which we stifle the more raw expression
of who we are. Sorting out these patterns of
Constraint means exploring the 'shoulds' and
'don'ts' which regulate our lives and deciding which of them provide useful and necessary containers and which of them we wish
to reject because they stifle our true expression of vibrant aliveness.

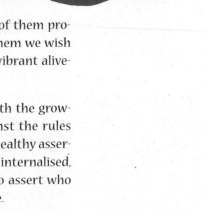

Constraint arises from the relationships we have with the growing edges of our being as we shape ourselves against the rules
imposed by family, authority and culture. Wherever healthy asser-
tion of aliveness is chronically suppressed and then internalised,
patterns of constraint will develop as we struggle to assert who
we are against the 'controller' we have taken on inside.

As patterns of Constraint penetrate deeper they can become patterns of Qi Stagnation, with increasingly physical manifestations.
This is the second level of manifestation. For many people, the origin of a physical problem is in a much earlier psychological
struggle which becomes buried, hidden from awareness; the
symptom is seen as dissociated from their emotional life. Irritable
bowel syndrome, for example, is normally caused by feelings that
have become deeply hidden in the bowels of the body, in the shad-
owy realms of the unconscious, and which are reactivated by
stress. The cure is rarely just dietary: it involves an exploration of
our reaction to stress and sometimes the full uncovering of its
psychological roots.

*Running water is never
stagnant and a door-
hinge never gets worm-
eaten. This is what
motion is all about…
If the body does not
move then the Jing will
not flow. And if the
Jing does not flow
then Qi stagnates*

Lu Shi,
Spring and Autumn Annals

All patterns of Stagnation have some emotional root and are ultimately connected to the Liver whose role is to smooth the flow of
Qi through the bodymind. Physically there is frequently a pattern
of diaphragmatic tension, a holding of the breath and the suppression of internal movement. There may also be pain, usually a pain
that comes and goes with stress.

Recognising Stagnation

Stagnation of Qi is generally recognised by the following signs:

abdominal distension, wandering distending pains, depression and irritability, volatile moods and frequent sighing. The Liver is the most commonly affected Organ but the Qi of other Organs may also become Stagnant. Stagnation of Blood is recognised by: pain which is stabbing and fixed in one location, purple lips and tongue, fixed abdominal lumps, bleeding with dark blood and a tendency towards blood clots, pain and clotting at the onset of menstruation. Again, the Liver is the most commonly affected Organ but the Heart and Uterus are also frequently affected.

Clearing Stagnation

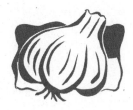

Stagnation requires movement. At the psychological level this means transforming the stuck places in the psyche through whatever means we may: relationship, ritual, therapy. At the physical level we simply need to move both in ways that are expressive and in ways that break through subdued patterns of shallow breathing and muscular tension. This can mean dancing, running, swimming, playing sport, any activity which galvanises the system into action and breaks away from inertia.

Of course, patterns of Stagnation are self-perpetuating because they also serve us in some way. So breaking out is risky and takes some persistence. It may help to develop a structure so that movement becomes integrated into daily life, perhaps a subscription to the local gym, joining a sports club or finding a friend to move with. Success is usually dependent on the 'F' word: fun! If an activity is fun, we are likely to continue it.

Stagnation can be helped through creative projects: painting, sculpting, woodworking, singing, any activity through which we can express the natural creativity at our core. Many people are also helped by Tai Ji, Qi Gong or martial arts which help to channel the disruptive and stuck Qi appropriately and release our patterns of holding into freeing movement.

Dietary Approaches

The dietary approach is to eat lightly and simply, to pay particular attention to posture and tension whilst eating and to avoid difficult food combinations. Herbs and spices which aid the digestion are helpful too. A clean liver is a good physical support to dealing with Stagnation, so plenty of fruit and vegetables and a moderate amount of whole grains are important (a classic high-roughage diet). It is helpful also to become aware of patterns of 'comfort eating' – eating to suppress emotions – and all the addictive behaviours that keep us 'stuck' in one place. The recommended recipes are therefore generally light and make free use of the aromatic herbs and spices which stimulate the system to break down food and resolve the build-up of fermentation.

The practice of 'food-combining' is sometimes useful for regulating a tendency towards Stagnation. The habit of making meals too complex increases the likelihood of competing demands on the digestion resulting in congestion. An absolute and dogmatic following of food-combining principles can be over-restrictive and generate neurosis, anxiety and guilt, none of which are helpful to good digestion nor to the basic enjoyment of food. A more simplified, general approach, however, can be very useful. Try these key guidelines: keep sugar and fruit separate from meals which emphasise starch (i.e., avoid sugary desserts and consider eating fruit either as a snack or as a whole meal); avoid combining dairy produce with meat; avoid combining too many protein-rich foods in one meal; combine rich foods with lighter, easily digestible foods (e.g., meat with greens and low-starch vegetables rather than grains or potatoes).

For Stagnation affecting the Stomach and Liver, bitter herbs are effective. Though not necessarily pleasant to the western palate, these can become more acceptable over time. We have mostly lost the tradition of aperitifs whose bitterness stimulates the digestive juices and prepares the digestive system to better process the food. There are several alcoholic and non-alcoholic bitters commercially available. Alternatively, simple teas such as wormwood can be taken. A segment of grapefruit serves a similar function, especially when eaten without sugar.

The pungent flavour, provided it is not used to excess, will stimulate the system out of Stagnation. Mildly pungent foods such as the onion family, fennel and pungent leaves such as mustard greens or watercress are good choices. Tangerine or other citrus peel, which combine both bitter and pungent flavours, are well known for their Stagnation-resolving action. Try adding a little citrus peel to grain dishes or teas. The sweet flavour will also encourage circulation of both Blood and Qi so sweet root vegeta-

A mouthful of food less at dinner time can help you live 'til 99

Chinese saying

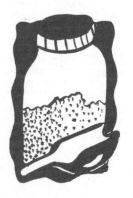

bles, squash, chestnuts, pine nuts and sweet rice are appropriate. However, as a general rule, the more starchy the grain or vegetable the more it supplements the Qi and the less its ability to move the circulation.

Carrot is a simple and effective remedy for digestive Stagnation. Eaten as a soup, flavoured with a gentle pungent herb such as fresh coriander, carrot nourishes and soothes the digestive tract and eases Stagnation. It is an ideal food for babies, nourishing without being congesting, and mildly stimulating the circulation of both Blood and Qi.

After or with a meal, simple teas such as fennel, jasmine, aniseed, dill or chamomile help reduce the tendency to Stagnation. Following a meal with a small helping of pickles is also suitable. When the Large Intestine is affected and its Qi is sluggish a useful remedy is a glass of warm water with a teaspoon of molasses on rising in the morning. Warm water alone is one of the best stimulants for bowel movement and is a simple remedy for babies experiencing constipation. Rhubarb, figs and cabbage are also good helpers.

When the Liver Qi is Stagnant, a condition at the root of most patterns of Stagnation, a glass of warm water with cider vinegar and honey can be drunk on rising, or simply warm water with a twist of lemon. The sour flavour can be used to move and cleanse the liver. Olive oil with lemon juice and cayenne pepper can be used as a salad dressing or it can be taken in small doses as a general stimulant to the Liver Qi. A warm bath with lavender oil can be helpful as can a massage with rosemary oil. Rosemary, spearmint or dill seed can also be drunk as tea and sour fruits such as gooseberry, plum and prune are helpful.

Because Qi and Blood are closely interdependent it is probably too fine a distinction to list foods separately for conditions of Qi and Blood Stagnation. What moves the Qi will move the Blood and vice-versa. Perhaps an exception to this is aubergine which specifically moves the Blood in the Uterus and is helpful in all menstrual conditions involving Stagnant Blood. Vinegar is also commonly used.

To stimulate the circulation of both Qi and Blood a tea can be made of equal parts cinnamon, ginger and tangerine peel. The tea is simmered until a third of the fluid has evaporated.

Ultimately, Liver depression and Qi Stagnation are emotional issues which need to be addressed primarily on that level. If one with such an imbalance becomes fixated on diet, they miss the point of their diagnosis, for in the end, the key piece of advice to such persons is to kick back and relax

Bob Flaws,
Arisal of the Clear

Essence

Essence describes the inanimate physical substances that give rise to life itself. Just as organic life needs a particular composition of carbons and gases to begin on a planet, so too the human body needs certain conditions and materials to grow and thrive. When the Essence is strong, life can thrive.

Essence is partly inherited from parents. This 'prenatal' Essence is the root stock or the genetic inheritance which predisposes each person to certain patterns of growth and development and gives support throughout life. It is considered finite. This precious substance may become exhausted through wasteful lifestyles and Chinese medicine insists that it must be conserved if a person is to remain strong and vital. It is stored in the Kidneys and transformed through the interaction of the three Jiao or burning spaces referred to as the Triple Heater.

Essence may also be accumulated through storing the subtle nourishment available from food and all the sources discussed in the previous chapters. This is called 'post-natal' Essence. A weak constitutional inheritance can be considerably improved by persistent attention to receiving high-quality nourishment and leading a balanced lifestyle. The more weak the inherited Essence the more need there is to practice containment and nourishment.

Nourishing the Essence

The approach to nourishing this most precious substance is twofold. The first is to conserve. This means having good quality sleep and learning how to be effective with the least overspending of energy. Overdoing both physical and mental work calls deeply on the body's resources and will result in premature aging if allowed to continue for too long. Conservation of Essence also means avoiding substances which deplete it. These are excessive use of alcohol, caffeine, recreational drugs, chemicals and preservatives used in food processing. Damage to the Essence is also possible through the consumption of genetically manipulated food; a special section at the end of this book discusses this danger.

Yellow Emperor:
I do not wish to
make love any more.

Simple Girl:
As human beings, we
must not do anything
that contradicts
nature. Now, your
majesty wishes to
refrain from sexual
intercourse and that
is entirely against
nature. When Yin
and Yang are not in
contact, they cannot
complement and
harmonise each other.
We breathe in order to
exchange stale old air
for fresh new air. When
the jade stem is not
active, it will atrophy.
That is why it must be
exercised regularly.
If a man can learn to
regulate and control
his ejaculations
during sex, he may
derive great benefit
from this practice.
The retention of semen
is highly beneficial to
man's health

Classic of the Simple Girl
(Su Nu Ching)

For men, conserving Essence may also mean ejaculating less frequently, a discipline covered extensively in old Taoist texts. In a book known as the *Classic of the Simple Girl*, the Emperor is taught by three women the secrets of longevity through correct sexual practice. Although withholding the semen is the best-known practice, it is little understood and can even be dangerous if practised rigidly and unskilfully. It is worth noting that lack of ejaculation is also sometimes seen as damaging to health.

To become a master of Taoist bedroom arts takes dedication and guidance. For most men the following guidelines are sufficient: the most depleting ejaculations occur when under the influence of alcohol or strong drugs, when exhausted and when there is no love between the sexual partners. Energy lost through ejaculation when the heart is open can flow back when the Yin and Yang polarities of each partner are aligned.

The emphasis on regulating the amount of semen lost through ejaculation also has a basis in western science. Vital minerals are concentrated in semen and need replenishment when lost. Zinc, for example, is highly concentrated in semen and its lack has been identified as contributing to male infertility. Although women do not lose such concentrated fluids as men, dietary and lifestyle neglect can also diminish Essence and lead to problems in the reproductive system. Childbirth creates massive demands on a woman's body and special attention to nourishment and rest needs to be given to avoid Essence depletion.

The first principle, then, is to conserve. The second is to nourish through food, drink and air. The subtle energy extracted from the air is grasped by the Kidneys and is partly used to replenish and invigorate the Essence. Therefore, learning to concentrate the breath into the Dan Tian of the lower abdomen is a way of nourishing the Essence. Meditative breathing practices are the primary way that Essence is nourished and even a few minutes every day of attentive breathing will bring long-term benefits.

Dietary Approaches

Food which nourishes Essence encompasses all the vitamins, minerals, amino acids, enzymes and trace elements essential for life, so a wide diet is called for. Some foods, however, are especially useful. Seeds, which contain all the elements necessary for the growth of plants and trees, are good tonics for the Essence. So too are plants from the sea, the origin of human life, which are rich in essential minerals. Bone marrow, which is itself produced from Essence, is deeply tonifying, so meat stock made from the bones of animals is a good source. Other special foods include ghee (clarified butter), almonds, pollen, microalgae, artichoke leaf and nettle. A little raw milk is also helpful and animal organs provide concentrated nutrition that can nourish Essence.

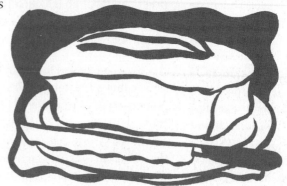

Chapter Five

Yin and Yang

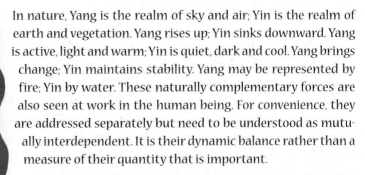

In nature, Yang is the realm of sky and air; Yin is the realm of earth and vegetation. Yang rises up; Yin sinks downward. Yang is active, light and warm; Yin is quiet, dark and cool. Yang brings change; Yin maintains stability. Yang may be represented by fire; Yin by water. These naturally complementary forces are also seen at work in the human being. For convenience, they are addressed separately but need to be understood as mutually interdependent. It is their dynamic balance rather than a measure of their quantity that is important.

In the human body, Yang can be described as the field of activity of the sympathetic nervous system and the adrenal medulla. The sympathetic nervous system mobilises our resources for action, responds to stimuli, gets us ready and moving. Yin can be seen as the complementary field of activity of the parasympathetic nervous system and the adrenal cortex which governs the more inner world of nutrition, maintenance and storage. Yin/Yang balance can be seen as the relative balance within these two branches of the nervous system, a dynamic relationship.

Yang tonics tend to stimulate the sympathetic nervous system, exciting the body to generate warmth, sensation and movement. Yin tonics by contrast tend to be sedative and soothing, calming the overactivity of Yang and encouraging regeneration and rest. In our diets, the Yang is supported by warming and stimulating foods, the Yin by cooling, soothing and moistening foods. We can find this principle at work in many classical meals: a warming, drying curry balanced by moistening and cooling yoghurt, hot lamb balanced by mint sauce, cool watermelon sprinkled with hot ginger.

Yin provides the stillpoint, the anchor for activity, the resting place of regeneration. It is the quiet pool inside to retire to and refresh ourselves. We connect with the Yin aspect through meditation and quietness, through turning the attention inward. It is nourished by adequate rest and relaxation and may be diminished by overstimulation and nonstop activity. In the caffeine-driven culture of the USA where I am currently sitting to write this section of the book, Yin Deficiency is common; there is an absence of stillpoint and of ground, of real substance and relation to soul. In physical terms this appears as all sorts of exhaustion, as mineral depletion, as restlessness and an unsettled spirit. In a culture where the earth is being stripped to desert and worked to exhaustion it is not surprising to find this mirror in the health of its people.

Yang is connected to will, the motivating force within us. Yang provides the fire for all metabolic processes, just as it provides the fire that drives our lives and gives birth to our assertiveness in the world. It is nourished through movement and activity, through having a goal, through stimulation. Deficiency of Yang is frequently tied into patterns of Spleen and Kidney Qi Deficiency and patterns of Cold, Damp and Stagnation, so it needs to be addressed against this background. When the Yin becomes deficient for a long time then the Yang may also collapse through lack of fuel. This is typical in the deeper, more long-term patterns of exhaustion that are prevalent in today's culture.

Abundant Yang energy manifests as physical warmth and vitality, strong metabolism and a strong back. Sexual desire is strong, the willpower is assertive and there is fire and determination in the way a person engages with life. There is an ability to move forward through life, to rise to challenges and to find motivation easily. Deficient Yang energy is characterised by coldness, low energy and lack of motivation. The metabolism will also be slow and there will be a tendency towards Stagnation and the accumulation of Dampness.

Yin energy is contained within the fluid substances of the body: the intercellular fluids carrying nutrients and messages around the whole body, the joint-lubricating fluids, the sexual fluids. Abundant Yin energy manifests as deep physical reserves and the ability to continually replenish the body's physical and mental energy. The body is fertile, the mind calm and receptive. There is an ability to withdraw deep inside the self to visit and replenish the internal 'well of nourishment', both in sleep and daily activity. Deficient Yin energy is characterised by loss of the ability to calm and soothe the system. Exhaustion is deep-rooted and the nervous system 'strung out'. There may be a tendency towards the build-up of Heat and Dryness.

The best doctors in the world are Doctor Diet, Doctor Quiet and Doctor Merryman

Jonathan Swift

Yang Deficiency

Yang becomes deficient through inactivity, through the repeated intake of cold foods and substances, through exposure to cold weather or to cold generally, and through weak constitution.

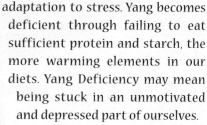

Yang may also collapse in the later stages of adaptation to stress. Yang becomes deficient through failing to eat sufficient protein and starch, the more warming elements in our diets. Yang Deficiency may mean being stuck in an unmotivated and depressed part of ourselves.

These three areas – lifestyle, diet and emotions – are always considered when we explore the etiology of a health condition. Today's lifestyle within industrialised countries is more likely to create conditions of Yang Deficiency than the more agriculturally-based way of life we recently left behind us. A lack of physical exercise and raw physical challenge is compensated for by reliance on stimulants to create that Yang quality of fiery aliveness. Stimulants tend to exhaust the body's ability to generate Yang and, though they mimic the experience of vitality, they do not achieve the burning off of waste material and the creation of true inner fire that supports the functioning of metabolism. It is therefore common to see Yang stimulants such as coffee failing to transform the accumulation of fat and congestion.

The dietary picture that contributes to conditions of Yang Deficiency frequently occurs amongst raw food eaters. Raw food is perfectly nutritious and health-enhancing for some people, but where a tendency to Yang Deficiency exists, raw food, which is energetically cold, will aggravate this tendency. Erratic eating and low starch or low protein diets are also less appropriate for people tending towards Yang Deficiency. Overwhelming the body's fire with too much liquid may also weaken the Yang. (Generally thirst is the best indicator of the need for fluids but at mealtimes it is better not to drown the food with too much liquid intake.)

Emotionally, patterns of Yang Deficiency are connected with depression and lack of motivation. In childhood Yang is

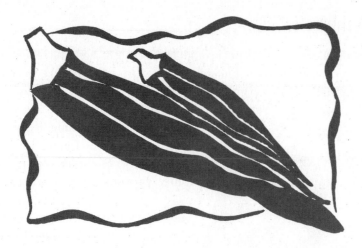

constrained by parental overprotection or overcontrol during the will-developing phase ('the terrible twos') and becomes reckless if not given sufficient boundary and containment against which to shape itself. This may set up patterns of Yang Deficiency or reckless Yang in later life. Yang may also be constrained in adulthood by life situations that feel too limited, without space to stretch and be expressive.

Psychologically Yang Deficiency describes states of fearful paralysis, withdrawal from life and inability to assert the will. To strengthen the Yang means to learn to stand on our own two feet, assume responsibility for our lives and take our place in the world. *Feel the Fear and Do It Anyway*[26], the title of a popular book in the early 1990's, is a rousing summons to our Yang. Henry V's 'Once more unto the breech' speech before the gates of Harfleur is another[27]. The message is 'triumph over fear's paralysis'.

Recognising Yang Deficiency

Yang Deficiency is recognised by the following general signs and symptoms: all manifestations of Qi Deficiency plus feeling cold, cold limbs, lack of thirst, a desire for hot drinks, a pale face, loose watery stools and frequent pale urination. The most commonly affected Organs are the Kidney, Spleen and Heart.

Nourishing the Yang

To work with a condition of Yang Deficiency we need to bring warmth and activity into our lives. It is difficult to get the Yang moving without moving the body. So any exercise at even the most limited level, from jogging to toe-wiggling is part of the programme. Keeping warm is important, especially around the waist and digestive area. Stimulating the back and sides of the body through rubbing, brushing and slapping will also help.

To stimulate the Yang we can also challenge ourselves, do something to get the adrenalin moving. The physical challenge of climbing a rock face or canoeing white water, or the challenge of confronting a difficult situation that demands physical action, or the challenge of getting up a few minutes earlier to do some stretching or movement before starting the day – all these can help develop the power of Yang.

It is helpful to protect the body from cold. One of the most useful practices, especially in cold weather, is to wear a thin silk or cotton scarf around the waist, protecting the kidneys, lower back, belly and bladder. Heat can also be applied directly by the use of moxa, especially around the lower waist, or rubbing warming oils into the body. The penetrating heat of a sauna or a sweat lodge is also effective, warming the core of the body and removing water and toxins. (This is very un-Chinese, whose culture values sweat as a precious substance to be contained, but seems to me to be a valuable time-honoured western practice.) Although it may seem contradictory, a short cold shower or plunge in the river, followed by a vigorous rub and exercise will also stimulate the Yang.

Yang is constrained by fear. To unleash Yang potential requires transforming the places of fear within the psyche, liberating them into action. We may do this through entering our fears in psychotherapy, ritual or creative expression. We may also look for sources of inspiration. A life that is passionately inspired is a life that transforms fear. The source of inspiration may be a political cause, a competitive sport, a romantic love, anything which engages the positive force for life more strongly than our resistance to it. Ultimately, the object of our desire will become more and more firmly located within.

The question for the Yang Deficient person is often 'How can I step into my power?' or 'How can I take charge of my life?' or 'How can I move from this stuck place?' The archetype which can be called on is the Warrior. We can summon the inner warrior through activities such as martial arts or competitive sport. We can summon it by embarking on an adventure. We can summon it by setting our sights on a passionately-desired goal. Whatever the situation, this summoning of the inner warrior is the core shift needed to rouse Yang.

Dietary Approaches

The choice of foods in conditions of Yang Deficiency seeks to correct the tendency towards cold and inertia. Helpful foods are therefore warming and stimulating. Warmth is derived both from the inherent nature of a food and the method of its preparation. Red peppers, for example are a warm food by nature. Their effect will be to warm us up inside. A dish of potatoes, though quite neutral in temperature, can be made more warming by long, slow cooking methods such as baking and roasting, and by combination with warming herbs and spices such as cayenne and black pepper.

So to correct Yang Deficiency we favour foods that are energetically warm by nature and cooking methods that deeply imbue the food with warmth. In this respect there is no comparison between a dish of roasted vegetables that has sat at the back of an old rayburn oven for a couple of hours and a dish taken out of the microwave after a few minutes. The microwaved food is no more warming than when it went in, with the added bonus of being nutritionally wrecked, whereas the oven baked dish will fill us with a sustaining heat for several hours.

The flavour of Yang-fortifying foods is most often sweet and/or pungent. The sweet flavour is an indicator of a food's sustaining nutritional power and the pungent flavour provides a stimulus to the metabolism. A spice such as cinnamon is both sweet and pungent, heating from the inside out and encouraging the flow of energy through the body. Cinnamon joins ginger, cardamom and clove as magical Yang stimulants. The dishes recommended for Yang Deficiency will warm the body and develop the power of Yang but they should not overheat to the point of provoking sweat. If sweating is provoked the body is cooled and heat is lost.

When working to fortify the Yang there are a few things to avoid. It is better to reduce raw and cold food especially in cold weather. It is also advisable to avoid cold drinks and not to flood the digestive system at mealtimes with too much fluid. Because Yang Deficiency easily leads to the accumulation of Dampness in the body we need to be wary of congesting ourselves with too much stodge and fat. How much exactly will depend on the depth of the Deficiency and how it is manifesting in the body.

Fruit, because of its generally cool nature, should be featured a little less in the Yang strengthening diet. It is better to be very moderate with cold fruits such as bananas and watermelon. However it would be a mistake to avoid fruit altogether as it has many properties that will benefit all conditions. Dried fruit tends to be energetically warmer and is more suitable for Yang Deficiency. Some fruit such as cherry, raspberry and apricot are at the warmer end of the fruit spectrum. Baking or cooking fruit with spices will moderate its cool nature.

The pattern of Yang Deficiency is normally only talked about in terms of the Kidney, Spleen and Heart. The Kidney is seen as the root of the whole body's Yang, fuelling both the digestive fire of the

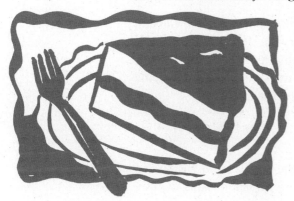

Spleen and the circulatory fire of the Heart. By implication, if the Yang is weak, then the dynamic activity of all the Yang Organs will also be impaired. The Yang of the Liver is more commonly in Excess and the Yang of the Lung is subsumed under the Yang of the Heart.

Kidney Yang Deficiency

Kidney Yang Deficiency manifests as the general symptoms of Yang Deficiency with additional Kidney signs such as aching lower back, cold and weak knees, weak bladder, oedema in the lower body, impotence in men and infertility in women.

A warming diet with the inclusion of Kidney specific foods is called for. These include the onion family (especially garlic), chicken, lamb, trout, salmon, lobster, shrimp, prawn, mussel, black beans, walnuts, chestnut, pistachio, raspberry and quinoa.

Warming and pungent spices include dried ginger, cinnamon, cayenne, clove, fenugreek and black pepper. Star anise and fennel seeds also make excellent tea. Rosemary is a very good Yang tonic and can safely be used over a long period of time. Juniper is helpful and can also be used as an essential oil in the bath or in massage oil.

Spleen Yang Deficiency

Spleen Yang Deficiency manifests as poor digestion with watery stools, low appetite, bloating and tiredness after eating as well as other signs of general Yang Deficiency such as chilliness and oedema. Guidelines for Spleen Yang Deficiency are the same as for Kidney Yang Deficiency with an emphasis on avoiding foods that congest the digestive system and on including warm Spleen Qi tonics such as oats and chicken.

Oats, chestnut, lamb and chicken are both warming and nourishing to the Spleen. All foods which nourish Spleen Qi mentioned in the last section are helpful and raw food is best kept to a minimum.

Horseradish makes a good warming accompaniment to meals and the warm aromatic spices high in essential oil such as cardamom, aniseed, ginger, black pepper, clove and fennel are also helpful. Jasmine and fennel tea can be drunk with meals and a 'chai' could be made from any combination of these spices.

Heart Yang Deficiency

Heart Yang Deficiency manifests as the familiar cold feeling and tiredness of Yang Deficiency together with palpitations, discomfort around the heart, depression, cold hands and some sweating. At the root of Heart Yang Deficiency is commonly a Deficiency of Heart Qi and Deficiency of Kidney Yang so these sections should also be read.

In addition to the Yang-strengthening foods and herbs mentioned earlier, lamb's heart is specifically recommended and cinnamon is the herb of choice. Ginseng may also strengthen Heart Yang but should be taken only under supervision from a herbalist.

Yin Deficiency

As Yin is nourished by rest and by deep nutrition, the causes of its decline have to do with exhaustion. Yin becomes depleted when we overspend our resources through overwork or overactivity. Lack of sleep and lack of restful spaces in the day mean that our Yin is not fully replenished and we begin to 'run on empty'.

Chronic febrile illness, the loss of body fluids through dehydration, childbirth, the overuse of sweating or purging therapies such as sauna, or diaphoretic or purgative herbs, enemas, etc., that cause 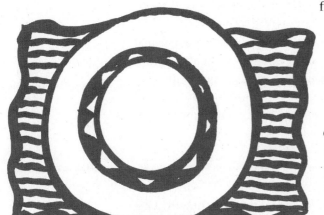 fluid loss may all contribute to weak Yin. Nutritionally, a diet low in minerals and vitamins such as one dependent on the impoverished foods currently adorning Western supermarket shelves, grown in depleted soils, or a diet making too much use of hot spicy flavours which tend to dry one up, may eventually lead to depletion of Yin. Genetically manipulated foods also seem likely to weaken the Yin.

Constant exposure to dry environments, including air-conditioned and centrally-heated spaces, can lead to dryness and depletion of fluids. Exposure to sources of electric and electromagnetic energy such as computer terminals also play their part. Too much television or time spent at a computer in childhood, which exposes the body to rapidly alternating electromagnetic fields, can set up a tendency to Yin Deficiency. The tendency towards Yin Deficiency will be aggravated by the use of stimulants and any products which leach the body of vital nutrients.

Yin may also be depleted through overspending sexual energy and loss of sexual fluids. For men, semen is a highly concentrated substance rich in minerals such as zinc, which in many oriental practices is retained and reabsorbed during sex. These practices are discussed in various books and cannot be addressed here. Although there is no such obvious equivalent for women, replenishment of fluids lost through sexual activity and menstruation is important. The key factor is not abstinence from sex or from orgasm, but the rechannelling and recycling of sexual energy, the containment and building of sexual energy rather than its waste.

Yin Deficiency arises simply when we are overfocused into the Yang aspect of being. Living constantly in 'doing' mode without attending to 'being' mode sets up patterns of stress which eventually lead to exhaustion and depletion of Yin. From the perspective of the nervous system, when the system is 'jammed' in sympathetic mode, the parasympathetic functions are constrained and sufficient renewal becomes impossible.

Recognising Yin Deficiency

Deficiency of Yin classically manifests as low-grade fever especially a sensation of heat in the afternoon, feelings of heat in the palms, soles of the feet and the upper chest or face, night sweats, dryness of the throat at night and insomnia. In addition to these general manifestations, there may be other signs which point towards Yin Deficiency affecting specific Organs.

Nourishing the Yin

The key to replenishing Yin is rest and deep nourishment. This means deep sleep, learning how to relax, meditation. All activities which are calming and turn attention inward can be said to be Yin-nourishing. Meditation and bodywork practices which connect us to the subtle rhythms of our fluids or tune us into the cellular regeneration within the bone marrow are Yin replenishing practices.

Psychologically, Yin is expressed as acceptance of oneself, an inner calm and strength, an ability to simply be, and the cultivation of deep-rooted presence. The work of cultivating Yin is therefore reflective and quiet in nature. Through meditation we can build the ground of our being, the root strength and anchorage in the self; and through contemplation we can reach a place of acceptance and an ability to move gracefully with the flow of our lives.

Rest is also important. This may mean giving time to ourselves during the day to sit or lie down. It may take the shape of receiving a massage, going for a quiet reflective walk in nature, taking time to watch the sunset or listening to Gregorian chanting. Whatever way we take our rest, the key quality is the shift into a more inner, receptive state of being. Listening to music and turning the focus inward connects us to the place of Yin.

Replenishing the Yin means turning away from stimulation. Watching the view, a corner of the garden or a burning candle will be more effective than watching television. Active watching tends to be too stimulating and can encourage too much mental activity. The English romantic poet William Wordsworth described the eye as an 'intellectual' organ that can block us from true seeing. In the language of Yin and Yang, looking is more Yang in nature, seeing more Yin. To see means to receive and be nourished through the eye rather than to use the eye to search and analyse.

Dietary Approaches

A Yin-nourishing diet is mineral- and vitamin-rich. It includes many foods from the sea such as seaweeds and fish, many seeds and beans which are full of the concentrated nourishment a plant needs for growth, a wide range of fruit and vegetables, dairy and a little meat. The more nutritious grains such as wheat and oats are appropriate choices. To nourish the Yin means to pay attention to the wide spectrum of minerals, vitamins, amino acids and trace

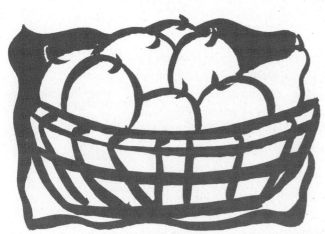

elements which form the ground of good health. Yin nourishing food needs to penetrate deeply into the body. Yin is like a well which must not run dry, a reserve of nutrients which form the basis of growth and the fuel for all physiological activities.

Yin nourishing meals typically combine a small amount of high quality protein with a wide range of vegetables and fruit. Yin tonics are typically sweet and cool and often include salty or sour flavours. The drying bitter flavour and the stimulating pungent flavour are less used. This diet is not very different from the Blood-nourishing diet, and recipes from these two sections of this book are happily complementary.

When Yin Deficiency includes Dryness, more lubricating foods are used. These are foods with high water and mucilage content such as marrow and sweet lubricating fruits such as pear. Demulcent herbs such as slippery elm are also appropriate. Of all the Deficiencies, Yin Deficiency calls for the highest use of fruit and all fruits are appropriate.

The restraints of the Yin nourishing approach have to do with stimulants, especially the more drying stimulants such as coffee, very hot spices and alcoholic spirit. These will exhaust the Yin and dehydrate the fluids. Red meat may also be too warming. In conditions of Yin Deficiency it is also important not to overdo rich Yin tonics which, for all their nutritional value, may congest the function of the Stomach and Spleen and generate Dampness.

All fruit and vegetables, seaweeds, fish, seeds and nuts, dairy, eggs, beans, pork, duck are all useful for Yin Deficiency. Rosehip and hibiscus make helpful teas. The mineral rich comfrey and nettle are also well suited to Yin Deficiency. Moistening herbs such as mullein, borage, marshmallow, slippery elm and aloe are helpful when there is Dryness. Royal Jelly is a very nutritious supplement when the condition needs extra help. Geranium and rose are useful as essential oils for the bath and massage oil.

Kidney Yin Deficiency

Kidney Yin Deficiency often underlies other patterns of Yin Deficiency. It manifests as a collection of Kidney-related symptoms which include dizziness, low frequency ringing in the ears, memory loss, heat in the 'five palms' (soles of the feet, palms of the hand and upper chest or face), night sweats, aching lower back and deep ache in the bones.

Kidney Yin Deficiency is addressed by following the guidelines above for general Yin Deficiency and including several foods specific to the Kidney. These include barley and millet, tofu, string bean, asparagus, all dark-coloured beans, dark fruits such as blackberry, mulberry and blueberry, all seaweeds, and animal products including fish, eggs, dairy produce, duck and pork.

Tonics such as spirulina, kelp and wheatgrass are appropriate. Marshmallow, comfrey and slippery elm are excellent for providing both moisture and nourishment.

Liver Yin Deficiency

It is common for Kidney Yin Deficiency to occur with the pattern of Liver Yin Deficiency with additional symptoms from the Liver's realm. These include disturbed sleep, irritability, dry stools, numbness in the limbs and scanty or absent menstruation.

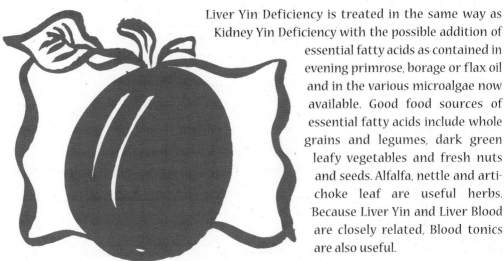

Liver Yin Deficiency is treated in the same way as Kidney Yin Deficiency with the possible addition of essential fatty acids as contained in evening primrose, borage or flax oil and in the various microalgae now available. Good food sources of essential fatty acids include whole grains and legumes, dark green leafy vegetables and fresh nuts and seeds. Alfalfa, nettle and artichoke leaf are useful herbs. Because Liver Yin and Liver Blood are closely related, Blood tonics are also useful.

Stomach Yin Deficiency

Stomach Yin Deficiency frequently arises from long-term neglect of the need to eat. A history of erratic hurried eating with late night binges is typical. Usually there will be no appetite, dryness in the mouth and throat but little desire to drink and often pain in the epigastrium.

The condition of Stomach Yin Deficiency is improved by the use of watery soups and mucilaginous vegetables such as summer squash. Barley and millet are helpful grains and tofu, mung beans, spinach, chard, alfalfa, asparagus, sweet potato and chickweed are good choices.

Demulcent herbs such as slippery elm and comfrey are also useful.

Lung Yin Deficiency

Lung Yin Deficiency manifests with many of the classic signs of Yin Deficiency accompanied by a dry or tickly throat and an irritating but unproductive dry cough.

Useful foods include all the foods already recommended for Yin Deficiency with the inclusion of extra fruit such as apples, pears, peaches, bananas and oranges. Pine kernels are a specific tonic, chickweed can be eaten in salads and comfrey, mullein and borage can be drunk as tea.

Heart Yin Deficiency

In this case the general symptoms of Yin Deficiency are present with palpitations and a feeling of restlessness. The approach to Heart Yin Deficiency is broadly the same as for Kidney Yin Deficiency.

Mung bean and wheat berry are helpful foods and, as with Lung Yin Deficiency, chickweed is supportive. Borage tea helps calm anxiety as well as nourish Yin. All calming teas will help ease the anxiety generated by Heart Yin Deficiency.

Chapter Six

The Climates

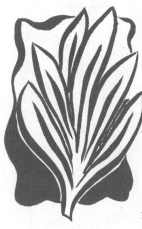

The bodily landscape, just like any ecosystem, has its own climate and, within certain limits, change is natural and healthy. When the system is out of harmony, natural changes in climate can become disruptive. Many of the pathological events and processes of the bodymind are described in terms of weather and its effect on a person. The common climates which can arise in a person are known as Heat/Fire, Cold, Dampness, Dryness and Wind.

When the Organs and Substances are flourishing and vibrant, a healthy climate will normally reign and all will be well. When the Organs and Substances are not functioning well, the internal climate can change and become damaging. When the internal climate loses its balance in this way, pathological conditions arise. These are named according to their nature and location and are recognised by their signs and symptoms. For example, symptoms of irritability and sudden outbursts of anger might indicate Heat in the Liver; a stomach ulcer might indicate Heat in the Stomach; constipation might indicate Heat in the Intestines.

The various adverse climates of Heat, Cold, Dampness, Dryness and Wind are known as patterns of Excess. A pattern of Cold, for example, means that too much Cold is present in the system; a pattern of Dampness, too much moisture and so on. The treatment of Excess conditions is different from the treatment of Deficiency. Whereas Deficient conditions call for nourishment and supplement, Excess conditions call for reduction and removal of the aggravating force.

This section deals with adverse climates that arise internally and are known, not surprisingly, as internal conditions. They are the result of weaknesses in the system compounded by lifestyle factors such as diet, living and working conditions, and emotions. 'Stormy weather' may also arise in response to invasion by external climates. In this case they are called external conditions and are dealt with in the next section.

Heat

Warmth is necessary for all physiological functions but its excessive presence spells trouble. The pattern of excess Heat refers to a condition of overactivity and strain causing Heat, possibly with inflammation and dryness. If we think about what happens when we apply heat to something, the symptoms of Heat become obvious: movement and agitation, redness, perhaps moisture being pushed to the surface, thirst. Empty Heat, which arises from a Deficiency of the cooling and lubricating qualities of our Yin, is discussed under Yin Deficiency. Heat may also combine with Dampness and this combination is discussed later.

How do we become Hot?

Excess Heat accumulates in the system from pent-up emotion, from the intake of too many heating foods or substances, or from the residual effect of pathogens lodged and unresolved within the system. Heat may also be a response to environmental toxins accumulated in the body. It may also lodge locally as the result of injury or repeated strain in the muscles and tendons. In this last case, topical rather than systemic remedies are applied.

Hot Blood will often erupt as skin rashes or bleeding. The Stomach, Liver, Intestines and Lung are also common sites of excess Heat. Emotional stress usually manifests eventually as Heat in the Heart with a characteristic red tipped tongue and possible accompanying signs of anxiety and palpitations.

An excessive intake of hot stimulants such as spicy foods and alcohol produces Heat, as does the excessive intake of certain B vitamins and amphetamines.

Recognising Heat

As one might expect, Heat is generally recognised by redness, inflammation, thirst, red eyes, burning sensations, scanty urination and constipation. The tongue may show a yellow coating and the pulse usually feels slightly rapid. The location of Heat is established by the other presenting signs and symptoms.

Clearing Heat

The simple answer is 'cool down'. We need first to identify the source of the Heat. If the source is emotional then we are looking at stress management, relaxation, going to the heart of what troubles us. If the source has to do with the inappropriate intake of heating substances then these are reduced: tobacco may be causing dry Heat in the Lungs, caffeine causing Heat in the Liver, spicy and greasy food causing Heat in the Stomach/Liver and so on. If the source is infection chronically lodged in the body then it is best to enlist the help of a herbalist, as is the case with toxic poisoning.

Dietary approaches

The dietary approach is simply to include more cooling and soothing foods in the diet and to reduce heating foods. A cooling diet is high in fruits and vegetables, low in fried and fatty foods. Steamed vegetables, soups and boiled foods are favoured over other heating methods. Overcongestion of the system through overeating or poorly combined foods is also avoided. Stimulants, alcohol and sugar are high on the don't list. When there is nervous agitation, then calming herbs are included. Raw foods are also helpful provided the digestion is strong enough. Bitter, sour and salty flavours are favoured over sweet and pungent.

When there is excessive Heat in the Stomach a simple remedy is to eat a small bowl of grated white radish (daikon) with a splash of soya sauce. Mung bean soup is a classical remedy, and moistening fruits such as banana, strawberry and melon are appropriate. Cabbage is both soothing and cooling and wide use can be made of the bitter salad vegetables such as endive and lettuce. Peppermint is ideal as a tea.

When the Liver is more affected the recommendations are similar to those for Stomach Heat as these are usually related. Cucumber, celery, alfalfa, lemon, purslane and spinach could be added to the list and dandelion coffee is a useful drink. Heat in the Blood can be helped by spinach, chard, bamboo shoots, chickweed and lemon; rose petals and chrysanthemum can also be taken as tea. In general, many foods listed as nourishing the Yin will also be appropriate.

Cold

The accumulation of Excess Cold in the system refers to obstruction and overburdening of the system with Cold. Too much cold energy will cause the system to slow down with the result that functions are obstructed. This may manifest as painful contraction, as the retention of excess fluid, as obstruction in the meridians and as a slowing down of functioning.

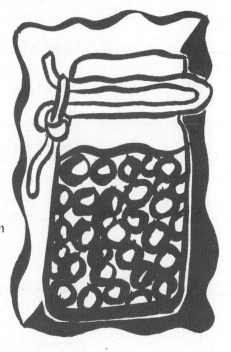

Cold is often a factor in obstruction of the menstrual cycle and generally within the realm of sexual functioning. Cold in any part of the system will create there a sensitivity to further aggravation by cold, and this is taken as one of the diagnostic signs of its presence. Cold Lung for example will be more prone to catch cold, Cold Bladder will be more prone to chills and so on. Cold can painfully obstruct the meridians causing congestion in the local tissues.

Except where pathogens are a key cause, Cold may be treated as Yang Deficiency. Excess Cold and Deficient Yang commonly co-exist. A condition of Excess Cold, insofar as we can distinguish it from Yang Deficiency, will usually involve the accumulation of mucus and fluid in the body and of toxins, perhaps accompanied by a tendency towards overweight. It will generate heaviness, slowness and Stagnation. Because Cold obstructs there may also be pain, especially in the abdomen, and discomfort when the painful area is pressed.

How do we become Cold?

We become Cold through the intake of cold substances, through inactivity or through exposure to cold environments. Excessive use of energetically cold foods, of refrigerated or raw foods, and excessive consumption of chilled drinks can eventually cause Cold to accumulate. Some drugs such as anaesthetics, antibiotics, tranquillisers, diuretics and antacids are also Cold in nature.

Emotionally, Cold is caused by chronic fear which causes contraction and the inhibition of our responses. Cold is also found as the residue of unresolved pathogens lodged in the system. If there is the suspicion that the Cold is caused by residual pathogens it is better to consult a herbalist to ensure that the pathogens are dislodged and moved out of the system.

Recognising Cold

The presence of Cold manifests as chilliness, a desire for warm places, food and drink, abdominal pain that feels worse for pressure, lack of thirst, loose stools and abundant clear urination. There may be a white coating on the tongue and the face may appear pale or blue-tinged.

Clearing Cold

Cold is treated quite simply by the opposite principle of warmth. At the local level, where Cold is causing painful obstruction of the circulation, massage and the local application of heat are called for. Typically this would be the use of moxa, but warming and invigorating essential oils may be used, as can compresses. The intention is to invigorate the circulation and disperse Stagnation.

Cold also needs movement and activity. Vigorous breathing techniques can bring warmth to the internal regions, as can exercise which focuses on alternating contraction and expansion. These techniques invigorate the area and break through Stagnation. Exposure to warmth, especially sunlight, and the use of sauna can help to expel Cold.

The use of warming essential oils such as juniper which stimulate circulation can be helpful, and massage oils can be infused with ginger. At a more systemic level, where Cold has penetrated the Organs, internal remedies are needed. This is the realm of food and herbs.

Dietary approaches

Warming foods and warming cooking methods are used to drive out the Cold and transform Stagnation. For the purposes of this book, conditions of internal Cold and Yang Deficiency are treated in the same way. Please refer to the section on Yang Deficiency for further guidelines.

Dampness

Dampness refers to the accumulation of fluid, mucus and phlegm in the body. As its name suggests, its nature is heavy, sticky and obstructive. Some of the most stubborn western ailments including candida, allergies, thrush, eczema, asthma, arthritis, tumours and being overweight are frequently seen as involving patterns of Dampness in Chinese medicine. Usually a person will already be predisposed to Dampness and this tendency is aggravated by factors such as a heavy, fatty and sweet diet; lack of exercise; the use of certain drugs, in particular antibiotics, steroids, birth control pills; and exposure to Damp environments.

Dampness can manifest both systemically and locally. Locally there is painful obstruction of the meridians and tissues and a buildup of deposits and toxins. The muscles may feel numb, heavy, tired or achy. Joints may be painful and swollen. In these cases it is common for symptoms to worsen in damp or humid weather. Fungal infections of the skin are also in the realm of Dampness as are any moist or sticky discharges. Dampness can even lodge in the head making the thinking fuzzy and the head heavy.

Systemic Dampness is likely to cause Stagnation, clogging up the works and causing swamp-like conditions in the lower belly. In the digestive system this is experienced as fermentation, bloating, discomfort after eating and difficulty processing dense or complex foods. Actually, the nature of Dampness, as with all forms of Stagnation, is that it likes to perpetuate itself, so people commonly find themselves craving the very thing which congests their system.

Phlegm is a more congealed stage of Dampness resulting from fluids failing to be transformed. Phlegm behaves differently according to where it is manifesting. In the Lungs it manifests as sputum, bronchial obstruction or nasal discharge; in the Spleen appearing as tiredness, vomiting, mucus in the stool or lack of appetite; in the Heart the manifestation is often more mental, causing confusion or possibly palpitations, even coma.

Dampness may also be present as oedema, the retention of water in the body. The transformation and movement of fluids through the body is dependent on the Kidney, Spleen and Lung. The location of oedema is an indication of which Organ is most involved: oedema in the face and upper body reflects a failure of the Lung to disperse the fluids; oedema in the belly reflects a weakness of Spleen Qi; and oedema in the lower body, such as swollen ankles, reflects failure of the Kidney Qi. Oedema in the lungs reflects a serious failure of the Kidney Yang.

Because patterns of internal Dampness usually involve a failure of the Yang and weakness in the Qi of the Spleen, Lung and Kidney, it would therefore be useful to read those sections of this book. Dampness also combines easily with Cold and Heat.

How do we become Damp?

Dampness is the result of the body's failure to burn off or transform moisture. A sedentary lifestlyle and overconsumption are primary causes. Poorly digested food that is eaten hastily and not chewed well also contributes to the build up of Dampness. Too much nutrition, especially in the form of fats, starchy or glutinous foods and sugars, will overburden the system and when the system is overwhelmed a backlog of unprocessed food builds up. This is clearly seen in babies and infants who quickly develop catarrh, ear infections or weepy eyes in response to too much Damp food, a general pattern known as 'accumulation disorder'.

Dampness is a kind of congestion frequently resulting from an inability to transform food and drink. Many people with weak digestive systems and a lack of fire will be prone to accumulate Dampness. The key word is 'transformation'. A strong digestive system can transform most foods, provided we don't chronically overeat. Much is also due to combining foods poorly, either by making meals too heavy or too complex, or by combining foods that tend to ferment together. Eating large meals late in the evening will also tend to cause congestion; and overwhelming a meal by drinking too much water with it will also aggravate a tendency towards Dampness. Poor quality food such as synthetic, chemically grown food, food which is stale, food which is overcooked and food which is old and reheated more than once will also contribute somewhat to the perpetuation of Dampness.

Sometimes Dampness may have a pathogenic rather than a dietary cause. A simple example is an infection in the digestive system with 'damp' symptoms of nausea and heaviness. Infectious hepatitis is an example of a deeper problem where a pathogen has attacked the

Liver and triggered a 'damp' reaction (usually described as Damp Heat affecting the Spleen or Gall Bladder). In these cases it is important to drive out the pathogen; otherwise more problematic conditions may become established as the external Dampness becomes an internal condition. Conditions such as M.E. (myalgic encephalitis) are often precipitated by a Damp pathogen left unresolved in the system.

Western medicine is sometimes responsible for the establishment of chronic Dampness in our systems. The overuse of antibiotics frequently results in fungal overgrowth in the intestines, sometimes to the extent that dietary remedies alone cannot reestablish balance. Steroid creams which inhibit conditions such as weeping eczema will tend to drive the Dampness deeper into the body, as will steroids used to suppress asthma. Birth control pills which inhibit the menstrual cycle also block the body from discharging Dampness from the reproductive system and this may lead in turn to more hardened accumulations of Dampness in the form of cysts.

There is also an emotional climate which helps to create an environment for Dampness to set in. Lingering feelings of guilt and shame, or of self-disgust, are common accompaniments to physical manifestations of Dampness, especially in the Intestines. Worry is also known to knot the digestive system and it can interfere with the Spleen's transformative process. Wherever in the psyche there are feelings which fester and cannot be transformed, the psychological ground for Dampness is laid.

Lastly, environmental factors play their part too. Living in a damp climate or a damp house makes it more likely to be penetrated by Dampness. Sleeping on damp ground, we are likely to wake up feeling heavy and achy and over time such exposure may allow Dampness to become lodged in the joints and muscles. This external manifestation of Dampness does not necessarily imply a more internal weakness of the Organs.

Recognising Dampness

The manifestations of Dampness will vary widely according to which part of the bodymind is affected and whether it is combining with other influences such as Heat and Cold. The general manifestations are a feeling of bodily heaviness, lack of appetite, a feeling of congestion in or just below the chest, difficulty passing urine, a sticky taste in the mouth and dirty or sticky discharges.

Clearing Dampness

Dampness, with its resultant Stagnation, needs movement. This requires exercise, especially if we are living in a damp environment. Stretching muscles both lengthways and across their fibres will help eliminate Dampness from the muscles. Exercise will also stimulate the Yang to begin burning off accumulated moisture. Massage, especially with Damp-transforming essential oils (such as sage for the lungs, sandalwood for hot conditions, juniper for cold conditions or cardamom for the digestion) is also helpful.

Sometimes deep psychological work is needed to break through emotional 'bogginess'. Going down into the dark and swampy parts of our being is rarely fun, so taking a good light and a sense of humour with us can make all the difference.

Dietary Approaches

With regard to food, regular eating will support the elimination of Dampness. Generally it is better to eat richer, more nutritious foods in smaller quantities, well distributed throughout the day. It is also advisable not to eat heavily, especially in the evening. We also, of course, need to moderate consumption of the Dampening foods. These include dairy produce (sheep and goat products are less Dampening), fatty meats and fried foods, saturated fats, sugar and sweeteners, wheat, bread, beer, and concentrated foods such as concentrated orange juice or tomato purée. Hydrogenated oils, which interfere with enzyme production in the liver and increase cholesterol levels, are Dampening. Too many nuts will also be Dampening but sunflower seeds, pumpkin seeds, walnuts and almonds are somewhat less congesting.

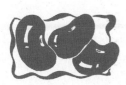

Dampness is not just a matter of pointing the finger at a list of offenders. There are positive steps to take. The essential principles of working with a condition of Dampness through diet are to eat a relatively low-fat wholefood diet and to include some drying and draining foods. Whereas sweet foods will tend to worsen conditions of Dampness, bitter and pungent flavours will be helpful. The moderate use of sour foods can help break down congestion but too much will tend to increase retention of moisture, especially when combined with the sweet flavour.

Foods with draining qualities such as aduki beans and alfalfa sprouts are especially useful in resolving Dampness in the lower abdomen, affecting the genitourinary system and colon. Dampness in the middle zone of the body which includes the Liver, Gall Bladder and Stomach can be helped by bitter foods which dry Dampness such as endive and dandelion and pungent foods which break through Dampness such as the onion family. In the upper body, Phlegm in the Lung can be helped by pungent foods such as radish, garlic or mustard greens.

Fruit is generally moistening but certain fruits have decongesting qualities that can benefit Dampness. Papaya, pineapple and pears can be useful helpers. Papaya enzymes have sometimes been used to increase the digestibility of meat, and pineapple is a natural accompaniment to cheese. It would be a mistake, and a shame, to cut out fruit; rather, more care needs to be taken not to cause fermentation though combining fruit with starchy foods. It is the more lubricating fruits such as banana and the tropical fruits that are most likely to aggravate Dampness; although, where Cold and Dampness combine, all raw fruit intake needs to be very restricted.

The treatment of Dampness depends on how and where it is manifesting. It may be combining with Heat or Cold and focused in the Gall Bladder or manifesting as Phlegm in the Lung. Generally speaking all bitter flavoured herbs will be helpful. For example, a cup of dandelion coffee after a meal can help the breakdown of food and when Dampness is affecting the skin, burdock is a good remedy. Barley water is an excellent general counter to Dampness (see recipe section). It is customary in China to serve jasmine or green tea with a meal to reduce its Dampening effects. Sage is also recommended as a general remedy for all Damp conditions.

Pungent, decongesting foods can be used to accompany rich foods such as meat. Mustard and horseradish are particularly useful in damp and cold climates such as northern Europe's. These are native plants, ideally suited to the civilisations they live with.

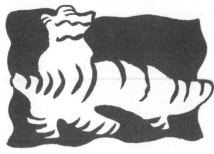

Dampness in the Spleen and Intestines

Dampness in the Spleen's realm may affect the whole digestive system, the muscles, and even the power of concentration. It is the strength of the Spleen and the power of the Yang which transform moisture in the body and prevent Dampness from accumulating. Therefore it would be helpful to read those sections of this book too. When the Spleen Qi is very weak and unable to transform food, digestive enzymes are sometimes helpful as a supplement.

Spleen Dampness is addressed by strengthening the Spleen Qi and by stimulating the Spleen's action through the use of bitter and aromatic flavours. This makes aromatic basmati rice the rice of choice, especially when flavoured by aromatic herbs and spices such as basil, thyme and fennel. Most beans have a strengthening as well as a drying action: broad bean, which is somewhat aromatic, and chickpea are especially helpful. Corn-on-the-cob and pumpkin provide both Spleen-nourishing and Damp-resolving actions. The combined condition of Cold and Dampness affecting the Spleen can be countered by the inclusion of warm and pungent herbs such as horseradish, cardamom, ginger, clove and black pepper.

Porridge made from millet will help remove Damp Heat from the Stomach and Spleen whilst strengthening the Kidney at the same time. It is also common to find conditions of Damp Heat in the Intestines. Here both cooling and draining qualities are called for. Rice and barley are mildly diuretic grains which will help as will the diuretic actions of aduki and mung beans and the draining action of celery, seaweed or watercress. When blood is present in the stool, aubergine can be helpful. The bitter nature of pumpkin seeds is also useful.

Dampness in the Stomach, Liver and Gall Bladder

When Dampness combines with Heat and affects the Stomach, Gall Bladder and Liver this may manifest as nausea, discomfort around the lower ribcage, a bilious taste in the mouth and reactiveness to foods with moist and hot energies such as fried and fatty foods. Bitter foods are called for here and foods which cool the system and drain moisture. Judicious use of sour foods such as unsweetened pickles will also help to decongest the Liver.

Such bitter leaves as chicory and endive are helpful; rye and roasted barley are helpful grains; mung beans will cool and drain moisture. A soup of mung bean and seaweed or watercress soup would be appropriate. A dish of barley and lightly cooked cabbage also has a reputation for helping this condition. Useful herbs include include purslane, wormwood, goldenseal, gentian and dandelion root.

Dampness in the Bladder

Dampness in the Bladder can combine with either Heat or Cold. Its characteristic symptoms are difficult, frequent and cloudy urination. Heat or Cold are distinguished by the colour of the urine: more yellow in cases of Heat and more pale in cases of Cold. This pattern frequently occurs as a result of exposure to cold or damp environments. The appropriate dietary approach is to drain the Dampness and resolve the Heat or Cold.

Diuretic foods such as aduki bean or peas are helpful for all conditions of Dampness in the Bladder. Where Heat is present, more cooling foods such as celery, cranberry, seaweed, melon, alfalfa, aduki or mung bean are good choices; goldenseal, celery seed or cornsilk (the tassles on the end of a corncob) are very effective as tea, and barley water is a classic remedy (see recipe section). Where Cold is present, some warming spices such as fennel, fenugreek or ginger can be added to support the Kidney Yang.

Dampness in the form of oedema needs the help of diuretic remedies: useful herbs include dandelion (whose leaf can be added to salads), elderflower and, a weed understandably hated by gardeners, couch grass root.

Phlegm in the Lung

When Dampness collects in the Lung it forms Phlegm. This usually results from a weakness of the Spleen failing to transform moisture and manifests as mucus and congestion. A dietary approach is to favour the pungent and bitter flavour to draw out, transform and break through the mucus. Phlegm in the Lung easily combines with Cold or Heat so foods are chosen according to temperature.

In cases of Hot Phlegm such cooling, bitter and/or pungent foods as radish, watercress and seaweed are appropriate. Where there is Cold, more warming foods such as garlic, onion, horseradish, mustard greens or kohlrabi can be chosen. A simple dish of grated turnip can be used as a remedy for both Hot and Cold Phlegm.

Expectorant herbs such as mullein, coltsfoot, eucalyptus and elderflower help to resolve conditions of Hot Phlegm. An effective and pleasant tea can be made from equal parts coltsfoot, mullein and licorice. Thyme, hyssop, basil and winter savory can be used to resolve Cold Phlegm and tangerine peel is excellent in tea. Nettles provide a useful tonic for the Lung and help resolve all conditions of Phlegm.

Moderating the effects of Dampening foods

To moderate the Dampening nature of wheat, wheat bread can be toasted; or less Dampening flours such as rye can be used. Caraway, dill seed or other decongesting spices and herbs can be added when making your own bread. In the case of pasta, use pesto, garlic, peppers, onions or walnuts to create a decongesting sauce. Pizza can be served with toppings of anchovy, garlic, onion, tuna, sweetcorn and olives, flavoured with Damp-resolving herbs such as basil and thyme and accompanied by a small bitter salad.

If using dairy, try goat and sheep, soured dairy products, soya milk and unpasteurised raw milk and consider combining them with some Damp-resolving spices. Hard cheese can be eaten with apple or onion; cottage cheese, which is a less Dampening option, can be accompanied by chives, garlic or pineapple. Rye crackers make a more drying base.

Beef and heavy meat can be served with horseradish or mustard and accompanied by green leafy vegetables or a bitter salad. Beer drinkers can favour more bitter varieties, organically produced and served at room temperature. Nuts can be dry roasted gently to lessen the effects of rancidity. Sugar 'fixes' can make use of less refined sweeteners such as molasses, malt extract, date syrup, amasake or honey.

The absolute avoidance of Dampening foods isn't fun. When Dampening food is consumed try to limit the amount, avoid overeating and offset the food's Dampening nature with foods that have Damp-resolving properties.

Wind

Wind, as might be imagined, is a disruptive climate. As in nature, its behaviour is unpredictable, mostly affecting the upper parts of the body with symptoms that wander around and interfere with the smooth functioning of the bodymind. Two kinds of Wind are distinguished: internal and external.

The condition of internal Wind is normally a secondary complication of other conditions such as Deficient Blood or excessive Heat in the Liver. Internal Wind often disrupts the brain and may cause headaches, vertigo, confusion and all manner of spasms and neuromuscular disturbance. Internal Wind can be seen in such disorders as Parkinson's Disease or epilepsy.

The dietary approach is to eat a fairly bland diet, nourish the Blood and keep the Liver clear. Some foods have a particular reputation for subduing Liver Wind. These include coconut, black soya beans, sage, chamomile, hops, passionflower and skullcap. Some foods are also reputed to agitate Wind: these are eggs, crab and buckwheat.

Wind is known as the 'spearhead of the hundred diseases'[28] and it is as an external invader that it is most commonly encountered. External Wind can be the precursor of more serious problems and needs to be properly cleared from the system. Neglecting to rest and drive out the invasion of Wind can allow a relatively minor problem to penetrate the interior of the body where more serious harm can be done. The condition of external Wind is discussed in the next chapter of this book.

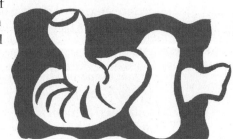

Chapter Seven

Invasion and Defence

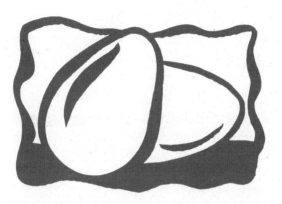

When a person receives pernicious influences on his body, there must be a place where they are granted entrance. These influences have gone there because they responded to a summons. As long as a person's essence and spirits are complete and strong, no external evil will dare to offend that person

The Yellow Emperor

We are exposed to viruses and bacteria all the time. Normally, the presence of these pathogens poses little challenge to the healthy person and illness does not follow. When the conditions of the time make a person vulnerable, or when the pathogen is particularly strong, a fight begins between the pathogen and the person's defensive energy.

An important distinction is made between adverse climates that arise from within the body and those which occur as a reaction to external events such as the invasion of a virus or literal exposure of the body to extreme environments. The last section explained how adverse climates that arise from inside are known as internal conditions. Adverse climates that arise from invasion of the body by pathogens or environmental factors are known as external conditions. A good rule of thumb is that external climatic conditions are almost always distinguished by their sudden onset.

An external condition is one where the progression of illness has not penetrated beyond the outer layers of the system. The invading force is being engaged in combat by the defensive energy and the internal Organs are not affected. Only the Lung, which is the most vulnerable Organ, will be disrupted, giving rise to some of the typical signs of invasion such as runny nose or sneezing.

This is important in practice. Adverse internal climates are treated simply by food and herbs of their opposite nature, e.g., the use of Cold substances to treat Hot conditions. When the condition is external the same principle applies but pathogens must also be pushed out of the body. This is done through use of the pungent flavour. So a Hot invasion is countered with a cool and pungent substance such as elderflower; a Cold invasion is countered with a hot and pungent substance such as ginger.

Invasion of Wind

An invasion of Wind would be described in western medicine as the first stage of a bacterial or viral infection such as the common cold, influenza, laryngitis or an upper respiratory tract infection. Its symptoms mimic the behaviour of Wind in nature: sudden onset, wandering pain and agitation mostly affecting the upper parts of the body. Wind is usually also marked by an aversion to wind and cold, reluctance to go outside, chilliness, occipital ache and a runny nose or sneezing.

A Wind invasion is always characterised by its sudden onset. It rarely appears by itself and usually brings the forces of Heat, Cold or Dampness with it. Wind Heat, Wind Cold and Wind Damp are descriptions of the acute stages of the body's invasion by pathogens (bacteria and viruses). Their characteristic symptoms of chills, aches, stiffness and fever can be seen as the struggle between the body's defensive Qi and the invading forces.

The intensity of the symptoms reflects both the power of the individual immune response and the power of the pathogen itself. Generally, if the defensive Qi is weak, the pathogen will enter the body with fewer symptoms and possibly penetrate more deeply. Strong defensive Qi will often put up a dramatic fight. If the defensive Qi fails to throw off the invading forces, then the illness moves from an acute to a chronic stage and begins to penetrate the interior.

At the initial stage of Wind invasion, diet can serve to block the immune response or assist it in its resistance. It is always best to simplify and reduce the diet, cutting out all mucus-forming or potentially obstructive foods such as meat, dairy, fatty foods and bread. A short fast, drinking only fluids for a day or so, frequently speeds the passage of the illness. The best foods are vegetables and lightly cooked fruits with only a few simple grains and proteins. Herbal remedies which assist the defensive Qi are called for. These are known as herbs which 'release the exterior' and are generally pungent in flavour.

Invasions of Wind are not exclusively caused by pathogens. They may also occur literally as the response to strong climatic conditions such as wind, heat and cold. Regardless of their cause, these patterns are approached in the same way and the body will need help to reduce or expel their influence.

Invasion of Wind Heat

When the onset of infection is characterised by moderate fever, inflammation and pain with sensations of heat predominating over sensations of cold, the diagnosis is Wind Heat. The dietary approach is to cool the body, circulate the defensive Qi and push the invaders back out again. This is achieved by eating cooling simple

foods, usually as soup, flavoured with pungent and cool spices and herbs. Vegetable soup flavoured with mint, marjoram or lemon can be supported by herbal teas which provoke sweating such as elderflower. Some fruit which is cool and moist is also helpful.

The pungent flavour of turnip, Chinese cabbage and watercress makes them good choices for soup. Apples and pears can moisten, soothe and cool the Lung and grapes provide good support for the Qi. Chrysanthemum, mulberry leaf, peppermint, elder, lime, catnip, spearmint, lemon balm, boneset and vervain make helpful teas. A classic tea for the onset of Wind Heat is a combination in equal parts of peppermint, elderflower and yarrow. Mint combines well with chrysanthemum to bring relief. Pot barley water can also be drunk as a tea with peppermint.

Although it may seem contradictory, some of the warm pungent herbs can also be helpful, notably ginger. Adding a little garlic or fresh ginger to these recipes is appropriate. When the throat is affected a gargle of salt water or sage and honey tea can soothe and reduce inflammation. A bath with essential oil of lavender can also help shift the invasion.

Wind Heat may also be a description of allergic reactions such as allergic rhinitis, hay fever or urticaria. Treatment usually means attending to both internal and external aspects of the condition. Internally patterns of Liver congestion, Dampness, Deficient Kidney and Lung or Spleen weakness usually provide the ground for allergies to take hold. Externally, the various triggers need to be identified and reduced as much as possible. A diet free of sugar, and low on fat and stimulants is necessary.

Invasion of Wind Cold

When the onset of infection is characterised by chills, aches and pains, stiffness and little or no fever, the diagnosis is Wind Cold. The dietary approach is to warm the body, circulate the defensive Qi and push the invaders back out again. This is achieved by eating warming foods, usually as soups, flavoured with pungent and warm spices and herbs supported by herbal teas which provoke sweating. The onion family, which combines warmth with pungency, is ideal; both garlic and scallions are particularly effective. Black pepper is excellent and cinnamon and ginger, or ginger and spring onions, combine well as a tea to expel Wind Cold.

A mustard water footbath and the use of eucalyptus, pine, 'Olbas' and ginger oils, inhaled or added to a hot bath, provide useful support. Wind Cold may obstruct the pores and the body will need extra encouragement to sweat. The use of diaphoretic (sweat-inducing) herbs can be supported by sweating therapies such as sauna or simply by having a hot bath, then wrapping up well and going to bed. A hot whisky or brandy 'toddy' before going to bed is also a time-honoured cure.

Wind Cold also combines frequently with Dampness to produce acute interference with the harmonious flow of Qi and Blood in the meridians. This manifests as pain which is the experience of obstructed flow. The guiding principle for treatment is essentially the same as that for Wind Cold, with the addition of some Damp-resolving herbs and foods. A massage oil made from 2 parts juniper, 1 part cypress and 1 part cinnamon oil can be rubbed into the body or the oils used in a bath. Thyme oil may also be helpful.

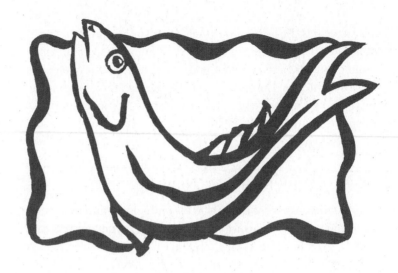

Invasion of Wind Damp

When Wind combines with Dampness the classic symptoms of Wind appear alongside the symptoms of Dampness. Wind Damp usually invades the meridians, joints and skin causing itchy skin and rashes which move from place to place, painfully swollen joints and aching muscles. Symptoms are worse for humidity and there may be a general feeling of heaviness. Food and herbs that combine pungent and Damp-resolving properties are called for.

Juniper is a specifically useful herb and can be drunk as tea or used in massage oil. It should not be used if there is Heat or during pregnancy. Peppermint, basil, spearmint or tangerine peel can be drunk as tea. Pungent and Damp-resolving foods such as the onion family, kohlrabi, mustard greens, turnip and radish are all appropriate.

Invasion of Cold

Cold easily rides on the back of Wind but may also enter alone. This is usually as a result of exposure to actual environmental cold. External conditions of Cold are characterised by feeling cold, contraction, sharp pain and stiffness. The onset is quicker than internal Cold and the location is most commonly the muscles, meridians and joints. However Cold can also penetrate directly through the skin and accumulate in the Uterus, Bladder, Stomach and Intestines.

The treatment is the use of direct heat, such as moxa, and warm circulatory stimulants such as cayenne, cinnamon, ginger, juniper or rosemary. Any of these can be used as tea or as essential oils and rubbed into the skin. The approach to eating described as strengthening the Yang would also be appropriate and it is important not to aggravate the condition by the intake of cold energy foods.

Invasion of Dampness

External Dampness is characterised by acute onset and the general symptoms of heavy sensations and ache. Its behaviour will vary according to its location, with a tendency to invade the lower part of the body first, flowing upwards into the pelvis and intestines. Here it can cause vaginal discharge, turbid urine or loose stools. If it invades the joints it can cause swelling and ache.

External Dampness soon transforms into internal Dampness. Foods and herbs which resolve Dampness, stimulate Qi circulation and open the surface of the body to expel the invader are chosen. The onion family and pungent herbs such as ginger or peppermint are good choices.

Part Three
Recipes for Self-Healing

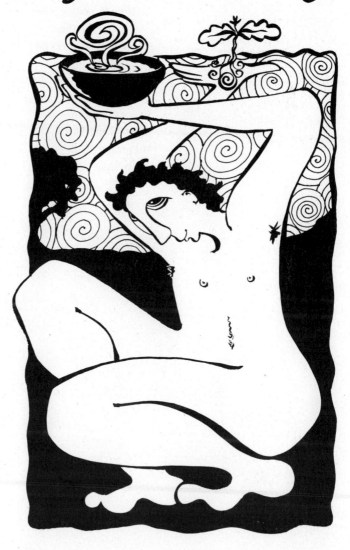

Above all, take
satisfaction in the
cooking and joy in the
eating. If cooking is no
more than time-
consuming drudgery and
eating nothing better
than fear, denial and the
observation of dietary
guidelines, then we
subvert and deny one of
the great pleasures of our
kind. Enjoy!

Elisabeth Rosin,
The Universal Kitchen

Nutrition East and West

Nutritional information in the West is usually presented in terms of quantity. Each food contains a specific amount of certain nutrients. The side of a packet of cornflakes will tell you that it contains x amount of niacin, vitamin C, iron, carbohydrates, fat, etc. Often there is a measure of its caloric value to tell you how fattening it is. In Chinese medicine we talk about food not in terms of quantity but of quality. Each food has certain qualities which describe its effect on the human system. A western assessment of a food's nutritional value is achieved by measurements carried out in a laboratory. A Chinese assessment is achieved by observing the effect of food on the human being. Understanding this distinction is vital for understanding the material presented in this book.

Example: Carrot

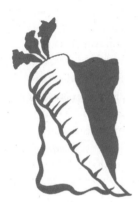

Western description: an alkaline-forming vegetable, containing protein, calcium, phosphorus, silicon, beta-carotene, vitamins B1 & B2, anthocynanidin, fat, oil, and a volatile oil. From this it may be deduced that carrots help clear acidic blood; have useful anti-oxidant properties (a function of beta-carotene); strengthen the connective tissue and aid calcium metabolism (functions of silicon); assist against pinworms (a function of its essential oil).

Energetic description: vegetable possessing a neutral temperature and sweet flavour whose essence travels to the Spleen, Lung and Liver and whose action is to mildly nourish Qi and Blood and stimulate Qi circulation. From this we can say that a carrot neither heats nor cools the body so is appropriate for all conditions; that it is strengthening (a function of the sweet flavour) and that this strength will primarily support the Spleen, Lung and Liver, thereby strengthening digestion, improving respiration, nourishing the skin, stimulating waste elimination, improving Blood quality and smoothing the flow of Qi; and that it will mildly counteract Stagnation.

Chinese nutritional science is the study of vibration and resonance. This is energy medicine, closer to the western practice of homeopathy than conventional allopathy. Each food has a vibrational resonance that affects the bodymind in various ways: heat it up or cool it down; create moisture or dryness; stimulate or sedate; nourish specific organs or functions; move up, down, in or out. These qualities are referred to as **temperature, flavour, action and route**.

The **temperature** of a food describes its action after entering the body. Some foods are more warming, some more cooling. A cold person will naturally benefit from more warming foods, a hot person from more cooling foods. Often these principles are naturally balanced within a meal: warming lamb is cooled by mint sauce, curry is cooled by yoghurt, watermelon warmed by ginger. Temperature is one of the most important factors in our individual choice of food.

The **flavour** of a food describes other aspects of its action. Five principle flavours are distinguished: sweet, pungent, salty, sour and bitter. A food's flavour tells you something of what it does in the body: sweet flavours are nourishing[29] and moistening, pungent flavours dispersing and stimulating, salty flavours softening and sinking, sour flavours astringent and cleansing[30], bitter flavours drying and draining.

Each flavour also has an affinity for a particular Organ, a resonance which carries the action of a food into that Organ's realm. The sweet flavour affects the Spleen, the pungent flavour affects the Lung, the salty flavour affects the Kidney, the sour flavour affects the Liver and the bitter flavour affects the Heart. A chronic craving for a particular flavour is indicative of an imbalance in the associated Organ's function[31].

The type of flavour is established mostly according to its taste on the palate but also according to a food's energetic action. In the case of herbs there are general correspondences between the flavours and their chemical components: pungent herbs tend to contain high levels of volatile oils, bitter herbs tend to contain alkaloids and glucosides, sweet herbs tend to contain high levels of amino acids and sugars, sour herbs tend to contain high levels of tannins and organic acids, salty herbs tend to contain high levels of organic salt, sodium sulphate and iodine[32].

The other categories of **route** and **action** describe where in the body each food particularly resonates and what activity it supports. Foods may strengthen a substance or function, described as tonifying the Qi, Blood, Yin or Yang; or foods may regulate what disrupts or obstructs the harmonious flow of energy, described as regulating the forces of Heat, Cold, Damp and Stagnation.

How we cook our food will affect the moisture and energetic temperature of a meal. Lighter and more watery methods such as steaming or boiling are generally less warming than frying or roast-

> If people pay attention to the five flavours and blend them well, their bones will remain straight, their muscles will remain tender and young, breath and blood will circulate freely, the pores will be fine in texture, and consequently breath and bones will be filled with the Essence of life
>
> *The Yellow Emperor*

Sour travels to the
tendons, Pungent
travels to the Qi, Bitter
travels to the Blood,
Salt travels to the
bones, and Sweet
travels to the flesh

Lingshu

ing. Longer and slower cooking methods will tend to impart more deeply penetrating heat into a food. To cook food is to add fire and begin the digestive process outside of the body, lessening the work on our digestive system and making nutrients more easily available.

Some Guidelines for Eating

The digestive system is supported by offering it well-harmonised flavours and easily digestible food. Here are some simple guidelines for supporting the digestive system to effectively transform food into nourishment:

- **Eat simply.** Too many ingredients poorly combined make hard work for the Spleen (the Organ governing the digestive process in traditional Chinese medicine). Simple food will help support easy digestion as well as an inner sense of clarity.

- **Eat lightly.** Overeating will congest the Spleen's function and is a major cause of Stagnation and Dampness. The art is to stop just before becoming full. If we can do this we will find that we have much more energy available.

- **Reduce sugar.** Sugar and all highly sweet foods can easily overwhelm the Spleen. The over-consumption of sugar easily leads to intestinal fermentation and creates a happy home for intestinal parasites. It also weakens the Blood and destabilises energy levels.

- **Include a few naturally fermented foods** in the diet such as natural sauerkraut, dill pickles or natural yoghurt. These are good helpers to the digestive process.

- **Separate sweet foods and fruit from the main meal.** For many people this helps reduce digestive fermentation and supports the Spleen's action of sifting and sorting.

- **Drink between rather than with meals.** The Spleen is easily overwhelmed by too much fluid. It is generally better to limit intake to a cupful of water or tea at meals so as not to over-dilute the digestive juices.

- **Avoid too much cold food.** Cold food overwhelms the digestive fire and can slow down the digestive process.

- **Chew well.** Chewing starts the digestive process in the mouth. Well-chewed food presents less work for the stomach and intestines.

- **Relax and sit comfortably when eating.** When we are tense, twisted or slumped we compress the digestive organs and make it more difficult for digestion to work. It is important to create physical space below the ribcage, especially between the ribcage and navel, where most of the digestive organs are situated. A few calm breaths just before eating will be helpful.

- **Trust your body.** The body knows what nourishes it. We need to take time to listen and to find our way skilfully beyond our neuroses and beyond the relentless misinformation and subliminal prompting of advertising. Once we are deeply connected to our own inner knowing we can throw away all our health and diet books (except this one of course!).

- **Enjoy your food.** This is probably the most profound piece of advice anyone can give. A deep appreciation and enjoyment of food can open one's whole being to receive nourishment. This advice is the only commandment in this book.

Enjoying your food is very important, because to enjoy something is how we connect to the world, to one another, to our inner being. When you enjoy your food, you will be happy and well nourished by what you eat

Ed Brown,
Inquiring Mind Magazine

Choosing Ingredients

If you are reading this book you are probably already of the persuasion that modern chemical farming is damaging to the health of this planet and its people. Not only does organically grown food taste better, it is also more nutritious[33]. One contribution we can make to the reversal of this damage is to support in whatever way we can the practices of organic husbandry. This may mean choosing to buy organic produce[34], growing some of our own food and/or supporting environmental organisations.

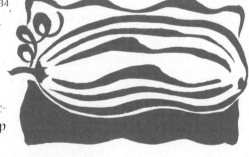

It is possible to feel genuinely committed to the healing of the planet but unable to find or afford organic produce. Where these two factors collide, the following information may help in making educated choices about spending.

Recent British research into pesticide residues in foods shows that some foods tend to retain higher concentrations of pesticides than others. Carrots, potatoes and lettuce were found to be the highest concentrators of pesticides, with strawberries, grapefruit and apples also showing high concentrations (apple juice, interestingly, showed much lower concentrations than fresh apples). At the other end of the spectrum some foods showed much lower concentrations. These were asparagus, green cabbage, cauliflower, cucumber, garlic, leek, marrows, frozen peas, pumpkins and squashes[35].

In the USA, similar studies list the twelve most commonly pesticide-contaminated foods in the following order: strawberries, bell peppers, spinach, US cherries, peaches, Mexican cantaloupe, celery, apples, apricots, green beans, Chilean grapes and cucumbers. The twelve least contaminated are listed as: avocado, corn, onion, sweet potato, cauliflower, Brussels sprouts, US grapes, bananas, plums, green onions, watermelons and broccoli[36].

Today's domestically grown food travels on average 1300 to 1800 miles and changes hands up to six times before reaching the table. This is often true even if that table is right back in the community where the food was grown

National Catholic Reporter, Feb 99

The first consideration in shopping for vegetables should therefore be to give priority to buying organic products where contamination is most likely i.e in carrots, potatoes and lettuce. A second consideration is the possibility of removing some of the toxins from food at home. Washing fruit and vegetables in a bowl of water with a good splash of cider vinegar will remove some, but not all, harmful residues. Leave the food to soak for a quarter of an hour before scrubbing.

At the time of writing this book there are movements in the world's food market which are more threatening to our lives than even radioactive pollution. I am referring to the genetic manipulation of plants. Despite the claims of scientists working in this field, it is far from an exact science and its consequences are irreversible. A special section is included at the end of this book to explain the dangers. An absolute avoidance of genetically modified food is recommended.

Another possibility is the growing of some of our own food. For those without land, the simple practice of sprouting seeds in jars or in a sprouter can be a way of bringing fresh organic produce into the diet. A few herbs can be grown in pots on the windowsill or in an outdoor window box. Even a small courtyard, imaginatively designed, can be a source of fresh food as well as lots of fun.

Lastly, it is worth considering the inclusion of some wild foods among our groceries. Perhaps the most useful of these are the bitter greens such as dandelion leaf, wild cress, chickweed or sorrel. Seasonal nuts or berries are also easy to find. These wild foods have a quality of aliveness lacking in so much of our commercially-grown produce.

The Energetics of Food

This section is a brief overview of food energetics. The energetic properties of food are listed in more detail in the companion book *Helping Ourselves: A Guide to Traditional Chinese Food Energetics*. Also available is a wallchart describing the energetic properties of most foods (see ordering details at the end of the book).

Grains

Grains form the foundation of diet in most cultures and are the basis of Qi and Blood. Their essential sweetness nourishes the body, their fibrous husks scour the intestines; regular consumption of grains helps us remain calm and centred. They supply the complex carbohydrates lacking in modern refined diets, providing a steady release of energy into the system. Grains are the major food of the Earth element[37], the most important nourisher of the Spleen.

An increasingly wide variety of grains is now available. There are slight differences among them in energetic make-up, which means that each person can select a range of grains well-suited to his or her individual constitution. The most nourishing way to eat grains is whole, either cooked or sprouted. Eaten plain they help us distinguish and appreciate the flavours of accompanying dishes. Grains ground into flour have a tendency to oxidise and go rancid after a while.

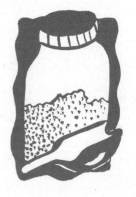

Rice

The sweet flavour and neutral temperature of rice make it a balanced food, which means that we can't really have too much of it. Over time, rice strengthens and calms the digestive system and moderates the excessive influence of more extreme foods. Rice strengthens the Spleen, harmonizes the Stomach and boosts the Qi.

Rice porridge (congee) is traditionally used in China for almost any condition; it is very easy to digest and gently strengthening. To make rice porridge mix one part rice with seven or eight parts water and cook on the lowest possible heat until it is completely soft and sweet. A slow cooker is helpful, as this process may easily take six hours or more. Small amounts of other food such as meat, vegetables or herbs may be added at the beginning according to the desired effect. In some shops it may be possible to purchase a product known as amasake culture which will produce mildly cultured and sweetened rice in much the same way as one makes yoghurt.

Oats

Oats are sweet and warming. They are a magnificent Qi tonic much loved by the Spleen, with additional benefits to the Heart and nervous system. Over time, regular consumption of oats will increase the resistance of joints to Dampness and Cold. They are the ideal grain for all Deficient conditions, nourishing Qi, Blood and Essence. Sometimes oats will be poorly tolerated in gluten-sensitive people and those with very Damp conditions and this can be slightly alleviated by dry roasting the grains. As there is also a mild tendency for oats to generate Phlegm in the Lung it is inadvisable to combine them with Phlegm-forming foods such as milk and sweeteners.

Oat porridge is a traditional start to the day for many people. Its warming and energising effect may last for several hours. Oat porridge is usually better if soaked overnight. Adding salt or miso will direct its action more towards the Kidney and lower abdomen; adding molasses will increase its Blood-nourishing ability; and adding tahini will increase its ability to nourish the Yin. Oats combine well with dates to make an excellent energy tonic.

Barley

Barley, like all grains, nourishes Qi and Blood and has the additional property of counteracting/draining Dampness. It is a good tonic for all Deficient conditions and is an excellent choice when Dampness and Heat need to be drained from the body.

The old European habit of drinking barley water has been sworn by thousands to be the secret of their good health. Barley water can be made by adding an ounce of barley, dry-roasted, per pint of water and simmering the liquid until it has reduced to a slightly thickened texture. Barley is especially good in soups and stews.

(Note that pearl barley is a partially refined grain lacking the full nutritional value of pot barley.)

Rye

One of the more bitter grains, rye also has Damp-resolving ability and rye bread is often the bread of choice in Damp conditions. Rye crackers are especially drying and form the perfect accompaniment to cheese and other rich and Dampening spreads. The

Eating three grains of rice with full consciousness, chewing them carefully and extracting every element of nutrition may be just as nourishing as grabbing a sandwich as we rush from one meeting to another

Sandra Hill

heaviness of some rye breads can be relieved by including caraway and other strong tasting seeds. The hardness of rye grain lends itself to sourdough baking and a true sourdough ryebread will both counteract Dampness and help resolve Liver Qi Stagnation.

Wheat

Wheat is moist and cool with a special affinity for the Heart and Kidney. Its versatility as a flour is probably the reason it has been so widely adopted in the west as the primary grain. However, this has been at the expense of other native grains such as oats, barley and rye. An increasing number of people are now experiencing problems with wheat, signifying that something is out of balance. The problems are probably due to overconsumption and the intense selection practices of the growers, leading to a huge loss of variety and a greatly diminished gene pool. There is also anthropological evidence to suggest that signs of arthritic problems in human skeletons coincide with the advent of wheat as a staple grain. Wheat flour is also quick to turn rancid.

Modern strains of wheat are significantly lower in nutritional value than the wheat grown fifty years ago (Kansas wheat of the 1930's consisted of 30% protein, whereas today its protein levels measure about 12%).[38] The hard wheats used to make pasta appear to be energetically somewhat stronger, as is spelt, an earlier form of wheat, now more easily available in the shops. Spelt is highly recommended by the mystic Hildegard von Bingen as the staple grain for a healthy diet. Wheat's benefits are probably best received by eating the whole grain (wheat berry) either cooked whole or sprouted.

Given the state of affairs with commercial wheat, it seems especially important to eat organic varieties if we want to benefit from wheat's nutritional gifts. An excellent way of eating wheat is as sprouted wheat bread, a deliciously sweet and moistening bread that is easy on the digestion and nourishes the Heart and Kidney Yin.

Other grains

Millet is an easily digestible alkaline grain, slightly cool with a sweet and salty flavour, strengthening to the Spleen and Kidney. It is particularly helpful when the digestion is weak and is a good grain for young children. It is a staple grain in many parts of Africa.

Amaranth and **quinoa** are both exceptionally high in protein, making them unusually nutritious grains. Amaranth is slightly cool in nature, quinoa slightly warm; otherwise their properties are broadly similar. Quinoa has a special reputation in supporting lactating mothers and is one of the few foods reputed to directly nourish the Pericardium.

Buckwheat nourishes the Intestines and stimulates Blood circulation. In cases of Wind and Heat, buckwheat is best avoided. It is not recommended for infants and very young children.

Corn is a somewhat incomplete grain and needs to be eaten as part of a wider diet. Traditionally corn is prepared with lime or ash through a special process discovered by the ancient civilisations of South America, to increase the uptake of niacin in which it is exceptionally low. It is useful in drying Dampness and it strengthens the Kidney and Heart.

Vegetables

A diet high in vegetables will keep most people in good health and keep the Qi strong. Combined with grains, their nourishment potential is enhanced. Dark green leafy vegetables are especially helpful in building strong Blood and activating the Liver. Root vegetables are good builders of Blood and Qi and their sweetness is nourishing to the Spleen. Vegetables of the onion family are pungent and warming. Watery vegetables such as marrow and cucumber are generally cooling and moistening. The squash family nourish the Spleen and are good for the Intestines.

Greens

Mildly sour and bitter, greens have a gentle cleansing action on the Liver and contain nutrients vital for the Blood. It is not really possible for a vegetarian to be in full health without leafy greens. The simple principle of eating something green every day deserves a place in our diets alongside the old principle that 'an apple a day keeps the doctor away'. Meat eaters receive some of the benefit of greens already transformed into flesh.

The cabbage family nourishes the bone marrow, moistens the Organs, nourishes the Heart and strengthens the bones and sinews. Cabbage has a long history in the treatment of stomach and duodenal ulcers and is generally soothing to the digestive tract. The darker green leaves are rich in chlorophyll which helps the formation of haemoglobin in the blood. Pickled cabbage is helpful for the Liver. Chinese cabbage is a little more cooling and is especially helpful in conditions of Damp-Heat. Spinach and watercress both build and cleanse the Blood, and spinach has a lubricating effect on the Intestines.

Root Vegetables

Root vegetables are essentially sweet and will strengthen both Qi and Blood. They benefit the Spleen and Lung, are easy to digest, mildly warming and drying and therefore helpful in conditions of Dampness. Carrot, for example, is a simple sweet food that nourishes Blood and Qi and it is one of the easiest foods for an immature or weak digestive system to accept. It is an ideal food for babies. As well as being comforting to the Spleen, carrot benefits the Liver, strengthens the Lung and helps maintain healthy bacteria in the intestines.

Potatoes are useful Qi tonics. Sweet potatoes and yam are highly regarded for their strengthening effect on the Spleen Qi; yam also strengthens the Kidney. Other root vegetables such as parsnips, swede, kohlrabi, Jerusalem artichokes and turnip have some action against Dampness as well as a warming and mildly stimulating action on the circulation. Beetroots provide a rich source of nourishment for the Blood and are helpful in conditions of stagnant Liver Qi.

Squash

The deeply orange flesh of pumpkin is legendary for its ability to strengthen the Spleen. Its sweet flavour, yellow/orange colour and round shape all resonate with the Earth element and make pumpkin of special value. As well as nourishing the Spleen, pumpkin will soothe the digestive tract and help to drain Dampness. The greener- or paler-fleshed squash tend to be a little cooler but share the same general properties.

Onion family

The onion family, which includes leek, garlic, chive, spring onion and shallot, is warming and pungent. All this family will break through Stagnation, prevent the accumulation of Dampness and

When you prepare food... maintain an attitude that tries to build great temples from ordinary greens, that expands the buddhadharma through the most trivial activity... Handle even a single leaf of green in such a way that it manifests the body of the Buddha. This in turn allows the Buddha to manifest through the leaf

Dogen and Kosho Uchiyama, *Zen Kitchen to Enlightenment*

help in the breakdown of rich food. The hottest of the onions, garlic, has strong antimicrobial properties and assists the Lung in throwing off colds and flu. Onions bring movement to a meal and stimulate digestion.

Salad greens

Lettuce and many of the salad greens have a bitter flavour and will therefore help drain Dampness and stimulate digestion. Not long ago it was common practice to eat a sprinkling of wild bitter greens with a meal, a practice which deserves resurrection. Parsley merits special mention as a great Blood nourisher. It also has a strong affinity for the urinary system and is useful in nearly all urinary problems. Radishes should be mentioned too for their ability to cut through Mucus. They are helpful in all Stagnant conditions and in cooling Heat.

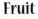

Fruit

Fruit tends to be both moistening and cooling. The sweet flavour of many fruits is combined with sourness and will generate fluids in the body. This makes fruit very supportive of the Yin and the body's fluids. Most fruit will also benefit the Qi and Blood. When the Yang is Deficient, fruit is usually better dried which makes it both warmer and less Dampening. Some fruits, such as apricot, cherry and raspberry are slightly warm in nature and can be favoured by those who are Yang Deficient.

Fruit is also cleansing and will help reduce Stagnation. For all people tending towards Excess and those eating meat-rich diets, fruit is very helpful in preventing accumulation of Heat and Stagnation. For Deficient and Cold conditions fruit is best cooked and the colder tropical fruits best avoided. For Damp conditions it is often better to moderate the intake of fruit, reducing oranges and bananas in particular. For those prone to constipation most fruit is naturally laxative (dark berries such as raspberry and blackberry are exceptions, as are pineapples).

Artificially ripened fruit may not be as easily digestible as fresh tree/vine ripened fruit. The acids and sugars have not properly matured and some people have adverse reactions. Fruit which has been imported or picked immature should be left to ripen at room temperature. Generally it is best to eat native seasonal fruit and to eat tropical fruit mostly in the summer months. Moist, cooling tropical fruits are inappropriate for cool temperate winters.

Queen of all fruits, the apple is much loved by the Stomach and Heart. It is sweet and slightly sour in flavour and cool in temperature. Apple suits virtually all conditions except deep-seated Coldness and can be eaten throughout the year. It benefits Damp conditions by inhibiting fermentation; it increases appetite and is excellent in all low blood sugar conditions.

Grapes are also a useful general tonic, strengthening the Blood and Qi and cleansing the Liver; they are helpful in treating rheumatism and arthritis. Pears have a special affinity with the Lungs, reducing Heat and Mucus; plums have an affinity for the Liver, cooling Heat and benefiting degenerative conditions such as cirrhosis; peach is excellent for moistening the Intestines and soothing dryness in the Lung; cherries are a good choice when there is Coldness, especially when the joints are painful, and they also nourish the Blood. The oily fruits such as avocado and banana are lubricating for the Intestines and nourishing for the Yin. Citrus fruits increase the body fluids; their peel, on the other hand, is very useful for resolving Dampness. 'Pippy' fruits such as blackberry, raspberry and strawberry generally have an affinity for the Kidney and Liver, strengthening the urinary system through their astringent action. The melon family are all very cooling, thirst quenching and mildly diuretic.

The seeds, pips and skins of several fruits have additional uses. Citrus peel counteracts Stagnation and resolves Dampness; citrus pips destroy parasites; and watermelon seeds strengthen the Kidney and promote diuresis. Fruit juices are even more cleansing than the whole fruit and should be used cautiously.

Beans and Pulses

Beans are essentially sweet which means that they strengthen Deficiency. The concentrated nourishment of legumes makes them useful Blood and Yin tonics. Though rich in nourishment they are not Dampening and many beans, such as chickpeas, broad beans and aduki beans, are particularly helpful in draining Dampness. They combine well with grains and vegetables.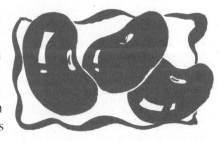

Late-onset diabetes is often markedly improved by regular consumption of beans. Those for whom beans generate intestinal gas will find that thorough soaking and rinsing, then cooking the beans with a few cloves or carminative spices such as cardamom will ease the problem. Alternatively they can be presoaked in bicarbonate of soda, then rinsed, or cooked with a few strips of seaweed.

The darker beans such as kidney and black beans have an affinity with the Kidney. Soya beans can be difficult to digest but when processed to make tofu, or fermented to produce tempeh, miso or soya sauce they are easily digestible and a very rich source of nutrition, higher in protein than milk and rich in essential fatty acids. Lentils and peas are excellent Qi tonics and are generally easier to digest than other beans.

Nuts and Seeds

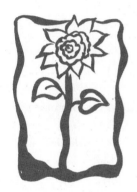

Like beans, nuts and seeds contain highly concentrated nourishment and most will strengthen the Yin, Blood and Qi. They contain all the nutrients necessary for a plant's first stages of growth. A few nuts, such as pistachio, chestnut and walnut also have Yang strengthening properties. The oily nature of nuts makes many of them somewhat Dampening and it is better to eat only small quantities at one time.

A few nuts, such as walnut, almond, chestnut and hazel are less Dampening than the oily brazil or cashew. Nuts and seeds are prone to oxidation, which can make them rancid and irritating to the digestion. To reduce this, it is best either to buy them in their shells or to store nuts and seeds in dark glass jars in cool places. Storing nuts and seeds in plastic risks a toxic reaction between the plastic and the oils.

Nuts and seeds are excellent lightly toasted and sprinkled over a meal or eaten as a snack. Roasting somewhat counteracts the effects of rancidity. Some seeds can also be sprouted which may make the nutrients more easily accessible. We need to give special attention to thoroughly chewing nuts and seeds to get the full benefit from them.

Peanuts, though they are, strictly speaking, a legume, are renowned for their tendency to generate Phlegm or allergic reactions in some people. They are also subjected to intense spraying against pests and synthetic treatment of their soil. Chemically grown peanuts are also more susceptible to contamination with aflatoxin, a carcinogenic fungus. For these reasons only organically grown peanuts are recommended.

Dairy

Dairy foods are deeply nourishing. They are sweet and moistening, making them excellent Qi and Yin tonics, with a special affinity for the Lung. However, their richness means that they are also very Dampening with a strong tendency to generate Phlegm and anyone with a Yang Deficient or Damp condition should treat them with caution. Pasteurised cow's milk is especially problematic. It is probably the pasteurising process itself which is responsible for some of the problems associated with dairy. The enzymes present in raw milk that are necessary for its digestion are destroyed in the pasteurisation process. Raw milk is usually better tolerated and a lot more tasty.

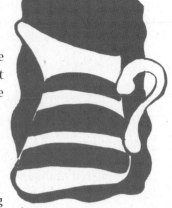

Sheep and goat's milks have few of the problems associated with cow's milk and are more suited to human consumption. They are less Dampening and allergic reactions are rare. Cow's milk is more beneficial when it has been mildly soured as in yoghurt or cottage cheese and will benefit the Intestines, whereas pasteurised cow's milk tends to putrefy. However, given that cow's milk is so much part of our culture, I would advocate that it be drunk warm with a few spices such as cardamom to make it more digestible. It is important not to mix milk with meat as they demand opposite reactions from the Stomach: meat needs the acidic environment of the Stomach which milk will neutralise. The result is Dampness and food Stagnation. Not mixing these two is also a key principle of kosher practice.

How can you expect to govern a country that has 246 kinds of cheese?

Charles de Gaulle

There is a longer discussion about dairy products in the last section of this book.

Meat and fish

Meat is generally warm and sweet and is the most Blood-nourishing of all foods. Liver and red meat are especially strong tonics for the Blood. Being so nutritious, it is of course also Dampening, espe-

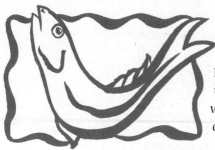

cially the fattier and heavier meats such as pork. This means that small portions are beneficial but too much will easily cause congestion and Dampness. Chicken is something of an exception to this and is even slightly drying. When the Spleen is weak, meat needs to be well cooked to be easily digestible; stews or casseroles are easy methods.

The basic principle concerning meat is that a little is good for most people and too much may be damaging. The meat of choice for Yang Deficiency is lamb which is very warming and energising. For Qi Deficiency chicken is excellent and its stock will increase the Qi-nourishing potential of any meal; for Yin Deficiency pork, which is moist and cool, is often chosen; and for Blood Deficiency liver is effective. The bones of meat make excellent stock and it is worth boiling them for a long time to extract the deep Yin and Essence-nourishing substances from the marrow.

Fish is normally cooler than meat. It is a good tonic for the Kidney and the Yin and and will strengthen all conditions of Blood Deficiency and general weakness. For those prone to Heat or to Dampness, fish is often a better choice than meat. However, with the prevalence of over-fishing of our seas, only moderate consumption of fish can be responsibly encouraged.

Shellfish and crustaceans provide very concentrated nourishment. Although foods from the sea are generally cool, many of these creatures are actually quite warming to the Kidney Yang. Shrimp and prawns, for example, are renowned Kidney Yang tonics. Care must be taken in selecting the source of these foods, as shellfish filter sea water and easily concentrate pollutants in their flesh. Many shellfish are considered to be very heating in traditional Chinese medicine and may cause 'hot' reactions such as skin rashes.

Seaweed is a salty-flavoured cooling food providing a rich source of nourishment for the Yin and Blood. It also has detoxifying and Damp-resolving actions. A little seaweed makes an excellent addition to any meal.

Herbs and Spices

Herbs and spices[39] are used to improve the digestibility of foods and to create certain energetic effects. Aromatic flavours stimulate the Spleen, bitter flavours counteract Dampness, the pungent herbs and spices counteract Stagnation; some herbs and spices can increase the energetic temperature of a meal, some cool it; and the actions of foods can be directed, through herbs and spices, towards certain areas of the body.

Spices such as cinnamon, cayenne, ginger, clove and garlic increase the warming quality of a meal. Carminatives such as caraway, dill, aniseed, fennel, cardamom and cumin ease the digestion. Marjoram and mint bring coolness to a dish; thyme, rosemary and sage bring warmth. Horseradish breaks down the rich nutrition in meat, pepper helps resolve Dampness and turmeric stimulates the circulation.

Traditional cooking from all cultures uses herbs and spices to balance and invigorate the diet. Mint sauce is served with lamb to cool it down, horseradish with beef to break through its heaviness, ginger is sprinkled on watermelon to moderate its coldness, mustard goes well with cheese and counteracts its Dampening effect, fennel brings warmth to fish, saffron introduces movement to rice and so on. The skilled cook uses herbs and spices to point a meal in the energetic direction most suited to their needs.

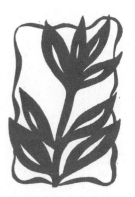

Many herbs can be drunk as tea and have helpful digestive properties. Jasmine, fennel, cinnamon, ginger, cardamom and star anise are warm in nature, support the digestive fire and help resolve Dampness. Peppermint is a more cooling digestive tea helpful in conditions of Dampness and Heat. Chamomile is neutral in temperature and will soothe all digestive systems and help resolve Dampness.

Ordinary black tea helps break down rich food and eliminate sputum from the Lung (there is a discussion of black tea at the end of this book). The various milder teas such as bancha, kukicha and green tea are also helpful and less stimulating to the adrenals. Citrus peel is a very helpful ingredient in teas for its power of breaking through Stagnation.

Wild Foods

Wild foods, which have asserted their place in the environment without help from gardener or farmer, are energetically stronger than domesticated foods. The same is true for wild animals. In an

age where the nutritional value of foods has been weakened by commercial growing practices it is helpful, perhaps vital, to occasionally include some wild foods in the diet. Wild greens can provide the bitter flavours missing in modern diets, fungus can provide rare minerals and berries can provide concentrated vitamins.

Dandelion is beneficial to the Liver and Gall Bladder, clearing Heat and Stagnation. Its bitterness makes it a useful digestive stimulant and it is well known as a diuretic, draining excess water from the system. From a western viewpoint it is high in potassium and vitamins A and C. Dandelion can be found almost everywhere. Its roots, gathered in late summer, can be roasted and prepared like coffee; they have a powerful diuretic and Damp-resolving effect on the organs of elimination.

Nettle is a rich tonic which nourishes the Blood and the Liver Yin and helps rid the body of toxins. Gardeners will tell you that nettles growing on your land indicate that the soil is rich. This much-maligned weed with a powerful sting is actually a remarkably mineral-rich food. It can be drunk as tea or cooked like spinach. The top few leaves of the plant taste best. Nettle is especially good as a tonic drunk daily for three weeks during Spring.

Chickweed is a cooling and moistening leaf useful in conditions of Heart and Lung Yin Deficiency. It is also soothing to the digestive tract. It is a mild-tasting herb that goes well in any salad; it is easily found in meadowland or on rough ground in autumn.

Comfrey is used by gardeners as a rich food for other plants. Its broad range of nutrients makes it a good Yin and Blood tonic. Its moist, demulcent nature gives it soothing properties for any inflammation of the digestive system. It is also famous for its tissue healing effects. It is best drunk as tea as its rough hairy leaf can be off-putting in salad. Comfrey can commonly be found in damp ground.

Yarrow is a useful herb for vitalising the Blood and it has a reputation as a general gynaecological remedy. It is helpful in conditions of Liver Qi Stagnation. A little yarrow can enliven a salad and it may also be drunk as tea. Yarrow can easily be found in grassland.

Bittercresses are common in lawns and share the same properties as watercress. They are bitter digestive stimulants and they add a hot perkiness to salad.

Wild strawberry is a cool, sweet and sour fruit appearing earlier than commercial strawberries, very small by comparison but considerably more tasty. Strawberry moistens the Lung and stimulates the function of the Spleen. It is especially helpful for urinary problems.

Blackberry and **raspberry** have similar properties to each other. They have an affinity for the Liver and Kidney and are nourishing for the Blood. Their astringent flavour particularly affects the urinary system, strengthening the Bladder and reducing excessive urination. Raspberry leaf is the herb of choice for pregnancy and its moderate use is renowned for its strengthening effect on the uterus, preparing it for childbirth.

Hawthorn berry supports the functions of the Heart, nourishing its Yin aspect (much used in the treatment of hypertension) and regulating the activity of the whole cardiovascular system. They are rather sour tasting and dry. It is easy to find hawthorn in hedgerows and woodland edges.

Juniper berry is a spicy warming berry which can strengthen the Yang. It is helpful in conditions of Cold and Damp. A little juniper tastes wonderful cooked with cabbage. (Avoid juniper during pregnancy and do not eat regularly for more than six weeks at a time.)

Mushrooms are a good source of rare minerals such as germanium, and some are known to be immune-strengthening. They detoxify the body, remove Heat and are especially useful for meat-eaters with a tendency to overheat. They help resolve Phlegm in the Lung and generally benefit the digestion. Autumn is the most prolific time for wild fungus but they can still be found at other times of year. Very few wild mushrooms are poisonous but it is advisable to have a good field guide or, better still, a knowledgeable friend to help identify edible fungus.

Chestnut is a wonderfully strengthening nut, very sweet in nature and mildly warming. It strengthens the Stomach, Spleen and Kidney.

Hazelnut is an easily digested nut which can be strengthening to the Stomach and Spleen. It is useful in all conditions of Stomach and Spleen Qi Deficiency.

About the Recipes

The recipes that follow are for you to enjoy and be inspired by. They have been chosen for this book primarily because they are delicious. This is the first test they have had to pass before getting in. The second consideration in developing these recipes has been their appropriateness for various conditions and constitutions. The fact that they are good for this or that condition is important, but secondary to their deliciousness.

Some are traditional recipes adapted from various world cultures; some are derived from the inspiration of friends and a few recipe books that feel like friends; and many have been specifically created for this book. All have been developed and tested here in our own home kitchen. They taste and feel best when made with fresh organic ingredients and prepared with love.

If you wish, you can ignore everything else in this book and use it as a conventional recipe book. The recipes that you like the best and that feel good deep down in your body are probably the ones you need to eat. Otherwise, the unique feature of the recipe pages is that they offer you a way of tailoring your diet to your own personal energetic needs. My fondest wish is that they nourish you deeply and that they empower you on your personal journey towards wellbeing.

All recipes are built on the belief that somewhere at the beginning of the chain there is a cook who did not use them. This is the great nostalgia of our cuisine, ever invoking an absent mother-cook who once laid her hands on the body of the world for us and worked it into food. The promise of every cookbook is that it offers a way back onto her lap

John Thorne

Understanding the Recipe Pages

At the bottom of each page the various check-boxes give a quick guide to the principal actions of the recipe. These are not the only effects of the recipe, simply the most notable. They should not be taken to mean that there are no other actions. For example, if the 'Qi' box is not ticked, this does not necessarily mean that the recipe does not strengthen the Qi, but simply that this is not a major aspect of the recipe's action. Similarly, if the 'Kidney' box is not ticked, this does not mean that there are no benefits for the Kidney.

It is impossible to put the overall effect of any meal into rigid boxes so please take these as a loose guide only. These check-boxes exist to help choose recipes at a glance that particularly support the various substances, functions or Organs of the body-mind, or recipes which help resolve the various conditions of Dampness, Cold and so on. In this way you can choose recipes particularly beneficial for your own condition and constitution. Unless contraindicated, each recipe is also perfectly acceptable for all other conditions.

Bon appetit.

Measurements

All measurements are approximate and have either been rounded up or down. All spoon measurements are gently rounded and a cup is the size of an English teacup (about 6 fl oz).

Oven temperatures

Gas Mark 1 = 275°F = 140°C

Gas Mark 2 = 300°F = 150°C

Gas Mark 3 = 325°F = 170°C

Gas Mark 4 = 350°F = 180°C

Gas Mark 5 = 375°F = 190°C

Gas Mark 6 = 400°F = 200°C

Gas Mark 7 = 425°F = 220°C

Gas Mark 8 = 450°F = 230°C

Gas Mark 9 = 475°F = 240°C

Volume

2 fl oz = 55 ml

5 fl oz (quarter pint) = 150 ml

10 fl oz (half pint) = 275 ml

20 fl oz (one pint) = 570 ml

Weights

1/2 oz = 10 g

1 oz = 25 g

4 oz = 110 g

8 oz = 225 g

1 lb = 450 g

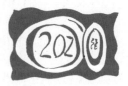

Equipment

The only piece of gadgetry I have in my kitchen is a hand-held electric whizzer, the kind you can stick straight into the saucepan and whizz most things to a smooth consistency. Some recipes call for the use of such a device but if you don't have one you can get by with a masher and a bit of muscle power on most recipes. Otherwise a good sharp knife, a chopping board, a wooden spoon and a few pots and pans is all you will need.

Language

Having spent time in the USA I am aware that, even though it sounds the same, American English is in some respects another language. It took me a long time to realise that coriander leaf is cilantro in American and even longer to discover that rocket is arugula. Below are a few translations for American readers.

UK	USA
Aubergine	Eggplant
Beetroot	Beet
Broad bean	Fava bean
Celeriac	Celery root
Chickpea	Garbanzo
Coriander leaf	Cilantro
Courgette	Zucchini
Rocket	Arugula
Spring greens	Collard greens
Spring onion	Scallion
Swede	Rutabaga

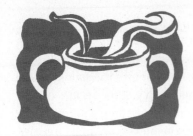

Aniseedy Cabbage Soup

This is a very soothing soup. It tastes sweet with a special pungency added by the aniseed. Even those who think that cabbage has been forever ruined for them by the sulphurous experiences of school dinners will like this soup. In fact, the first time I cooked it, no one guessed that cabbage was a main ingredient.

Preparation time: 15 mins
Cooking time: 30 mins
Serves: 4–6

Ingredients

12 ounces hard cabbage
8 ounces fennel
12 ounces carrot
4 ounces potato
1 ounce butter or ghee
1–2 teaspoons aniseed

2 pints water
1 teaspoon light miso

Method

Chop all the vegetables, melt the butter at the bottom of the pan and add all the ingredients including the aniseed. Cook slowly, turning occasionally for about 10 minutes or until the vegetables begin to reduce in size.

Add two pints of water, bring to the boil and simmer for another 20 minutes or until cooked. Add miso, stir well and partially liquidise.

Primary actions	Primary influences	Contra-indications
■ Qi ■ Blood	☐ Lung	☐ Qi def
☐ Yin ☐ Yang	■ Intestines	☐ Blood def
■ Damp	■ Stomach	☐ Yin def
☐ Phlegm	☐ Spleen	☐ Yang def
☐ Water	☐ Heart	☐ Damp
■ Qi stagnation	☐ Bladder	☐ Stagnation
☐ Blood stagnation	☐ Kidney	☐ Heat
	☐ Gall bladder	☐ Cold
■ Heat	☐ Liver	☐ Wind invasion
☐ Cold		
☐ Wind heat	**Temperature**	
☐ Wind cold	☐ Cooling	
☐ Wind damp	■ Neutral	
☐ Dryness	☐ Warming	

Energetics

Cabbage has an ability to cool Heat in the digestive system and is perfect for all ulcerative digestive conditions. Carrots nourish Blood and benefit the Liver as well as being mildly soothing. The fennel brings warmth and movement to the Intestines, stimulates the Spleen and moves Stagnation, properties shared by the aniseed.

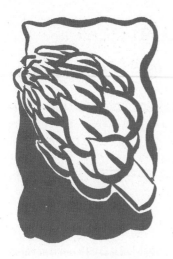

Artichoke and Bacon Soup

Our neighbour brought this soup round one day. It was a perfectly timed gift and so delicious that I knew it had to have a place in this book. Artichoke and bacon is one of those combinations made in heaven.

Preparation time: 10 mins
Cooking time: 20 mins
Serves: 4

Ingredients

4 slices bacon
2 onions
6–8 jerusalem artichokes
2 large leeks
2 teaspoons olive oil
Small knob of butter

2 pints water
1 teaspoon bouillon
4 tablespoons mashed potato
Salt and pepper

Method

Chop the onions, leeks, artichokes and bacon into small pieces. Gently fry the onions in the olive oil and butter, adding the leeks, bacon and the artichokes when the onions are softened and sweet. Stir for a while and allow them to sweat together.

Add water and the bouillon. Cook gently for 15 minutes or until done. Thicken with the mashed potato. Liquidise most of it but leave a few chunky bits. Add freshly ground black pepper to taste.

Primary actions	Primary influences	Contra-indications
■ Qi □ Blood	■ Lung	□ Qi def
■ Yin □ Yang	□ Intestines	□ Blood def
□ Damp	□ Stomach	□ Yin def
□ Phlegm	■ Spleen	□ Yang def
□ Water	□ Heart	□ Damp
□ Qi stagnation	□ Bladder	□ Stagnation
□ Blood stagnation	■ Kidney	□ Heat
□ Heat	□ Gall bladder	□ Cold
□ Cold	□ Liver	□ Wind invasion
□ Wind heat		
□ Wind cold	**Temperature**	
□ Wind damp	□ Cooling	
■ Dryness	■ Neutral	
	□ Warming	

Energetics

In China a general tonic is sometimes made from duck or chicken cooked with a pig's trotter, pork bones and artichokes. This soup is a distant relative of the Chinese recipe! Artichokes strengthen the Spleen, Kidney and Lung. The bacon nourishes the Kidney Yin. Altogether this is a Qi and Yin nourishing soup.

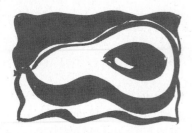

Avocado and Tomato Gazpacho

This is a colourful and refreshing summery kind of soup. It is served cool.

Preparation time: 10 mins
Cooking time: 10 mins
Serves: 6

Ingredients

1 cup unsweetened corn
6 tomatoes
½ cucumber
2 avocados
4 tablespoons lemon/lime juice
1–2 cloves garlic
2 teaspoons fresh mint
1 tablespoon fresh coriander
2–3 drops tabasco
½ teaspoon salt

Method

If available, this soup tastes best with fresh corn scraped direct from the cob and lightly blanched. Chop and purée the tomatoes with a little water, and grate the cucumber. Mash the avocado, crush the garlic, chop the herbs finely and combine all ingredients in a bowl, leaving to stand for at least an hour. Serve cool, garnished with extra coriander or mint leaf.

Primary actions	Primary influences	Contra-indications
☐ Qi ■ Blood	☐ Lung	☐ Qi def
■ Yin ☐ Yang	■ Intestines	☐ Blood def
☐ Damp	☐ Stomach	☐ Yin def
☐ Phlegm	☐ Spleen	☐ Yang def
☐ Water .	☐ Heart	☐ Damp
☐ Qi stagnation	☐ Bladder	☐ Stagnation
☐ Blood stagnation	☐ Kidney	☐ Heat
	☐ Gall bladder	■ Cold
■ Heat	■ Liver	☐ Wind invasion
☐ Cold		
☐ Wind heat	**Temperature**	
☐ Wind cold	■ Cooling	
☐ Wind damp	☐ Neutral	
■ Dryness	☐ Warming	

Energetics

This is a cooling, cleansing soup for the Liver. Tomatoes relieve Liver Heat and avocados nourish Liver Yin and Blood. Cucumber moistens and cools the body and has some detoxifying properties. The cooling effects are mildly offset by the garlic and spices.

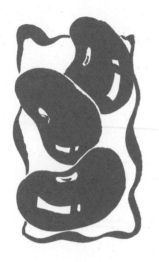

Black Bean and Celery Soup

A dark, smooth and deeply nourishing soup, perfect for a winter's day.

Preparation time: 15 mins
Cooking time: 30 mins
Serves: 4

Ingredients

½ pound dried black beans
A 6 inch strip wakame seaweed

3 sticks celery
1 onion
1 carrot
2 teaspoons fresh
(or 1 dried) savory
Zest of large orange

1–2 tablespoons miso
Juice of one lemon
Parsley to garnish

Method

Soak the beans overnight, discard the water and rinse. Cook with the wakame (or any other seaweed) until very tender.

Chop the vegetables, bring them to the boil in a separate pot and simmer until just softening. Add the beans with any remaining juice, the orange rind and the savory. Cook for a further 10 minutes or so. The beans should be thoroughly soft and splitting open.

Stir in the miso and partially liquidise the soup. Serve with plenty of fresh lemon juice and a garnish of parsley.

Energetics

Primary actions	Primary influences	Contra-indications
☐ Qi ■ Blood	☐ Lung	☐ Qi def
■ Yin ☐ Yang	☐ Intestines	☐ Blood def
▪ Damp	☐ Stomach	☐ Yin def
☐ Phlegm	☐ Spleen	☐ Yang def
■ Water	☐ Heart	☐ Damp
☐ Qi stagnation	■ Bladder	☐ Stagnation
☐ Blood stagnation	■ Kidney	☐ Heat
■ Heat	☐ Gall bladder	☐ Cold
☐ Cold	■ Liver	☐ Wind invasion
☐ Wind heat		
☐ Wind cold	**Temperature**	
☐ Wind damp	☐ Cooling	
☐ Dryness	■ Neutral	
	☐ Warming	

Black beans are a good tonic for the Kidney. They have diuretic properties, helping to resolve Dampness and Water. They also nourish the Blood and Yin. They are supported in their Damp resolving action by the celery which cools the system and removes Water. The seaweed nourishes Blood and Yin as well as draining Water; the carrot complements the Blood-nourishing action of the beans; and the onion provides warmth and movement. Miso brings the action of the soup into the 'lower burner'. Altogether this is a Blood and Yin nourishing soup with a strong action against Dampness.

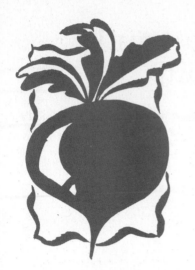

Borscht

If you appreciate colour in a meal then the deep purply red of this soup will delight you. Based on a traditional Polish soup, this version of borscht is velvet textured and perfectly captures the earthy distinctive taste of the beetroot. It touches like a lover and goes direct to the heart.

Preparation time: 15 mins
Cooking time: 40 mins
Serves: 2–4

Ingredients

1 small onion
½ pound beetroot
2 small potatoes
1 small carrot
2 pints vegetable stock

1 teaspoon dill
2 tablespoons cider vinegar
Yoghurt

Method

Finely chop the onion and fry it gently in a little oil until soft. Roughly chop all the other vegetables, add them to the onions and stir for a few minutes. Add the vegetable stock and let the soup cook for about 40 minutes.

Halfway through add the dill. When the soup is cooked, liquidise it and stir in the cider vinegar. Add more vinegar to taste and more water if the soup is too thick. Serve with a swirl of yoghurt and garnish with parsley.

Primary actions	Primary influences	Contra-indications
■ Qi ■ Blood	□ Lung	□ Qi def
□ Yin □ Yang	□ Intestines	□ Blood def
□ Damp	□ Stomach	□ Yin def
□ Phlegm	■ Spleen	□ Yang def
□ Water	■ Heart	□ Damp
■ Qi stagnation	□ Bladder	□ Stagnation
□ Blood stagnation	□ Kidney	□ Heat
□ Heat	□ Gall bladder	□ Cold
□ Cold	■ Liver	□ Wind invasion
□ Wind heat	**Temperature**	
□ Wind cold	□ Cooling	
□ Wind damp	■ Neutral	
□ Dryness	□ Warming	

Energetics

Beetroot nourishes the Blood and benefits the Liver and Heart. It is supported by the potato and carrot. The onion adds warmth and movement. The dill helps the digestion. The overall effect of this soup is to nourish the Blood and Qi and to uplift the Heart.

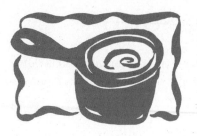

Caldo Verde (Green Soup)

This soup comes from Goa in its Portugese days. The twelve cloves of garlic are not a misprint! Try it and see.

Preparation time: 15 mins
Cooking time: 60 mins
Serves: 6

Ingredients

4 potatoes
1 onion
4 ounces kale
12 cloves garlic
1 teaspoon salt
2 ½ pints water

1 tablespoon olive oil
Black pepper
1 lemon
Grated carrot to garnish

Method

Chop all the vegetables coarsely. Put the potatoes, onion, garlic and kale in a pot with 2 ½ pints of salted water. Bring to the boil and simmer for an hour or so. Blend the soup until it is smooth.

Add the olive oil and freshly ground black pepper just before serving (a strongly flavoured olive oil is best). Add lemon and salt to taste and garnish with a twist of lemon and some finely grated carrot.

Energetics

Greens and potatoes are a well balanced combination and this simple soup nourishes both the Qi and the Blood. It is easy to digest and made quite warming by the addition of so much garlic.

Primary actions	Primary influences	Contra-indications
■ Qi ■ Blood	■ Lung	☐ Qi def
☐ Yin ☐ Yang	☐ Intestines	☐ Blood def
☐ Damp	■ Stomach	☐ Yin def
☐ Phlegm	■ Spleen	☐ Yang def
☐ Water	☐ Heart	☐ Damp
■ Qi stagnation	☐ Bladder	☐ Stagnation
☐ Blood stagnation	☐ Kidney	☐ Heat
☐ Heat	☐ Gall bladder	☐ Cold
☐ Cold	■ Liver	☐ Wind invasion
☐ Wind heat		
☐ Wind cold	**Temperature**	
☐ Wind damp	☐ Cooling	
☐ Dryness	☐ Neutral	
	■ Warming	

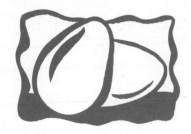

Egg Drop Soup

Shiitake mushrooms create a very special flavour, deep and earthy. They are revered in the east for their power to nourish the body.

Preparation time: 10 mins
Cooking time: 30 mins
Serves: 2–4

Ingredients

6 shiitake mushrooms
1 small leek
2 ounces fresh nettles
1 small carrot
2 teaspoons fresh ginger
2 tablespoons soya sauce
8 cups water

2 eggs
Toasted sesame oil

Method

If you are using dried mushrooms, soak them first in a cup of hot water. Chop the mushrooms into thin slices and bring them to the boil in a little water. Add the finely chopped leek, carrot, nettles and sliced ginger and the rest of the water. Add soya sauce and continue boiling until the liquid is reduced by nearly half.

Just before serving, beat the eggs together in a small jug. Use a wooden spoon to stir the soup until you get a strong spinning action like a whirlpool. Flow the eggs into this mixture so that the eggs form long strands. Add a splash of toasted sesame oil and soya sauce to taste before serving.

Primary actions	Primary influences	Contra-indications
■ Qi ■ Blood	□ Lung	□ Qi def
■ Yin □ Yang	□ Intestines	□ Blood def
■ Damp	■ Stomach	□ Yin def
■ Phlegm	□ Spleen	□ Yang def
□ Water	□ Heart	□ Damp
□ Qi stagnation	□ Bladder	□ Stagnation
□ Blood stagnation	■ Kidney	□ Heat
□ Heat	□ Gall bladder	□ Cold
□ Cold	■ Liver	□ Wind invasion
□ Wind heat	**Temperature**	
□ Wind cold	□ Cooling	
□ Wind damp	■ Neutral	
□ Dryness	□ Warming	

Energetics

The shiitake mushrooms and egg provide rich nourishment for the Blood, Qi and Yin. The leek helps break through the richness of the egg, and the carrots and nettles provide additional nourishment for the Blood. Ginger supports the Yang and many of the ingredients act against Dampness.

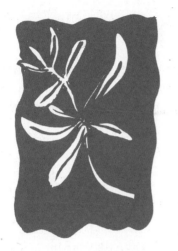

French Onion Soup

The art of making a good onion soup is to cook the onions slowly, preferably in a heavy cast iron pot. Beef stock is more traditional than the miso suggested in this recipe and may be substituted if preferred. Served with a good hunk of crusty bread it is almost irresistible.

Preparation time: 10 mins
Cooking time: 40 mins
Serves: 4

Ingredients

6 onions
2 tablespoons olive oil
1/2 teaspoon toasted sesame oil
1 teaspoon dried thyme
2 bayleaves
1/2 teaspoon dried rosemary

2 tablespoons tamari
4–5 cups water
2 tablespoons dark miso

Method

Slice the onion into thin strips. Heat the oil over a low flame and add the onion and all the herbs, stirring occasionally. Cook slowly for 30-40 minutes without burning the onions so that all the sweetness is brought out.

Add the water and tamari, bring to a boil and simmer for about five minutes. Scoop out a little of the soup into a cup, dilute the miso in this and then return it to the pot. Turn off the heat and stir for a few moments. Add extra tamari to taste. Voila! Serve with bread or croutons.

Primary actions	Primary influences	Contra-indications
☐ Qi ☐ Blood	■ Lung	☐ Qi def
☐ Yin ■ Yang	☐ Intestines	☐ Blood def
■ Damp	☐ Stomach	☐ Yin def
■ Phlegm	☐ Spleen	☐ Yang def
■ Water	☐ Heart	☐ Damp
■ Qi stagnation	☐ Bladder	☐ Stagnation
■ Blood stagnation	■ Kidney	■ Heat
☐ Heat	☐ Gall bladder	☐ Cold
■ Cold	☐ Liver	☐ Wind invasion
☐ Wind heat		
■ Wind cold	**Temperature**	
■ Wind damp	☐ Cooling	
☐ Dryness	☐ Neutral	
	■ Warming	

Energetics

Onion is warming and pungent with a special action on the Lung. Onion soup is excellent for all conditions of Dampness affecting the Lung and is helpful in moving Stagnation. The addition of thyme and rosemary give the soup Yang strengthening power and the miso brings the Damp and Stagnation resolving properties down to work in the intestines. This soup can also be used effectively to counter invasions of Wind Cold and Wind Damp.

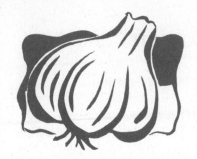

Garlic Soup

Here's a recipe for garlic fans. You may be surprised at the sweetness of the garlic when it is cooked in this way. Delicious and good for warding off vampires.

Preparation time: 10 mins
Cooking time: 35 mins
Serves: 4

Ingredients

2–3 bulbs garlic
1 onion
1 tablespoon olive oil
¹/₂ teaspoon toasted sesame oil

4 cups water
1 potato
3 bayleaves
¹/₂ teaspoon thyme
¹/₄ teaspoon oregano

6 tablespoons tamari
Pinch cayenne pepper

Method

Chop the garlic and onion and sauté together in the oil for about 20 minutes. Keep the heat very low.

Add the water, thyme, oregano, bayleaves and potato to the pot. Bring the soup to a boil then simmer until the potato is cooked.

Add tamari and a good sprinkle of cayenne pepper. Serve with croutons.

Primary actions	Primary influences	Contra-indications
☐ Qi ☐ Blood	■ Lung	☐ Qi def
☐ Yin ■ Yang	☐ Intestines	☐ Blood def
■ Damp	☐ Stomach	■ Yin def
■ Phlegm	☐ Spleen	☐ Yang def
☐ Water	■ Heart	☐ Damp
■ Qi stagnation	☐ Bladder	☐ Stagnation
■ Blood stagnation	☐ Kidney	■ Heat
☐ Heat	☐ Gall bladder	☐ Cold
■ Cold	☐ Liver	☐ Wind invasion
☐ Wind heat	**Temperature**	
■ Wind cold	☐ Cooling	
■ Wind damp	☐ Neutral	
☐ Dryness	■ Warming	

Energetics

Garlic is warm and pungent. This soup is an ideal remedy for all invasions of Wind Cold or Wind Damp and for any Phlegm conditions in the Lung. Garlic will also promote the circulation of Blood and Qi so this soup is well suited to all conditions of Stagnation and Cold.

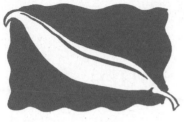

Indonesian Coconut Vegetable Soup

This is a version inspired by Elisabeth Rosin's recipe from 'The Universal Kitchen'. Lemon grass and coconut create an unmistakably Indonesian dish. A simple bowl of rice will be all that you need to accompany this soup.

Preparation time: 15 mins
Cooking time: 20 mins
Serves: 4–6

Ingredients

2 shallots
2 cloves garlic
1 tablespoon fresh ginger
¼ teaspoon chilli pepper
2 tablespoons olive oil

2 cups shredded white cabbage
1 stalk celery
1 carrot

2 pints chicken stock
¾ pint coconut milk
1 handful mungbean sprouts
1 handful mange tout peas
2 teaspoons lemongrass
(½ teaspoon if dried)
½ teaspoon turmeric
Salt
Lemon

Method

Finely chop the shallots, garlic and ginger. Cook in the oil together with the chilli for 5 minutes until the aromas are released.

Shred the cabbage, cut the celery and carrot into small strips and add to the pan, stirring for a few minutes.

Add the stock, coconut milk, mange tout, beansprouts, lemon grass and turmeric. Simmer until the vegetables are tender (about 15 minutes). Salt to taste and garnish with lemon. This soup is traditionally sprinkled with dried onion flakes.

Primary actions	Primary influences	Contra-indications
■ Qi ■ Blood	□ Lung	□ Qi def
□ Yin □ Yang	□ Intestines	□ Blood def
□ Damp	■ Stomach	■ Yin def
□ Phlegm	■ Spleen	□ Yang def
□ Water	■ Heart	□ Damp
□ Qi stagnation	□ Bladder	□ Stagnation
□ Blood stagnation	□ Kidney	■ Heat
	□ Gall bladder	□ Cold
□ Heat	□ Liver	□ Wind invasion
■ Cold		
□ Wind heat	**Temperature**	
□ Wind cold	□ Cooling	
□ Wind damp	□ Neutral	
□ Dryness	■ Warming	

Energetics

The basis of this soup is the chicken stock and coconut milk which both strengthen the Qi. The coconut has a special nourishing effect on the Heart and the chicken nourishes the Spleen. The various spices make this a warming dish. The vegetables, beansprouts and lemon garnish bring a cooling element to balance the overall warmth of the soup.

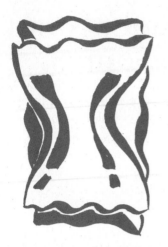

Minestra della Fattoria (Broccoli Soup)

This soup is a complete meal and needs only a chunk of gorgeous bread and a good sunset. As the name suggests, it captures the flavour of rural Italy.

Preparation time: 10 mins
Cooking time: 25 mins
Serves: 4

Ingredients

½ pound cooked cannellini or haricot beans
1 onion
4 tablespoons olive oil
1 head broccoli

6 cloves garlic
2 pints chicken stock
3 cups pasta
1 teaspoon dried oregano
2 teaspoons dried thyme
Salt & Pepper

Method

Soak and precook the beans and have them ready when you start to cook the soup. Chop the onion roughly and cook it slowly in the oil until it turns soft and golden. Meanwhile chop the usable parts of the broccoli stalk into small pieces and add to the onion, breaking up the rest of the broccoli head into 2 inch pieces and setting it aside.

Chop the garlic. Add the stock, garlic, cooked cannellini beans and pasta and bring to boil. Simmer for 10 minutes than add the broccoli and herbs, cooking for a further 5-10 minutes until the pasta is soft and the broccoli tender. Add salt and pepper to taste. Serve with hunks of crusty bread.

Primary actions	Primary influences	Contra-indications
■ Qi ■ Blood	■ Lung	□ Qi def
■ Yin □ Yang	■ Intestines	□ Blood def
□ Damp	■ Stomach	□ Yin def
□ Phlegm	■ Spleen	□ Yang def
□ Water	□ Heart	□ Damp
□ Qi stagnation	□ Bladder	□ Stagnation
□ Blood stagnation	□ Kidney	□ Heat
□ Heat	□ Gall bladder	□ Cold
□ Cold	□ Liver	□ Wind invasion
□ Wind heat		
□ Wind cold	**Temperature**	
□ Wind damp	□ Cooling	
□ Dryness	□ Neutral	
	■ Warming	

Energetics

This is a deeply nourishing soup suitable for all conditions. Chicken stock as a basis for soup brings nourishment to all the deficiencies (Yin, Blood, Yang and Qi). The beans nourish the Blood and Yin with some Damp resolving action. The pasta nourishes Qi and helps in the building of Blood with support from the broccoli. More moderation of Damp influences comes from the garlic and herbs. The combination of beans, grains and vegetables provides balanced nourishment.

Nettle Soup

In England, fresh stinging nettles can be found every-where. I let a few grow contentedly in a corner of the garden and use them for soup in the Spring and as fer-tiliser for the tomatoes when they are past their best. Pick only the top 4-6 leaves of each plant for a delightful earthy soup.

Preparation time: 10 mins
Cooking time: 20 mins
Serves: 4

Ingredients

1 onion
12 ounces potatoes
1 tablespoon sunflower oil

6 ounces nettles

2 pints vegetable stock
1 teaspoon nutmeg
Juice of 1 lemon
Salt and pepper
Soya sauce

Method

Cook the onion in the oil until golden then add the fine-ly chopped potato and stir frequently for about five minutes.

Add the nettles and a good splash of stock and let them sweat with the other ingredients for another 5 minutes.

Add the stock and simmer for about 15 minutes. Add the nutmeg just before the end. Liquidise and add the lemon, salt and pepper. Season with soya sauce and extra nut-meg and lemon if desired. Do not overseason, otherwise you will overpower the simple earthiness of this soup.

Primary actions	Primary influences	Contra-indications
■ Qi ■ Blood	■ Lung	☐ Qi def
■ Yin ☐ Yang	☐ Intestines	☐ Blood def
■ Damp	☐ Stomach	☐ Yin def
☐ Phlegm	■ Spleen	☐ Yang def
☐ Water	☐ Heart	☐ Damp
☐ Qi stagnation	■ Bladder	☐ Stagnation
☐ Blood stagnation	■ Kidney	☐ Heat
☐ Heat	☐ Gall bladder	☐ Cold
☐ Cold	■ Liver	☐ Wind invasion
☐ Wind heat		
☐ Wind cold	**Temperature**	
☐ Wind damp	☐ Cooling	
☐ Dryness	■ Neutral	
	☐ Warming	

Energetics

Nettles are an excellent tonic for the Blood, with a strengthening action on the Liver, Lung and Kidney. Nettles nourish the Liver Yin as well as helping resolve Phlegm in the Lung. The potato acts as a neutral, Qi-strengthening base for the nettle's action. The main action of this soup is to nourish Blood, support the Kidney and strengthen the Liver Yin.

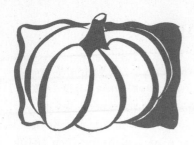

Pumpkin and Chestnut Soup

This is a smooth, creamy and completely delectable soup. It will leave you feeling as satisfied as a baby at the breast.

Preparation time: 10 mins
Cooking time: 50 mins
Serves: 6

Ingredients

1 cup dried chestnuts, soaked
2 onions
3 tablespoons olive oil
1 medium pumpkin

2 pints vegetable stock
2 cloves garlic
1 bayleaf
1 teaspoon rosemary
Splash of cider vinegar
Parsley to garnish
Pinch paprika

Method

Presoak the chestnuts overnight or use fresh chestnuts if available. Chop the onions roughly and fry in the olive oil until softened. Chop the pumpkin, removing the skin and seeds, and sweat with the onions, turning occasionally until it starts to soften.

Add the vegetable stock, chestnuts, crushed garlic, bayleaf and rosemary. Simmer for 40 minutes, remove the bayleaf and liquidise adding a splash of cider vinegar and a good twist of freshly ground black pepper. Serve garnished with parsley and a sprinkle of paprika.

Primary actions	Primary influences	Contra-indications
■ Qi ■ Blood	☐ Lung	☐ Qi def
☐ Yin ■ Yang	☐ Intestines	☐ Blood def
■ Damp	☐ Stomach	☐ Yin def
☐ Phlegm	■ Spleen	☐ Yang def
☐ Water	☐ Heart	☐ Damp
☐ Qi stagnation	☐ Bladder	☐ Stagnation
☐ Blood stagnation	■ Kidney	☐ Heat
☐ Heat	☐ Gall bladder	☐ Cold
■ Cold	☐ Liver	☐ Wind invasion
☐ Wind heat	**Temperature**	
☐ Wind cold	☐ Cooling	
☐ Wind damp	☐ Neutral	
☐ Dryness	■ Warming	

Energetics

Pumpkin nourishes the Spleen, strengthening the Qi and helping remove Dampness. Chestnuts also support the Spleen as well as warming the Kidney, strengthening Yang and gently stimulating Blood circulation. This recipe is ideal for the condition of Spleen Yang Deficiency.

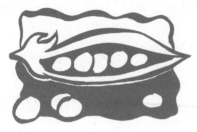

Split Pea Soup

You can use yellow or green split peas for this soup. It has something of an Indian flavour and I adapted it from a version in Madhur Jaffrey's encylopedic book of eastern recipes.

Preparation time: 10 mins
Cooking time: 80 mins
Serves: 6

Ingredients

10 ounces split peas
3 pints chicken or vegetable stock

Grated rind of 1 lemon
½ teaspoon turmeric
¼ teaspoon ginger
½ teaspoon salt
1 bayleaf
1 teaspoon black peppercorns
1 teaspoon whole cloves
1 teaspoon cardamom pods

Juice of 2 lemons

Method

Presoak the split peas overnight if possible, throwing away the soaking water and rinsing the peas. Bring the stock and soaked split peas to the boil.

Meanwhile wrap the cloves, bayleaf, peppercorns and cardamom in a piece of muslin or cheesecloth, slightly crush the seeds and drop the bag into the pot together with the turmeric, salt and the grated rind of one lemon. Simmer on a low heat until the peas are tender (this can be more than an hour), skimming the foam off the top for the first few minutes.

When done, remove the spice bag and squeeze its juices back into the pot. Add lemon juice to taste and serve immediately. It is good served with croutons as a garnish. If you are using vegetable stock, try adding a little light tahini to the soup.

Primary actions	Primary influences	Contra-indications
■ Qi ■ Blood	□ Lung	□ Qi def
■ Yin □ Yang	□ Intestines	□ Blood def
■ Damp	■ Stomach	□ Yin def
□ Phlegm	■ Spleen	□ Yang def
■ Water	□ Heart	□ Damp
□ Qi stagnation	□ Bladder	□ Stagnation
□ Blood stagnation	□ Kidney	□ Heat
□ Heat	□ Gall bladder	□ Cold
□ Cold	□ Liver	□ Wind invasion
□ Wind heat		
□ Wind cold	**Temperature**	
□ Wind damp	□ Cooling	
□ Dryness	□ Neutral	
	■ Warming	

Energetics

Peas are strengthening to the Stomach and have a mild action against Dampness. The peppercorns and cloves add warmth and improve the digestibility of pulses generally. The chicken stock provides a comprehensively nourishing base for the soup. This soup strengthens the Qi and is easy to digest.

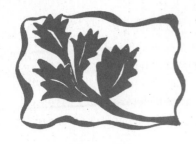

Tanov (Yoghurt Soup)

This is an unusual Armenian soup: silky, sour-sweet, lively and aromatic. Try serving it to friends and asking them to guess what is in it.

Preparation time: 10 mins
Cooking time: 25 mins
Serves: 4

Ingredients

1 pint yoghurt
1 pint water
1 ½ tablespoons white rice
½ teaspoon salt

2 teaspoons arrowroot
1 large egg

1 bunch spring onions
2 teaspoons dried dill
1 handful fresh coriander leaf
Black pepper
2 tablespoons yoghurt

Method

Combine the yoghurt and water, reserving half a teacup of the liquid. Pour the rest of the mixture into a saucepan adding the rice and salt and set on a low heat.

Meanwhile dissolve the arrowroot into the reserved liquid and beat in the egg. Add this to the soup, stirring continuously. Bring the soup to the boil then reduce to a simmer.

Chop the spring onions and add these with the dill after 15 minutes. Cook for another 5 minutes then add the coriander and cook gently for a further 5 minutes. The soup is ready as soon as the rice is cooked. Add a couple of tablespoons of fresh yoghurt just at the end. Add salt to taste and sprinkle with freshly ground black pepper.

Primary actions	Primary influences	Contra-indications
■ Qi ■ Blood	■ Lung	☐ Qi def
■ Yin ☐ Yang	■ Intestines	☐ Blood def
☐ Damp	☐ Stomach	☐ Yin def
☐ Phlegm	■ Spleen	☐ Yang def
☐ Water	☐ Heart	■ Damp
☐ Qi stagnation	☐ Bladder	☐ Stagnation
☐ Blood stagnation	☐ Kidney	☐ Heat
☐ Heat	☐ Gall bladder	☐ Cold
☐ Cold	☐ Liver	☐ Wind invasion
☐ Wind heat		
☐ Wind cold	**Temperature**	
☐ Wind damp	☐ Cooling	
☐ Dryness	■ Neutral	
	☐ Warming	

Energetics

Like all grains, rice nourishes the Qi and Blood. In combination with the yoghurt and egg, the Yin is also strengthened. The herbs increase the digestibility of the soup and the spring onions add warmth and movement, counteracting any tendency towards congestion.

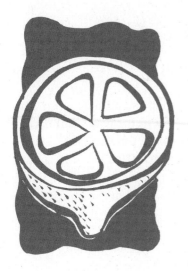

Turkish Lentil Soup

I first ate this soup in the pine forested mountains of southwest Turkey. I remember the sunset that evening, the laughter round our table and the local 'saz' player who wandered up the trail to make music for us. Unlike the wine we brought home which tasted disgusting out of its native habitat, the soup was every bit as good and evocative. If lentil soup sounds dull and pious to you, this recipe is guaranteed to redeem it.

Preparation time: 10 mins
Cooking time: 30 mins
Serves: 4

Ingredients

2 onions
3 tablespoons olive oil

2 or 3 medium potatoes
½ pound red lentils
2 pints water
1 bayleaf

1–2 teaspoons fresh mint
2 lemons
Salt

Method

Chop the onions finely and fry them in plenty of olive oil until soft and sweet smelling.

Meanwhile wash and chop the potatoes quite small. Add the lentils, stir for a minute then add the potatoes. Stir again. Add water and the bayleaf and bring to the boil. Simmer for about half an hour or until soft.

Add the chopped mint about halfway through and the lemon and salt at the end. When cooked, remove the bayleaf and mash or blend the soup a little.

Primary actions	Primary influences	Contra-indications
■ Qi ■ Blood	☐ Lung	☐ Qi def
☐ Yin ☐ Yang	☐ Intestines	☐ Blood def
■ Damp	■ Stomach	☐ Yin def
☐ Phlegm	■ Spleen	☐ Yang def
■ Water	☐ Heart	☐ Damp
☐ Qi stagnation	☐ Bladder	☐ Stagnation
☐ Blood stagnation	■ Kidney	☐ Heat
☐ Heat	☐ Gall bladder	☐ Cold
☐ Cold	☐ Liver	☐ Wind invasion
☐ Wind heat		
☐ Wind cold	**Temperature**	
☐ Wind damp	☐ Cooling	
☐ Dryness	■ Neutral	
	☐ Warming	

Energetics

This is a simple Qi strengthening soup. It is easy to digest and provides sustained release of energy. Lentils strengthen the Spleen and Stomach as well as benefiting both the Heart and Kidney. They also have a mild action against Dampness. The lemon and mint make this a slightly cool dish.

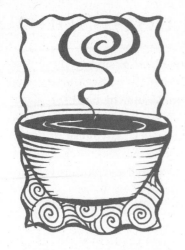

Wheat and Celeriac Soup

The wheat grains give this soup an unusual texture. This is a mild-tasting, hearty soup which is both soothing and satisfying. It needs a little more time and forethought than most recipes but is not difficult and definitely repays the effort. The idea for this recipe was inspired by Rose Elliot and Carlo de Pauli's 'Kitchen Pharmacy'.

Preparation time: 15 mins
Cooking time: 80 mins
Serves: 4

Ingredients

6 ounces wheat/spelt grains
2 ½ pints vegetable stock

1 onion
2 tablespoons olive oil
4 ounces carrots
½ pound celeriac

1 tomato
2 cloves garlic
4 tablespoons seaweed
1 ½ teaspoons dried dill
Juice of 1 lemon
Salt and pepper
Handful parsley

Method

Bring the wheat to the boil in the vegetable stock, turn off the heat and leave it to soak overnight if possible, or for at least one hour.

Chop the onion, carrot and celeriac into small pieces. Fry the onion in the oil until it softens, then add the carrot and celeriac, stirring frequently for 5-10 minutes.

Add the wheat and its liquid together with the chopped tomato, garlic and the seaweed (hijiki is good but any seaweed broken into small pieces will do). Cook slowly for an hour or more until the wheat is soft and breaking open. Add the dill about halfway through the cooking. Season to taste with lemon, and garnish with fresh parsley.

Energetics

Wheat is a cool and sweet grain which strengthens the Heart and Kidney, tonifies Yin and balances the nervous system. The seaweed also nourishes Kidney Yin and acts against Phlegm and Water. The carrot and celeriac benefit the Liver. The overall action is to strengthen these Organs, to nourish Yin and Blood, and to cool Heat.

Primary actions	Primary influences	Contra-indications
■ Qi ■ Blood	□ Lung	□ Qi def
■ Yin □ Yang	□ Intestines	□ Blood def
□ Damp	■ Stomach	□ Yin def
□ Phlegm	□ Spleen	□ Yang def
■ Water	■ Heart	□ Damp
□ Qi stagnation	□ Bladder	□ Stagnation
□ Blood stagnation	■ Kidney	□ Heat
■ Heat	□ Gall bladder	□ Cold
□ Cold	■ Liver	□ Wind invasion
□ Wind heat		
□ Wind cold	**Temperature**	
□ Wind damp	■ Cooling	
□ Dryness	□ Neutral	
	□ Warming	

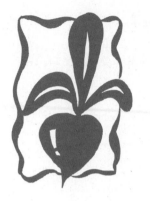

Beetroot Salad

The secret of this salad lies in the sweetness of the onion. Try to find a sweet one to make the most of the recipe. The pink colour is bright and unusual and the taste sweet and alluring.

Preparation time: 10 mins
Serves: 4

Ingredients

4 beetroot
1 cup goat yoghurt
1 teaspoon dried dill leaf
1 teaspoon powdered dulse (seaweed)
1 small sweet onion

Method

Grate the beetroot finely into a salad bowl. Mix together the yoghurt, dill, dulse and finely chopped onion. Pour it over the beetroot and allow it to sit a while.

Primary actions	Primary influences	Contra-indications
☐ Qi ■ Blood	☐ Lung	☐ Qi def
■ Yin ☐ Yang	■ Intestines	☐ Blood def
☐ Damp	☐ Stomach	☐ Yin def
☐ Phlegm	☐ Spleen	☐ Yang def
☐ Water	■ Heart	☐ Damp
☐ Qi stagnation	☐ Bladder	☐ Stagnation
☐ Blood stagnation	☐ Kidney	☐ Heat
	☐ Gall bladder	■ Cold
■ Heat	■ Liver	☐ Wind invasion
☐ Cold		
☐ Wind heat	**Temperature**	
☐ Wind cold	■ Cooling	
☐ Wind damp	☐ Neutral	
■ Dryness	☐ Warming	

Energetics

Beetroot nourishes the Blood and benefits the Liver. Yoghurt nourishes the Yin, benefits the Intestines and cools the system. Together they create a cooling, moistening salad.

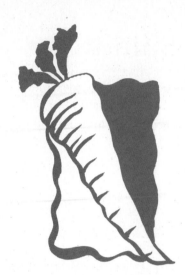

Carrot and Sauerkraut Salad

A simple and refreshing salad.

Preparation time: 10 mins
Serves: 4

Ingredients

3 cups grated carrot
1 cup sauerkraut
2 spring onions
½ teaspoon nori flakes
1 tablespoon olive oil
1 tablespoon lemon juice
Black pepper

Method

Grate the carrot finely. Wring the juice out of the sauer-kraut before chopping it. Chop the spring onions finely and combine all the ingredients in a salad bowl adding a good twist of fresh black pepper.

Primary actions	Primary influences	Contra-indications
■ Qi ☐ Blood	■ Lung	☐ Qi def
☐ Yin ☐ Yang	■ Intestines	☐ Blood def
☐ Damp	■ Stomach	☐ Yin def
☐ Phlegm	■ Spleen	☐ Yang def
☐ Water	☐ Heart	☐ Damp
■ Qi stagnation	☐ Bladder	☐ Stagnation
☐ Blood stagnation	☐ Kidney	☐ Heat
■ Heat	■ Gall bladder	☐ Cold
☐ Cold	■ Liver	☐ Wind invasion
☐ Wind heat		
☐ Wind cold	**Temperature**	
☐ Wind damp	■ Cooling	
☐ Dryness	☐ Neutral	
	☐ Warming	

Energetics

This salad benefits the Liver, is helpful for Qi Stagnation and is easy on the digestion. The sauerkraut is also bene-ficial for the Intestines.

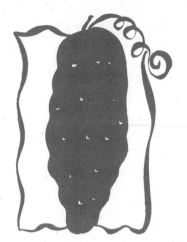

Cucumber Raita

This is a traditional Indian dish usually served as an accompaniment to curry. It is cooling and delicious.

Preparation time: 10 mins
Serves: 4

Ingredients

1 teaspoon cumin seeds
2 cucumbers
1 ½ cups yoghurt
¼ teaspoon salt

Method

Dry roast the cumin seeds until they are slightly browned then crush them with a rolling pin or mortar and pestle. Grate or finely shred the cucumber, combine with the other ingredients and let the mixture sit for half an hour or so before serving.

Primary actions	Primary influences	Contra-indications
☐ Qi ☐ Blood	■ Lung	☐ Qi def
■ Yin ☐ Yang	■ Intestines	☐ Blood def
☐ Damp	■ Stomach	☐ Yin def
☐ Phlegm	■ Spleen	■ Yang def
☐ Water	■ Heart	■ Damp
☐ Qi stagnation	☐ Bladder	☐ Stagnation
☐ Blood stagnation	☐ Kidney	☐ Heat
■ Heat	☐ Gall bladder	■ Cold
☐ Cold	☐ Liver	☐ Wind invasion
☐ Wind heat		
☐ Wind cold	**Temperature**	
☐ Wind damp	■ Cooling	
■ Dryness	☐ Neutral	
	☐ Warming	

Energetics

Cucumber is cool, sweet and cleansing and will relieve Heat throughout the body. Its moistening thirst-relieving nature will benefit Dryness and it has an uplifting affect on the Heart. Yoghurt is also moistening and cooling with special benefits for the Intestines. The cumin slightly moderates the coolness of this dish and counteracts the dampening nature of the yoghurt.

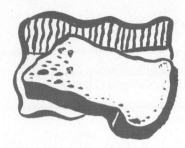

Frisée Lettuce and Bacon Salad

There is a delightful medley of textures in this salad. I first encountered it in Brittany and, whether or not the wine and company had anything to do with it, it has stayed in my mind ever since. Here's the version that emerged as I tried to recreate it in my own kitchen.

Preparation time: 20 mins
Serves: 4

Ingredients

2 eggs
4–5 slices bacon
1 ½ cups cubed bread

1 frisée lettuce
3 spring onions
3 tablespoons olive oil
3 tablespoons red wine vinegar
Salt and pepper

Method

Hard boil the eggs, peel and chop roughly. While the eggs are boiling, dice the bacon into bite-size pieces and fry it until it begins to crisp. Set it aside in a warm place and fry the cubed bread pieces in the bacon fat until browned, adding a little olive oil if needed.

Tear the lettuce, chop the spring onions, combine the oil and vinegar and turn all the ingredients in a bowl, tossing well. This salad is best if you can time it so that the cooked ingredients are still slightly warm. Serve with bread and perhaps a glass of white wine.

Primary actions	Primary influences	Contra-indications
■ Qi ■ Blood	☐ Lung	☐ Qi def
■ Yin ☐ Yang	☐ Intestines	☐ Blood def
☐ Damp	■ Stomach	☐ Yin def
☐ Phlegm	■ Spleen	☐ Yang def
☐ Water	☐ Heart	☐ Damp
☐ Qi stagnation	☐ Bladder	☐ Stagnation
☐ Blood stagnation	■ Kidney	☐ Heat
☐ Heat	☐ Gall bladder	■ Cold
☐ Cold	■ Liver	☐ Wind invasion
☐ Wind heat		
☐ Wind cold	**Temperature**	
☐ Wind damp	■ Cooling	
☐ Dryness	☐ Neutral	
	☐ Warming	

Energetics

Pork and eggs nourish the Yin. In this recipe their rich and somewhat dampening quality is nicely offset by the bitter lettuce, spring onions and the vinaigrette. Nevertheless, in severe cases of Dampness it is better to avoid this salad.

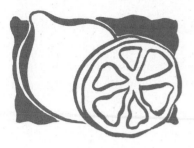

Green Bean Salad

This is a simple cooked salad that is easily prepared. The colours combine beautifully and the salad goes well with rice or fish dishes.

Preparation time: 15 mins
Serves: 4

Ingredients

³/₄ pounds string beans (haricot vert)
¹/₄ pounds carrots

2 tablespoons olive oil
1 ¹/₂ tablespoons lemon juice
1 clove garlic
2 teaspoons gomasio (see p. 235)
Small handful walnuts

Method

Top, tail and halve the beans and cut the carrots into thin strips of similar length. Steam for 5 minutes or until tender.

Meanwhile pour the olive oil, crushed garlic and lemon juice into a salad bowl and beat together until slightly thick. Turn in the beans and carrot while still warm, sprinkle with gomasio and lightly toasted walnuts. Serve at room temperature.

Primary actions	Primary influences	Contra-indications
■ Qi □ Blood	□ Lung	□ Qi def
■ Yin □ Yang	□ Intestines	□ Blood def
□ Damp	□ Stomach	□ Yin def
□ Phlegm	■ Spleen	□ Yang def
□ Water	□ Heart	□ Damp
□ Qi stagnation	□ Bladder	□ Stagnation
□ Blood stagnation	■ Kidney	□ Heat
□ Heat	□ Gall bladder	□ Cold
□ Cold	□ Liver	□ Wind invasion
□ Wind heat		
□ Wind cold	**Temperature**	
□ Wind damp	□ Cooling	
□ Dryness	■ Neutral	
	□ Warming	

Energetics

String beans strengthen the Kidney and nourish Yin. They are assisted in this by the sesame seeds and their action is reinforced by the salt. The walnuts broadly nourish the Kidney in both its Yin and Yang aspect. This salad may be considered a broad-based tonic for the Kidney Yin and Qi.

Green Tea Salad

This salad comes from Burma and is traditionally eaten after the meal. Don't be fooled by the tame title: this salad bites back.

Preparation time: 25 mins
Serves: 4

Ingredients

2 cloves garlic
2 tablespoons green tea
Juice of one lemon
1 tablespoon soya sauce
1 ½ tablespoons fish sauce
1 tablespoon grated ginger
¼ jalapeno pepper

2 tablespoons dessicated coconut
3 tablespoons chopped peanuts
1 tablespoon sesame seeds
1 cup shredded lettuce
½ cup chopped tomato
1 lemon

Method

Finely slice and gently fry the garlic for a minute or two without burning. Combine the garlic with the green tea, fish sauce, grated ginger, jalapeno pepper, lemon juice and soya sauce in a small bowl. Leave to soak for 20 minutes.

Meanwhile toast the dessicated coconut, sesame seeds and peanuts, crushing the peanuts a little first. Set to one side. Shred the lettuce into a salad bowl, chop the tomato and add that too. When the green tea mixture has soaked for twenty minutes, combine all the ingredients in the salad bowl. Garnish with lemon.

Primary actions	Primary influences	Contra-indications
☐ Qi ☐ Blood	☐ Lung	☐ Qi def
☐ Yin ☐ Yang	☐ Intestines	☐ Blood def
■ Damp	■ Stomach	☐ Yin def
☐ Phlegm	☐ Spleen	☐ Yang def
■ Water	☐ Heart	☐ Damp
■ Qi stagnation	☐ Bladder	☐ Stagnation
☐ Blood stagnation	☐ Kidney	☐ Heat
☐ Heat	☐ Gall bladder	☐ Cold
☐ Cold	■ Liver	☐ Wind invasion
☐ Wind heat		
☐ Wind cold	**Temperature**	
☐ Wind damp	☐ Cooling	
☐ Dryness	☐ Neutral	
	■ Warming	

Energetics

Green tea often accompanies a meal as a digestive aid. Here the benefits of the tea combine with the sharp flavours of the salad to improve digestion and counterbalance the congesting qualities of a meal.

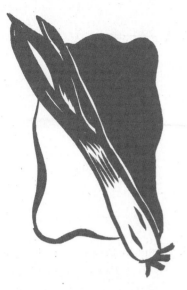

Leek and Seaweed Salad

Leeks have a subtle salty flavour that is enhanced by the seaweed and beautifully complemented by the nuttiness of sesame oil. This simple salad is very easy to make. A little finely sliced red pepper can look good with this salad and toasted walnuts can also be added.

Preparation time: 10 mins
Serves: 2

Ingredients

1 leek
Three 6-inch strips wakame seaweed
1 tablespoon cider vinegar
½ tablespoon sesame oil
Sprinkle gomasio (see p. 235)

Method

Soak the wakame for five or ten minutes and remove the tough central rib. Chop and steam the leek adding the sliced wakame for the last 30 seconds. Pour on the vinegar and oil, and sprinkle with gomasio. Serve warm or at room temperature.

Primary actions	Primary influences	Contra-indications
☐ Qi ■ Blood	☐ Lung	☐ Qi def
■ Yin ☐ Yang	☐ Intestines	☐ Blood def
■ Damp	☐ Stomach	☐ Yin def
■ Phlegm	☐ Spleen	☐ Yang def
■ Water	☐ Heart	☐ Damp
■ Qi stagnation	☐ Bladder	☐ Stagnation
■ Blood stagnation	■ Kidney	☐ Heat
☐ Heat	☐ Gall bladder	☐ Cold
☐ Cold	■ Liver	☐ Wind invasion
☐ Wind heat	**Temperature**	
☐ Wind cold	☐ Cooling	
☐ Wind damp	■ Neutral	
☐ Dryness	☐ Warming	

Energetics

Both leeks and seaweed help to resolve Dampness in the body. This dish will also move Stagnation, cleanse the Blood and nourish both Blood and Yin. Leeks and seaweed both act on the Liver and Kidney.

Moroccan Aubergine Salad

This summer salad goes well with tabbouleh and most egg or bean dishes. It is also known to increase the appetite for Mediterranean holidays.

Preparation time: 30 mins
Serves: 4

Ingredients

1 onion
2 medium aubergines
2 peppers (red and yellow)
2 courgettes
¼ cup olive oil
1½ teaspoons cumin
1 teaspoon ground coriander
1 teaspoon paprika
Salt and pepper

½ cup cashews, toasted
1–2 tablespoons lemon juice
1 cup coriander leaf
½ cup black olives
Dash chilli sauce
Cucumber, tomato, rocket to garnish

Method

Slice all the vegetables into strips and cut the onion finely. Cook all the vegetables slowly with the oil until they soften (about 15 minutes). Add the coriander, paprika, cumin, salt and pepper. Stir and cook for a further 5-10 minutes.

Meanwhile lightly toast the cashews. Remove mixture from the heat and stir in the fresh coriander, lemon juice, olives, toasted cashews and a dash of chilli sauce. Turn the mixture out into a salad bowl and allow to cool. Add additional lemon or salt and pepper as required. Garnish with slices of tomato, cucumber and leafy greens such as rocket.

Primary actions	Primary influences	Contra-indications
☐ Qi ■ Blood	☐ Lung	☐ Qi def
☐ Yin ☐ Yang	☐ Intestines	☐ Blood def
☐ Damp	■ Stomach	☐ Yin def
☐ Phlegm	■ Spleen	☐ Yang def
☐ Water	☐ Heart	☐ Damp
■ Qi stagnation	☐ Bladder	☐ Stagnation
■ Blood stagnation	☐ Kidney	☐ Heat
☐ Heat	☐ Gall bladder	☐ Cold
☐ Cold	■ Liver	☐ Wind invasion
☐ Wind heat	**Temperature**	
☐ Wind cold	☐ Cooling	
☐ Wind damp	■ Neutral	
☐ Dryness	☐ Warming	

Energetics

Aubergine has a reputation for moving Stagnant Blood in the Uterus and mildly easing Liver Qi Stagnation. It is energetically cool in temperature. Coriander leaf supports the Blood-moving action. The peppers and spices increase the warmth and Stagnation-moving effects of the recipe. This dish is recommended in all cases of Blood Stagnation. Aubergines, however, should not be overused in pregnancy because of their stimulating effect on the Uterus.

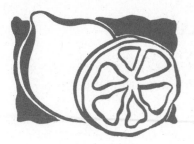

Papaya Salad

It would be hard to find a more simple salad that is also thoroughly exotic. This is best served as a starter, especially before a meat dish.

Preparation time: 5 mins
Serves: 2

Ingredients

1 papaya
1 tablespoon lime juice
Sea salt to taste

Method

Slice the papaya in half and scoop out the seeds. Cut it into bite-size pieces, peeling as you go. Salt it lightly then add the lime juice. Turn quickly to ensure it is well covered. Serve as a starter or alone.

Primary actions	Primary influences	Contra-indications
☐ Qi ☐ Blood	■ Lung	☐ Qi def
☐ Yin ☐ Yang	■ Intestines	☐ Blood def
■ Damp	■ Stomach	☐ Yin def
■ Phlegm	☐ Spleen	☐ Yang def
☐ Water	☐ Heart	☐ Damp
■ Qi stagnation	☐ Bladder	☐ Stagnation
☐ Blood stagnation	☐ Kidney	☐ Heat
☐ Heat	☐ Gall bladder	☐ Cold
☐ Cold	☐ Liver	☐ Wind invasion
☐ Wind heat	**Temperature**	
☐ Wind cold	■ Cooling	
☐ Wind damp	☐ Neutral	
☐ Dryness	☐ Warming	

Energetics

Papaya helps to resolve Dampness and Phlegm in the Lung, Stomach and Intestines and assists in the digestion of protein. It is a helpful food for digestive Stagnation.

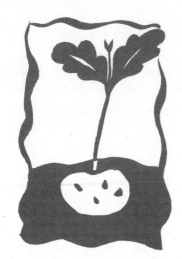

Potato Salad

Potato salad can sometimes be a little heavy. This version has a lively bite to it and nearly always has people coming back for more.

Preparation time: 10 mins
Cooking time: 20 mins
Serves: 4

Ingredients	Method
2 pounds new potatoes	Boil the new potatoes whole in slightly salted water.
½ cup yoghurt 4 tablespoons olive oil 1 tablespoon creamed horseradish 1 teaspoon cider vinegar	Combine the yoghurt, olive oil, horseradish and cider vinegar in the bottom of the salad bowl. When the potatoes are cooked, strain and tip them into the bowl with the dressing. Chop them a little and turn them.
½ cup parsley Bunch chives 2 tablespoons capers Salt and pepper	Chop the chives and parsley finely and add them with the capers to the salad. Turn once more and it's ready.

Primary actions	Primary influences	Contra-indications
■ Qi ■ Blood	■ Lung	□ Qi def
■ Yin □ Yang	□ Intestines	□ Blood def
□ Damp	■ Stomach	□ Yin def
□ Phlegm	■ Spleen	□ Yang def
□ Water	□ Heart	□ Damp
□ Qi stagnation	□ Bladder	□ Stagnation
□ Blood stagnation	■ Kidney	□ Heat
□ Heat	□ Gall bladder	□ Cold
□ Cold	□ Liver	□ Wind invasion
□ Wind heat		
□ Wind cold	**Temperature**	
□ Wind damp	□ Cooling	
□ Dryness	■ Neutral	
	□ Warming	

Energetics

Potatoes strengthen the Yin and the Qi. The parsley brings additional nourishment to the Blood and the horseradish, chives, capers and vinegar add warmth and movement. The yoghurt benefits the Intestines and the olive oil benefits the Liver.

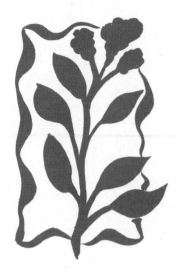

Tabbouleh

A Lebanese favourite which has now become an international classic, tabbouleh is a light salad with extraordinary amounts of parsley. Often there is more parsley than grain. Tabbouleh looks and tastes good served on cos (romaine) lettuce leaves and eaten like Mexican tacos.

Preparation time: 20 mins
Serves: 4

Ingredients

1 cup bulgur wheat	
3 bunches parsley	
1 handful mint	
Good pinch fresh thyme	
8 spring onions	
½ cucumber	
2 tomatoes	
4 tablespoons lemon juice	
4 tablespoons olive oil	
Salt and pepper	

Method

Soak the bulgur wheat for about 15–20 minutes in enough water to just cover it.

Meanwhile chop the herbs finely and cut the spring onions, tomatoes and cucumber into small pieces. Combine the chopped ingredients with the oil, lemon juice, salt and pepper in a salad bowl. Gently squeeze out any excess water from the bulgur wheat and toss the wheat into the bowl. Let the ingredients sit a while before serving.

Primary actions	Primary influences	Contra-indications
■ Qi ■ Blood	☐ Lung	☐ Qi def
☐ Yin ☐ Yang	☐ Intestines	☐ Blood def
☐ Damp	☐ Stomach	☐ Yin def
☐ Phlegm	☐ Spleen	☐ Yang def
■ Water	■ Heart	☐ Damp
■ Qi stagnation	■ Bladder	☐ Stagnation
■ Blood stagnation	■ Kidney	☐ Heat
☐ Heat	☐ Gall bladder	☐ Cold
☐ Cold	■ Liver	☐ Wind invasion
☐ Wind heat		
☐ Wind cold	**Temperature**	
☐ Wind damp	■ Cooling	
☐ Dryness	☐ Neutral	
	☐ Warming	

Energetics

Parsley is a fine tonic for the Blood. It also has a diuretic effect, draining Water from the body and supporting the Kidney. The wheat has a supportive action on the Kidney Qi as well as the Heart. The pungency of the mint and spring onions moves the Qi, and the olive oil/lemon combination stimulates the Liver. This is a good light salad for anyone who tends towards Stagnation.

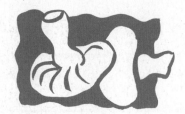

Barley and Mushroom Pilaf

Pilaf is a Middle Eastern dish that is commonly found anywhere from Armenia to India. Various grains can be used such as bulgur or rice with any number of nuts, meats, fish or other ingredients folded in. Cooked in a good stock, pilaf is very satisfying and once you have the hang of the basic method, you can reinvent this dish time and again.

Preparation time: 15 mins
Cooking time: 45 mins
Serves: 4–6

Ingredients

2 ounces fresh shiitake mushrooms
½ pound field mushrooms
1 onion
2 carrots
2 tablespoons butter
2 tablespoons olive oil

1 cup pot barley
3 cups chicken stock
Handful fresh parsley
½ cup walnuts
Soya sauce
Salt and pepper

Method

Chop the mushrooms, onions and carrots into strips. Sauté the mushrooms in a little of the olive oil and butter and set aside when browned.

Sauté the onion and carrots in the rest of the oil and butter for a few minutes, stir in the barley then add the stock. Cook for about 45 minutes or until the barley is tender, adding more stock if needed. Turn in the mushrooms and their juice and cook for a few more minutes. Toast the walnuts lightly, sprinkle with soya sauce and fold in. Chop the parsley and fold that in too. Season with soya sauce or salt and pepper and serve with some steamed greens.

Energetics

Barley is beneficial for the Stomach and Intestines and is very easily digested. It strengthens the Blood and the Yin whilst at the same time leaching surplus Water from the system. The mushrooms, like the barley, are slightly cooling and they help remove toxins and surplus Heat from the body. The overall effect of this dish is to reduce Heat, drain Water and nourish the Blood and Yin.

Primary actions	Primary influences	Contra-indications
■ Qi ■ Blood	■ Lung	☐ Qi def
■ Yin ☐ Yang	■ Intestines	☐ Blood def
■ Damp	■ Stomach	☐ Yin def
■ Phlegm	■ Spleen	☐ Yang def
■ Water	☐ Heart	☐ Damp
☐ Qi stagnation	☐ Bladder	☐ Stagnation
☐ Blood stagnation	☐ Kidney	☐ Heat
	☐ Gall bladder	☐ Cold
■ Heat	☐ Liver	☐ Wind invasion
☐ Cold		
☐ Wind heat	**Temperature**	
☐ Wind cold	☐ Cooling	
☐ Wind damp	■ Neutral	
☐ Dryness	☐ Warming	

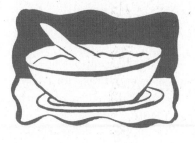

Coconut Rice

This is a sweet energising dish. The rice soaks up the coconut and the fat, tasting surprisingly rich. It tastes good with dal or most spiced Indian dishes and some simply cooked vegetables. It is quite sweet and oily so don't serve it with other rich food.

Preparation time: 10 mins
Cooking time: 30 mins
Serves: 4

Ingredients

3 cups cooked rice
2 ounces creamed coconut (unsweetened)
1 teaspoon black mustard seed
1 teaspoon garam masala
1 ounce butter or ghee
1 tablespoon honey

Method

Heat the ghee or butter in a frying pan over a moderate heat. Add the spices and coconut, cooking until lightly browned. Do not burn. Stir in the rice and honey and serve immediately.

Primary actions	Primary influences	Contra-indications
■ Qi ■ Blood	☐ Lung	☐ Qi def
☐ Yin ☐ Yang	☐ Intestines	☐ Blood def
☐ Damp	■ Stomach	☐ Yin def
☐ Phlegm	■ Spleen	☐ Yang def
☐ Water	■ Heart	■ Damp
☐ Qi stagnation	☐ Bladder	☐ Stagnation
☐ Blood stagnation	☐ Kidney	☐ Heat
☐ Heat	☐ Gall bladder	☐ Cold
☐ Cold	☐ Liver	☐ Wind invasion
☐ Wind heat	**Temperature**	
☐ Wind cold	☐ Cooling	
☐ Wind damp	☐ Neutral	
☐ Dryness	■ Warming	

Energetics

Rice is a simple sweet food that forms the basis of Qi and Blood. The addition of coconut increases its Qi strengthening properties; the spices increase its digestibility. Both the spices and the coconut are warm in nature. Coconut also has a tonifying effect on the Heart and a calming effect on the emotions.

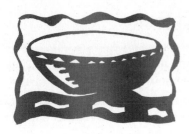

Congee

In China, Congee (or Jook as it should really be known) is a popular street-side snack, a favoured food for the old and sick and a soothing, easily-digested meal that is halfway between food and medicine. It consists simply of white rice cooked for a long time to a dilute porridge consistency with the addition of only one or two other ingredients. It is easy to create your own self-healing congee with a little knowledge of a food's properties.

Preparation time: 4–8 hours
Serves: 2

Ingredients

½ cup white rice
3–4 cups water

Method

Cook the rice in a pan on the lowest possible heat for about 4 hours, keeping the lid on. Alternatively use a slow-cooker or, better yet, a casserole dish and cook it in the oven overnight. The longer it cooks, the more nutritious it is considered to be.

Energetics

Congee is probably the most easily digested food in the world and is considered strengthening to the Spleen. Other ingredients are commonly added to guide its therapeutic action and their effects are easily assimilated into the body. Try adding small amounts (less than the rice) of the following: mung bean to reduce Dampness and Heat; chestnut to strengthen the Kidney; kidney with spring onion and ginger to counter Cold and strengthen Yang; pine kernel to nourish Yin, lubricate the Intestines and ease constipation (contraindicated for Spleen weakness); spinach to nourish Blood; or cook in chicken stock for a broad-based general tonic.

Primary actions	Primary influences	Contra-indications
■ Qi ☐ Blood	☐ Lung	☐ Qi def
☐ Yin ☐ Yang	☐ Intestines	☐ Blood def
☐ Damp	■ Stomach	☐ Yin def
☐ Phlegm	■ Spleen	☐ Yang def
☐ Water	☐ Heart	☐ Damp
☐ Qi stagnation	☐ Bladder	☐ Stagnation
☐ Blood stagnation	☐ Kidney	☐ Heat
	☐ Gall bladder	☐ Cold
☐ Heat	☐ Liver	☐ Wind invasion
☐ Cold		
☐ Wind heat	**Temperature**	
☐ Wind cold	☐ Cooling	
☐ Wind damp	■ Neutral	
☐ Dryness	☐ Warming	

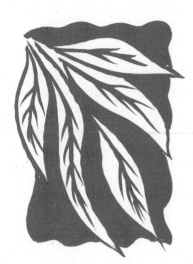

Herby Millet

This is a simple way to cook millet. It goes well with egg or cheese and with any vegetable dish.

Preparation time: 5 mins
Cooking time: 30 mins
Serves: 4

Ingredients

½ onion
2 cloves garlic
2 teaspoons fresh parsley
1 cup millet
2 ½ cups water
1 teaspoon nori flakes
1 teaspoon sage
¼ teaspoon thyme
Pinch salt

Method

Chop the onion, garlic and parsley fairly small. Then simply put all the ingredients in a pan, cover and bring to the boil. Simmer for 20-30 minutes adding more water if needed.

Primary actions	Primary influences	Contra-indications
■ Qi ■ Blood	■ Lung	□ Qi def
□ Yin □ Yang	□ Intestines	□ Blood def
■ Damp	■ Stomach	□ Yin def
■ Phlegm	■ Spleen	□ Yang def
□ Water	□ Heart	□ Damp
□ Qi stagnation	□ Bladder	□ Stagnation
□ Blood stagnation	■ Kidney	□ Heat
□ Heat	□ Gall bladder	□ Cold
□ Cold	□ Liver	□ Wind invasion
□ Wind heat		
□ Wind cold	**Temperature**	
□ Wind damp	□ Cooling	
□ Dryness	■ Neutral	
	□ Warming	

Energetics

Millet is a cool grain which nourishes the Kidney. It is also one of the few alkalising grains, making it easy to digest and strengthening to the Stomach and Spleen. The supportive action on the Kidney is reinforced by the garlic, parsley and nori whilst the sage and onion act against Phlegm in the Lung and the onion generates movement. This is a good recipe for Damp conditions.

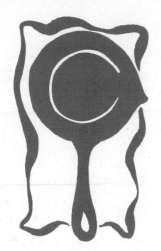

Kasha

This is a light and simple way to prepare buckwheat, Polish-style. Kasha can be used as an accompaniment to any vegetable dish and combines especially well with cabbage. It is also excellent with tofu or tempeh.

Preparation time: 5 mins
Cooking time: 25 mins
Serves: 4

Ingredients

1 onion
2 tablespoons olive oil
1 cup toasted buckwheat
1 egg, beaten

3 cups water or vegetable stock
2 teaspoons tamari

Method

Sauté the onions in the oil for a few minutes then add the buckwheat and stir for a little while longer. Remove the pan from the heat and quickly stir in a beaten egg. Return to the heat and stir again until the egg is cooked and the buckwheat grains separate.

Heat the water separately and when it boils pour it into the kasha. Add the tamari and simmer the kasha for about 20 minutes. Fluff it lightly before serving.

Primary actions	Primary influences	Contra-indications
■ Qi ■ Blood	□ Lung	□ Qi def
□ Yin □ Yang	■ Intestines	□ Blood def
■ Damp	■ Stomach	□ Yin def
□ Phlegm	■ Spleen	□ Yang def
□ Water	□ Heart	□ Damp
■ Qi stagnation	□ Bladder	□ Stagnation
■ Blood stagnation	□ Kidney	□ Heat
□ Heat	□ Gall bladder	□ Cold
□ Cold	□ Liver	■ Wind invasion
□ Wind heat	**Temperature**	
□ Wind cold	■ Cooling	
□ Wind damp	□ Neutral	
□ Dryness	□ Warming	

Energetics

Buckwheat has a cooling and strengthening effect on the Intestines. It helps remove Dampness and has a stimulating effect on the circulation of Blood and Qi. Those with symptoms of Heat or internal Wind may find that buckwheat aggravates their symptoms.

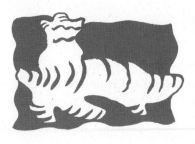

Kicharee

Kicharee is a traditional Indian dish translating roughly as 'hodge-podge'. Originally a simple combination of rice and lentils, Kicharee evolved to become 'kedgeree' with fish, rice and peas. Kicharee is one of those perfectly balanced meals that will feel right for almost everyone. It is very simple, very satisfying and very nutritious. It is to the Indian tradition what chicken soup is to the Jewish tradition, a recipe for every occasion. It is complemented perfectly by a bed of steamed greens. This meal will leave you with a feeling of satisfied calm.

Preparation time: 10 mins
Cooking time: 45 mins
Serves: 4

Ingredients

2 cups mung beans, presoaked
2 cups rice
1 onion
Small piece fresh ginger
½ teaspoon cumin
½ teaspoon turmeric
½ teaspoon coriander
4 tablespoons olive oil
Salt and freshly ground black pepper

Method

Soak the mung beans overnight. Rinse and cook together with the rice in 8 cups water until both are soft. When the rice and beans are underway, chop the onion finely and cook in the olive oil until soft. Add the spices and stir for a few minutes. Just before the rice and beans are cooked, turn the onions, oil and spices into the pot and stir well in. Continue cooking until the water is fully absorbed and season with salt and pepper.

Energetics

Together the beans and rice provide strong nourishment for the Qi and Blood. This combination will also help seep excess moisture from the body. Mung beans also nourish the Yin and support the Heart.

Primary actions	Primary influences	Contra-indications
■ Qi ■ Blood	□ Lung	□ Qi def
■ Yin □ Yang	□ Intestines	□ Blood def
■ Damp	■ Stomach	□ Yin def
□ Phlegm	■ Spleen	□ Yang def
■ Water	■ Heart	□ Damp
□ Qi stagnation	□ Bladder	□ Stagnation
□ Blood stagnation	■ Kidney	□ Heat
□ Heat	□ Gall bladder	□ Cold
□ Cold	□ Liver	□ Wind invasion
□ Wind heat	**Temperature**	
□ Wind cold	□ Cooling	
□ Wind damp	■ Neutral	
□ Dryness	□ Warming	

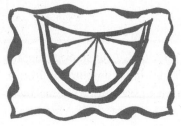

Lemon Rice

Basmati rice has its own distinct aroma which is enhanced by the delicate blend of lemon and spices. A dish of rice cooked this way will perfectly complement any vegetable or fish dish. The trick is not to burn the spices or let the rice go soggy.

Preparation time: 30 mins
Serves: 4

Ingredients

3 cups cooked basmati rice
3 tablespoons ghee or olive oil
½ teaspoon coriander seeds
½ teaspoon turmeric
½ teaspoon cumin
3 tablespoons lemon juice
Grated rind of one lemon
Salt

Method

Prepare the rice and set to one side. Heat the ghee or oil in a frying pan over a medium heat. Add the spices and cook until they pop, being careful not to burn them. Fold in the rice, lemon juice and lemon peel, stirring well. Add salt to taste and serve warm.

Primary actions	Primary influences	Contra-indications
■ Qi ■ Blood	☐ Lung	☐ Qi def
☐ Yin ☐ Yang	☐ Intestines	☐ Blood def
■ Damp	■ Stomach	☐ Yin def
☐ Phlegm	■ Spleen	☐ Yang def
☐ Water	☐ Heart	☐ Damp
■ Qi stagnation	☐ Bladder	☐ Stagnation
☐ Blood	☐ Kidney	☐ Heat
stagnation	■ Gall bladder	☐ Cold
☐ Heat	■ Liver	☐ Wind
☐ Cold		invasion
☐ Wind heat	**Temperature**	
☐ Wind cold	☐ Cooling	
☐ Wind damp	■ Neutral	
☐ Dryness	☐ Warming	

Energetics

Rice is a simple energy-building tonic for the whole body and, like all grains, is a basic building block for Qi and Blood. Basmati rice is particularly beneficial to the Spleen. The addition of the various spices and the lemon increases its digestibility and helps move Stagnation and Dampness from the system. This kind of dish is suitable for all conditions, especially Stagnation and digestive weakness.

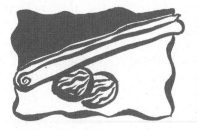

Porridge

OK, so what is porridge doing in a recipe book? After all, isn't it heavy and boring? Well, we don't think so. If you're not already a porridge devotee, try a few of these ideas to restore your faith.

Preparation time: 2 mins
Cooking time: 10 mins or overnight
Serves: 2

Ingredients

1 cup oats
2 ½ cups water
Molasses
Tahini
Marmalade
Miso
Dates
Apple
Ginger
Cinnamon
Walnuts

Method

Porridge oats can simply be cooked on top of the stove. You can also try soaking them overnight before cooking, or buy whole oats and use a slow cooker or low oven overnight. Here are a few suggestions for things to put in your porridge. Try it with molasses stirred in and sprinkled with toasted walnuts; or cooked with a little grated apple and with tahini and molasses stirred in; or stir in a dark and chunky no-sugar marmalade; or try it with miso and ginger; or cooked with dates and flavoured with cinnamon and ginger.

Primary actions	Primary influences	Contra-indications
■ Qi ■ Blood	□ Lung	□ Qi def
■ Yin ■ Yang	□ Intestines	□ Blood def
□ Damp	■ Stomach	□ Yin def
■ Phlegm	■ Spleen	□ Yang def
□ Water	□ Heart	□ Damp
■ Qi stagnation	□ Bladder	□ Stagnation
■ Blood stagnation	■ Kidney	□ Heat
□ Heat	□ Gall bladder	□ Cold
■ Cold	□ Liver	□ Wind invasion
□ Wind heat		
□ Wind cold	**Temperature**	
□ Wind damp	□ Cooling	
■ Dryness	□ Neutral	
	■ Warming	

Energetics

Oats are a warming tonic for the Qi. They strengthen the Spleen and benefit the nervous system and the bones. The various ideas for added ingredients can be used to supplement the porridge's action: molasses strengthens the Blood; tahini, molasses and apple together strengthen the Yin; marmalade moves Stagnation and helps resolve Phlegm; miso with ginger warms and strengthens the Kidney; dates with cinnamon and ginger nourish the Blood and strengthen the Yang.

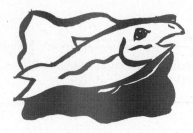

Sushi

Sushi take a little practice but they are not difficult and the effort is worthwhile. Sushi provide the perfect light meal or snack, keep for a day or two in the fridge and are a startling surprise to fish out of the picnic basket. They are very satisfying both to make and to eat and they are a complete meal in themselves. It's easy to vary sushi's ingredients and to be creative. Here are a few variations on what to put in the middle: pickled beetroot, anchovy, radish, smoked tofu, mushrooms, salmon, courgette, prawns, celery, avocado, pickled ginger.

Preparation time: 30 mins
Cooking time: 30 mins
Serves: 4–6

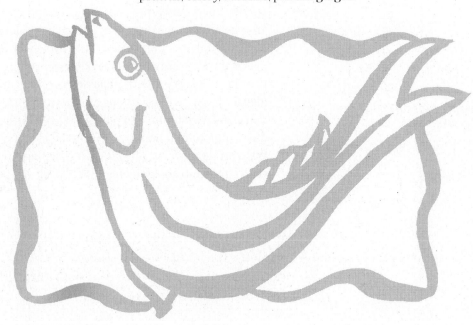

Primary actions	Primary influences	Contra-indications
■ Qi ■ Blood	□ Lung	□ Qi def
■ Yin ■ Yang	□ Intestines	□ Blood def
■ Damp	■ Stomach	□ Yin def
□ Phlegm	■ Spleen	□ Yang def
□ Water	□ Heart	□ Damp
□ Qi stagnation	□ Bladder	□ Stagnation
□ Blood stagnation	□ Kidney	□ Heat
	□ Gall bladder	□ Cold
□ Heat	□ Liver	□ Wind invasion
□ Cold		
□ Wind heat	**Temperature**	
□ Wind cold	□ Cooling	
□ Wind damp	■ Neutral	
□ Dryness	□ Warming	

Energetics

Sushi can be a complete food nourishing the Qi, Blood, Yin and Yang. The rice base nourishes the Qi and Blood. The warm ingredients such as the ginger and onion nourish the Yang. The mineral rich nori and the fish nourish the Yin. Damp resolving actions are also supplied by the ginger, onion, anchovy and nori. Variations in the energetic composition can easily be made by playing with the ingredients.

Ingredients	Method
2 cups short grain rice 2 teaspoons brown sugar 6 tablespoons cider vinegar	Cook the rice until just soft, stir in the brown sugar and cider vinegar and allow to cool. The rice is best rolled when it is still slightly warm.
4 teaspoons toasted sesame seeds	While the rice is cooking, lightly toast the sesame seeds and set aside.
$\frac{1}{4}$ avocado $\frac{1}{4}$ cucumber $\frac{1}{2}$ carrot $\frac{1}{4}$ long white radish 1 spring onion	Prepare the vegetables as late as possible to preserve their freshness, cutting them into thin 1 $\frac{1}{2}$ inch strips.
4 sheets toasted nori 6 teaspoons umeboshi paste A little anchovy, tuna or herring A little smoked tofu Pickled ginger to taste	Now it is time to lay out the nori sheets and roll the sushi. Using a sushi mat or a bamboo place mat, place the nori shiny side down. With wet hands spread a $\frac{1}{4}$" layer of rice over most of the nori leaving a half inch at top and bottom. Spread a teaspoon or so of umeboshi paste over the rice and sprinkle with sesame seeds. Make a groove in the rice about a third of the way away from you and lay in the sliced vegetables, pickled ginger and strips of fish or tofu. Be creative and vary your combinations.
	Now you are ready to roll. Begin at the near side rolling away from you, keeping the roll tight. When you reach the far side, moisten the exposed end of the nori sheet and seal the roll. Squeeze gently with your hand to ensure a good seal and leave the roll to one side until you are ready to serve. Repeat with the remaining three sheets.
	To cut the nori roll, use a sharp knife and wet it first. Each sheet will give six to eight pieces.
4 tablespoons soya sauce 1 tablespoon creamed horseradish 1 teaspoon fresh grated ginger 1 tablespoon cider vinegar 2 tablespoons water	Make the dipping sauce by combining the soya sauce, horseradish, ginger, vinegar and water. Alternatively, try a combination of shoyu, lemon juice, sake, water and ginger.

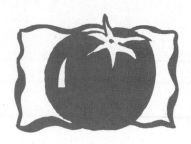

Baked Beans

Nowadays baked beans come in a tin. Here is a recipe that has probably been around in all sorts of permutations since way before canning was invented. The dark, sweet taste of these beans will take you back to ancestral times! It takes quite a long time to cook although the work is quite simple, so invite some friends round to share in the rewards of your labour. Vegetarians can omit the pork without damaging the balance of the recipe.

Preparation time: 10 mins
Cooking time: 4 hours
Serves: 6

Ingredients

½ pound haricot beans

4 ounces pork
1 pound tomatoes
1 onion
2 tablespoons molasses
1½ tablespoons red wine vinegar
2 cloves garlic
½ teaspoon freshly ground black pepper
1 teaspoon rosemary
1 teaspoon savory
3 bayleaves
1 tablespoon tamari
6 fluid ounces water

Method

The haricot beans need to be presoaked and washed, then boiled until tender. This will take about an hour.

Once the beans are underway, chop the tomatoes and cook them in an ovenproof dish until they have reduced by about half. Chop the pork into small cubes and add this. Chop the onion finely and add all the other ingredients, stirring together well until warmed. Drain the beans and add these. Cover the casserole with a tightly fitted lid and cook in the oven at a low setting for three hours or more. Serve with a simple grain and some greens, or offer them as 'beans on toast'.

Primary actions	Primary influences	Contra-indications
■ Qi ■ Blood	□ Lung	□ Qi def
■ Yin □ Yang	□ Intestines	□ Blood def
□ Damp	■ Stomach	□ Yin def
□ Phlegm	□ Spleen	□ Yang def
□ Water	□ Heart	□ Damp
□ Qi stagnation	□ Bladder	□ Stagnation
□ Blood stagnation	■ Kidney	□ Heat
□ Heat	□ Gall bladder	□ Cold
□ Cold	■ Liver	□ Wind invasion
□ Wind heat		
□ Wind cold	**Temperature**	
□ Wind damp	□ Cooling	
□ Dryness	■ Neutral	
	□ Warming	

Energetics

The beans and molasses are deeply nourishing to the Blood, which is the main focus of this dish. The pork nourishes the Yin. The vinegar, pepper, onion, garlic and herbs add warmth and movement. The tomato has a cooling action on the Liver and a cleansing action on the Blood, although its extreme coldness is moderated by the long and deep cooking method.

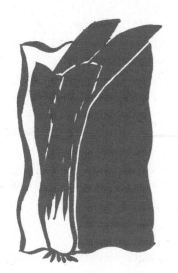

Brussels Sprouts with Horseradish

This way of cooking brussels sprouts has an earthy forcefulness which truly honours the tightly packed intensity of this fantastic winter vegetable. The strong, warming taste is perfect for a cold day and a good accompaniment to most meat.

Preparation time: 20 mins
Serves: 4

Ingredients

1 pound brussels sprouts
1 carrot
1 leek

2 tablespoons butter
3 tablespoons creamed horseradish
1 tablespoon cider vinegar
1 teaspoon dill weed
Salt and pepper
Small handful of chopped walnuts

Method

Roughly chop and steam the vegetables until tender. The brussels sprouts are best cooked whole with a cross nicked into the base to help them cook all the way through.

While the vegetables are steaming, melt the butter in a pan and add all the other ingredients, cooking gently for a minute or two. Serve the sauce poured over the vegetables and top with lightly toasted walnuts.

Primary actions	Primary influences	Contra-indications
■ Qi □ Blood	■ Lung	□ Qi def
□ Yin ■ Yang	■ Intestines	□ Blood def
■ Damp	□ Stomach	□ Yin def
□ Phlegm	□ Spleen	□ Yang def
□ Water	□ Heart	□ Damp
■ Qi stagnation	□ Bladder	□ Stagnation
■ Blood stagnation	□ Kidney	■ Heat
□ Heat	□ Gall bladder	□ Cold
■ Cold	□ Liver	□ Wind invasion
□ Wind heat	**Temperature**	
□ Wind cold	□ Cooling	
□ Wind damp	□ Neutral	
□ Dryness	■ Warming	

Energetics

Brussels sprouts are a warming vegetable, as are the leeks. The addition of pungent horseradish and cider vinegar increases the dish's heating and moving nature. The dill offsets an otherwise warming meal. This is a good dish for Yang Deficiency and for Stagnation. In serious conditions of Dampness, olive oil can be substituted for the butter.

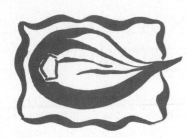

Cabbage in Chestnut and Walnut Sauce

Preparation time: 15 mins
Cooking time: 10 mins
Serves: 4

There is a lovely harmony between these two nuts and the humble cabbage. If you find cabbage boring, or if the horrible memory of school dinners still lingers in your body, this is the remedy. Goethe favoured another brassica, brussels sprouts, with his chestnuts and these could be used here too.

Ingredients

2 cloves garlic
Juice of 1 ½ lemons
¼ teaspoon dried ginger
2 cups pureed chestnuts
¾ cup olive oil
Salt and pepper

1 savoy cabbage
1 onion
1 teaspoon caraway seeds
1 cup walnuts, toasted

Method

To make the sauce, blend the garlic with the lemon juice and ginger, then add the chestnut purée. Beat in the olive oil gradually. Warm it through gently but do not boil. The final mixture should have the texture of mayonnaise.

Meanwhile shred the cabbage and slice the onion into thin rings. Place in a steamer sprinkling in the caraway seeds as you go. Steam for 5-8 minutes. Serve the cabbage, pour the sauce over the top and sprinkle with lightly toasted walnuts.

Primary actions	Primary influences	Contra-indications
■ Qi ■ Blood	■ Lung	☐ Qi def
☐ Yin ■ Yang	■ Intestines	☐ Blood def
■ Damp	■ Stomach	☐ Yin def
☐ Phlegm	☐ Spleen	☐ Yang def
☐ Water	☐ Heart	☐ Damp
☐ Qi stagnation	☐ Bladder	☐ Stagnation
☐ Blood stagnation	■ Kidney	☐ Heat
	☐ Gall bladder	☐ Cold
☐ Heat	☐ Liver	☐ Wind invasion
☐ Cold		
☐ Wind heat	**Temperature**	
☐ Wind cold	☐ Cooling	
☐ Wind damp	■ Neutral	
☐ Dryness	☐ Warming	

Energetics

Chestnuts and walnuts both support the Yang and help counteract Dampness. They are supported in this by the garlic whilst the lemon acts on the Liver and makes this dish more digestible. The cabbage helps strengthen the Blood and is especially beneficial for the Stomach and Intestines. The overall effect of this dish is to warm the body, clear Dampness, support the Kidney Yang and nourish the Intestines.

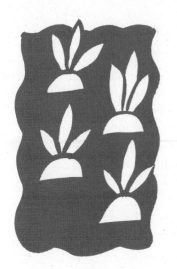

Carrot and Tofu Quiche

This is an unusual egg- and dairy-free quiche. The pale orange colour is beautiful and the taste is light, smooth and satisfying.

Preparation time: 20 mins
Cooking time: 40 mins
Serves: 4–6

Ingredients

4 carrots
1 pound tofu
Pinch of salt

1 small onion
1 clove garlic
½ teaspoon dill seed
1 teaspoon grated orange rind
3 teaspoons nori flakes
2 tablespoons fresh parsley
Sprinkle of sesame seeds
One 9 inch pastry caes

Method

Steam the carrots, strain and mash coarsely. Blend the tofu with some of the carrot water and the salt. Use enough water to give the tofu a creamy consistency.

Finely chop the onion and garlic and add them to the tofu together with the grated orange rind, the dill, nori flakes and the parsley. Stir in the mashed carrots and combine all the ingredients well. Turn the mixture into a 9 inch pastry case, sprinkle with sesame seeds and bake at 350°F/Gas Mark 4 for about 40 minutes or until set.

Primary actions	Primary influences	Contra-indications
■ Qi ■ Blood	■ Lung	□ Qi def
■ Yin □ Yang	□ Intestines	□ Blood def
□ Damp	■ Stomach	□ Yin def
□ Phlegm	■ Spleen	□ Yang def
□ Water	□ Heart	□ Damp
□ Qi stagnation	□ Bladder	□ Stagnation
□ Blood stagnation	□ Kidney	□ Heat
□ Heat	□ Gall bladder	□ Cold
□ Cold	■ Liver	□ Wind invasion
□ Wind heat		
□ Wind cold	**Temperature**	
□ Wind damp	□ Cooling	
□ Dryness	■ Neutral	
	□ Warming	

Energetics

The combination of tofu, carrot and parsley provide nourishment for the Blood and Qi. The onion, garlic, dill seed and orange rind give warmth and counter any Dampness and Stagnation arising from the richness of the pastry.

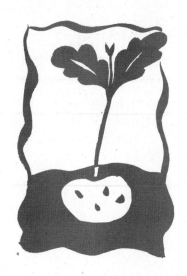

Celeriac Mash

Celeriac is often a somewhat neglected vegetable but its sweet subtle taste is perfect during the wintertime. Mashed celeriac can be eaten as a side vegetable, used as the topping for 'shepherd's pie' or served on a bed of greens and topped with a poached egg. Leftovers make an interesting addition to homemade vegeburgers.

Preparation time: 10 mins
Cooking time: 20 mins
Serves: 4

Ingredients

Method

2 pounds celeriac
2 pounds potatoes
Juice of ½ lemon

Chop and boil the celeriac and potatoes in water with the juise of half a lemon until tender, usually about fifteen minutes. Strain, keeping the juice for soup stock, and mash.

2 tablespoons dukkah (see p. 233)
Freshly gound black pepper
Juice of 1 ½ lemons

Add half the dukkah, liberal amounts of black pepper and the remaining lemon juice to the mash and fold in. Let the mash sit in a warm place for a while.

3 cloves garlic
5 tablespoons olive oil
2 tablespoons dukkah

Heat the olive oil and cook the garlic (crushed) for a few moments without burning. Pour the warm olive oil over the mash and sprinkle with the remaining dukkah.

Primary actions	Primary influences	Contra-indications
■ Qi □ Blood	□ Lung	□ Qi def
■ Yin □ Yang	□ Intestines	□ Blood def
■ Damp	□ Stomach	□ Yin def
□ Phlegm	■ Spleen	□ Yang def
□ Water	□ Heart	□ Damp
□ Qi stagnation	□ Bladder	□ Stagnation
□ Blood stagnation	■ Kidney	□ Heat
□ Heat	□ Gall bladder	□ Cold
□ Cold	□ Liver	□ Wind invasion
□ Wind heat		
□ Wind cold	**Temperature**	
□ Wind damp	□ Cooling	
□ Dryness	■ Neutral	
	□ Warming	

Energetics

Like most of the root vegetables, celeriac is sweet and slightly warming. It has a drying effect on Dampness. Combined with the potato, this dish is generally strengthening to the Qi and the Spleen. The various spices increase the digestibility and reduce any tendency towards Stagnation.

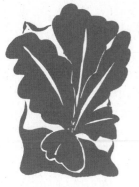

Leek and Chard Quiche

I like the dark moist green of the leaf inside the rich yellow of this quiche. Use a good mature cheddar for this recipe and, although powdered nutmeg is called for in the recipe, freshly grated nutmeg gives it an even more distinctive edge.

Preparation time: 20 mins
Cooking time: 30 mins
Serves: 6

Ingredients

Ingredients	Method
One 10 inch pastry case	Preheat the oven to 400°F/Gas Mark 6 and bake the pastry case for 5-10 minutes.
2 leeks 6 ounces chard or spinach 4 ounces mushrooms ½ tablespoon toasted sesame oil ½ tablespoon olive oil	Chop the leeks into half inch rings, cut the chard into thin strips and break the mushrooms into pieces. Fry the leeks gently in the oil for a few minutes then add the mushrooms. When the leeks are just starting to soften and the mushrooms have shrunk a little, add the chard and weight it all down with a plate or lid. Allow it to heat gently for a few minutes until the leaves have softened.
6 eggs 1 cup milk 2 teaspoons nutmeg ½ teaspoon salt Freshly ground black pepper 5 ounces mature cheddar cheese	Meanwhile beat together the eggs and milk with the nutmeg, salt and plenty of freshly ground black pepper. Grate the cheese. Remove the pastry case from the oven, fill with the vegetable mixture, pour in the beaten eggs and cover with the grated cheese. Bake at 400°F/Gas Mark 6 for 25-30 minutes.

Energetics

This rich dish is particularly nourishing to the Blood, as well as enriching the Qi and Yin. The nutritious nature of the eggs, milk and cheese makes them very dampening and this is somewhat offset by the leek, mushroom and nutmeg. The chard nourishes the Blood and lubricates the Intestines.

Primary actions	Primary influences	Contra-indications
■ Qi ■ Blood	■ Lung	☐ Qi def
■ Yin ☐ Yang	■ Intestines	☐ Blood def
☐ Damp	☐ Stomach	☐ Yin def
☐ Phlegm	☐ Spleen	☐ Yang def
☐ Water	☐ Heart	■ Damp
☐ Qi stagnation	☐ Bladder	■ Stagnation
☐ Blood stagnation	☐ Kidney	☐ Heat
☐ Heat	☐ Gall bladder	☐ Cold
☐ Cold	■ Liver	☐ Wind invasion
☐ Wind heat	**Temperature**	
☐ Wind cold	☐ Cooling	
☐ Wind damp	■ Neutral	
☐ Dryness	☐ Warming	

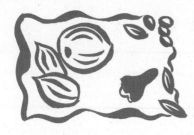

Lentil Parsnip Dal

This is a distinctly British variation on an Indian theme. Dal can be found all over India in as many different varieties as the French have cheese. Lentils combine well with sweet root vegetables and what better candidate than the parsnip. The best parsnips can be had after the first frost has bitten their tops. Don't be in a hurry when you cook them as they release more and more of their flavour as they absorb the oil and then sweat sweetly at the bottom of the pan.

Preparation time: 10 mins
Cooking time: 45 mins
Serves: 4

Ingredients

2 medium parsnips
2 tablespoons oil or ghee
1 teaspoon turmeric
¼ pint water

½ pound red lentils
1 bayleaf
1 short piece cinnamon stick
1 ¾ pints water

2 tablespoons oil or ghee
4 cardamom pods
2 teaspoons ground coriander
2 teaspoons ground cumin
2 onions
2 cloves garlic
Juice of one lemon
Salt and pepper
Fresh coriander to garnish

Method

Gently fry the parsnips with turmeric in oil until they start to soften and reduce in size. Add a little water, bring it to boiling and let the steam soften the parsnips a little more. Stir frequently.

Add the lentils with the bayleaf and cinnamon stick and the rest of the water. Bring to the boil, simmer and cook for 30 minutes or until tender.

Meanwhile fry the spices for 2 minutes in oil then add the onion and garlic, cooking for 10 minutes until well softened. Stir to avoid burning. When the lentils and parsnips are done, mash or blend them together and stir in the onion spice mixture with lemon juice to taste. Allow it to sit for a couple of minutes in a covered pan, removed from the heat, for the flavours to seep in. Season with salt and pepper. Garnish with fresh coriander and serve with rice and vegetables.

Energetics

Lentils are recommended for all conditions of Qi Deficiency, nourishing the Spleen and Kidney and strengthening the Heart. They also act against Dampness, an action shared by the parsnips. The sweet nature of parsnips also makes them nourishing to the Spleen and their mild pungency stimulates the Lung. The various spices bring warmth and movement and increase the action against Dampness.

Primary actions	Primary influences	Contra-indications
■ Qi ■ Blood	■ Lung	☐ Qi def
☐ Yin ☐ Yang	☐ Intestines	☐ Blood def
■ Damp	■ Stomach	☐ Yin def
☐ Phlegm	■ Spleen	☐ Yang def
■ Water	■ Heart	☐ Damp
■ Qi stagnation	☐ Bladder	☐ Stagnation
☐ Blood stagnation	■ Kidney	■ Heat
	☐ Gall bladder	☐ Cold
☐ Heat	■ Liver	☐ Wind invasion
☐ Cold		
☐ Wind heat	**Temperature**	
☐ Wind cold	☐ Cooling	
☐ Wind damp	☐ Neutral	
☐ Dryness	■ Warming	

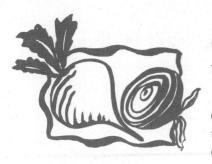

Oven Roasted Vegetables

Oven roasted vegetables are perfect for winter when there is an abundance of root vegetables to choose from. Cooked in this way the vegetables release their sweetness and warm the body all the way through. The dish is easy to prepare and can be varied according to whatever vegetables are available. The ingredients listed are simply suggestions.

Preparation time: 20 mins
Cooking time: 60 mins

Ingredients

Potato	Carrot
Swede	Turnip
Parsnip	Peppers
Squash	Beetroot
Garlic	Onion
Mushroom	Broccoli
	Cauliflower
	Tofu
	Toasted sesame oil
	Olive oil
	Rosemary
	Thyme
	Sesame seeds
	Nori
	Salt and pepper

Method

Chop the vegetables and tofu into large bite-sized pieces. Large onions can simply be quartered. Small onions, garlic cloves and mushrooms are best left whole. Mix up the oil with some sea salt and freshly ground black pepper, lay all the vegetables and tofu in a baking tray or earthenware crock, pour the oil over everything, turning thoroughly and sprinkle generously with sesame seeds, rosemary and thyme. Bake at 400°F/Gas Mark 6 for about an hour or until done. Keep the dish covered for the first twenty minutes and turn every now and then. Sprinkle with nori flakes and serve with a bitter green salad.

Primary actions	Primary influences	Contra-indications
■ Qi ■ Blood	☐ Lung	☐ Qi def
☐ Yin ■ Yang	☐ Intestines	☐ Blood def
☐ Damp	■ Stomach	☐ Yin def
☐ Phlegm	■ Spleen	☐ Yang def
☐ Water	☐ Heart	☐ Damp
☐ Qi stagnation	☐ Bladder	☐ Stagnation
☐ Blood stagnation	☐ Kidney	■ Heat
☐ Heat	☐ Gall bladder	☐ Cold
■ Cold	☐ Liver	☐ Wind invasion
☐ Wind heat		
☐ Wind cold	**Temperature**	
☐ Wind damp	☐ Cooling	
☐ Dryness	☐ Neutral	
	■ Warming	

Energetics

Roasting is a very warming method which benefits the Yang. Most root vegetables tend to be warm in nature and strengthening to the Qi. Whatever combination of vegetables is chosen, this dish is essentially Yang and Qi strengthening.

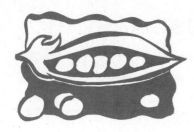

Potatoes with Peas and Fennel

This is a simple, sweet and lively dish that can happily be a meal in itself. It goes well with fish, chicken or a light omelette. It comes from Italy (via an idea in Nigel Slater's book, *The 30 Minute Cook*) so perhaps a glass of Italian wine is the perfect accompaniment.

Preparation time: 10 mins
Cooking time: 20 mins
Serves: 4–6

Ingredients

Ingredients	
2 pounds new potatoes	
¹/₂ pound fennel	
6 tablespoons olive oil	
6 tablespoons red wine vinegar	
1 ¹/₂ teaspoons mustard	
¹/₄ teaspoon salt	
1 pound peas	
3 tablespoons chives	
3 tablespoons fresh mint	
Black pepper	

Method

Scrub and boil the new potatoes.

Meanwhile finely shred or grate the fennel into a serving bowl. Mix together the olive oil, vinegar, mustard and salt and pour this over the fennel.

When the potatoes are done chop them into bite-size pieces and keep the water to lightly blanch the peas for a couple of minutes. Add the potatoes and peas to the fennel. Turn in the chopped mint and chives, sprinkle with freshly ground freshly ground black pepper and serve warm.

Primary actions	Primary influences	Contra-indications
■ Qi ■ Blood	□ Lung	□ Qi def
□ Yin □ Yang	□ Intestines	□ Blood def
■ Damp	■ Stomach	□ Yin def
□ Phlegm	■ Spleen	□ Yang def
□ Water	□ Heart	□ Damp
■ Qi stagnation	□ Bladder	□ Stagnation
□ Blood stagnation	■ Kidney	□ Heat
□ Heat	□ Gall bladder	□ Cold
□ Cold	□ Liver	□ Wind invasion
□ Wind heat	**Temperature**	
□ Wind cold	□ Cooling	
□ Wind damp	■ Neutral	
□ Dryness	□ Warming	

Energetics

Potatoes and peas are sweet and nourishing. They strengthen the Qi and benefit the Stomach and Spleen. Fennel moves Stagnation, mildly warms the middle Jiao and its aromatic flavour stimulates the digestive juices. Both peas and fennel also have an action against Dampness. This dish is a good general Qi tonic.

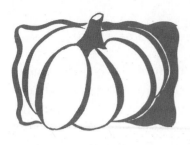

Pumpkin and Aduki Bean Stew

Preparation time: 20 mins
Cooking time: 3 hours
Serves: 4–6

This is a Japanese-style recipe that involves quite long cooking to reduce the volume and concentrate the flavours. If you want to be truly authentic you will need to find 'dashi broth' to use as stock or make your own by soaking and then simmering a few shiitake mushrooms and then straining the water. This stew needs little accompaniment but could go well with steamed greens and rice.

Ingredients

12 ounces aduki beans
2 strips kombu seaweed

1 small pumpkin or butternut/acorn squash
6 cups vegetable stock*

2 tablespoons soya sauce
1 teaspoon freshly grated ginger
¼ teaspoon salt
1 tablespoon honey
Black pepper

*If available dashi broth can be used to achieve the full Japanese flavour

Method

Soak the aduki beans overnight, rinse well then cook them in twice their volume of water with the kombu seaweed until they are soft.

Chop the squash fairly small, removing the seeds, and cook in the vegetable stock* until soft.

When both the aduki beans and the pumpkin are ready combine them with the soya sauce, ginger and salt and simmer slowly with the lid off until the liquid has reduced by half. Add the honey at the end, letting it blend in for a while without allowing the stew to boil, and season with freshly ground black pepper.

Primary actions	Primary influences	Contra-indications
■ Qi ■ Blood	□ Lung	□ Qi def
■ Yin □ Yang	■ Intestines	□ Blood def
■ Damp	■ Stomach	□ Yin def
□ Phlegm	■ Spleen	□ Yang def
■ Water	■ Heart	□ Damp
□ Qi stagnation	□ Bladder	□ Stagnation
□ Blood stagnation	■ Kidney	□ Heat
□ Heat	□ Gall bladder	□ Cold
□ Cold	□ Liver	□ Wind invasion
□ Wind heat		
□ Wind cold	**Temperature**	
□ Wind damp	□ Cooling	
□ Dryness	■ Neutral	
	□ Warming	

Energetics

This stew nourishes the Kidney and the Spleen and helps to drain Dampness. The aduki beans strengthen the Kidney Qi and Yin and have a diuretic action; the squash nourishes the Spleen Qi. This stew strengthens the whole body and can be used as the vehicle for other strengthening ingredients. Cinnamon, for example, can be added to strengthen the Yang, shiitake mushrooms to strengthen the Qi and seaweed to strengthen the Yin and Blood.

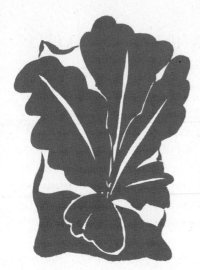

Spinach Bake

Spinach and cottage cheese are good companions. Traditional fillings for middle eastern pastries, they also combine well in this dish to make a taste and texture that will have you coming back for more.

Preparation time: 10 mins
Cooking time: 30 mins
Serves: 4

Ingredients

1 pound cottage cheese
2 eggs
½ teaspoon nutmeg
Salt
12 ounces spinach
2 tablespoons sesame seeds

Method

Beat together the cheese, egg, nutmeg and salt. Shred the spinach finely and fold it into the mixture. Turn it into a greased baking dish, sprinkle with sesame seeds and bake at 350°F/Gas Mark 4 for about 30 minutes.

Primary actions	Primary influences	Contra-indications
☐ Qi	■ Lung	☐ Qi def
■ Blood	■ Intestines	☐ Blood def
■ Yin ☐ Yang	☐ Stomach	☐ Yin def
☐ Damp	☐ Spleen	☐ Yang def
☐ Phlegm	☐ Heart	■ Damp
☐ Water	☐ Bladder	☐ Stagnation
☐ Qi stagnation	☐ Kidney	☐ Heat
☐ Blood stagnation	☐ Gall bladder	☐ Cold
☐ Heat	■ Liver	☐ Wind invasion
☐ Cold		
☐ Wind heat	**Temperature**	
☐ Wind cold	■ Cooling	
☐ Wind damp	☐ Neutral	
☐ Dryness	☐ Warming	

Energetics

The spinach, cheese and egg combine to make a rich tonic for the Blood and Yin. The dish is very moistening and is not well suited to Damp conditions.

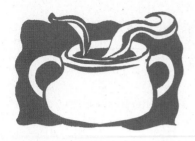

Stamppot

A traditional Dutch meal, stamppot is perfect family food: easy to make, comforting and filling. You can vary the ingredients for meat eaters by substituting bacon or smoked ham for the tofu.

Preparation time: 15 mins
Cooking time: 30 mins
Serves: 6

Ingredients

3 pounds potatoes
4 tablespoons butter
Salt
Good splash soya milk

1 pound sauerkraut
1 pound smoked tofu
Black pepper

Method

Boil the potatoes in a little salted water, drain and mash with butter and soya milk. Reserve the water for soup.

While the potatoes are cooking, gently heat the sauerkraut and the chopped smoked tofu. Fold them into the mashed potato and season with plenty of freshly ground black pepper.

Primary actions	Primary influences	Contra-indications
■ Qi ■ Blood	□ Lung	□ Qi def
■ Yin □ Yang	■ Intestines	□ Blood def
□ Damp	■ Stomach	□ Yin def
□ Phlegm	■ Spleen	□ Yang def
□ Water	□ Heart	□ Damp
□ Qi stagnation	□ Bladder	□ Stagnation
□ Blood stagnation	□ Kidney	□ Heat
■ Heat	□ Gall bladder	□ Cold
□ Cold	□ Liver	□ Wind invasion
□ Wind heat		
□ Wind cold	**Temperature**	
□ Wind damp	□ Cooling	
□ Dryness	■ Neutral	
	□ Warming	

Energetics

This simple meal nourishes the Blood, Qi and Yin. Both potato and tofu nourish the Qi and sauerkraut is very beneficial for the Intestines. Stamppot will be soothing to any digestive inflammation.

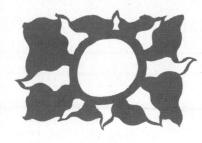

Spring Greens with Lemon

Simplicity is the key to enjoying fresh spring greens which are such a vital part of our diet. This way of cooking them is light and refreshing.

Preparation time: 10 mins
Serves: 4

Ingredients

1 pound spring greens
6 tablespoons olive oil
6 tablespoons lemon juice
Gomasio (see p. 235)

Method

Roughly shred the spring greens and steam them until just tender. Combine the olive oil and lemon. Serve the greens, pour on the dressing and sprinkle liberally with gomasio.

Primary actions	Primary influences	Contra-indications
☐ Qi ■ Blood	☐ Lung	☐ Qi def
☐ Yin ☐ Yang	☐ Intestines	☐ Blood def
☐ Damp	☐ Stomach	☐ Yin def
☐ Phlegm	☐ Spleen	☐ Yang def
☐ Water	☐ Heart	☐ Damp
☐ Qi stagnation	☐ Bladder	☐ Stagnation
☐ Blood stagnation	☐ Kidney	☐ Heat
☐ Heat	☐ Gall bladder	☐ Cold
☐ Cold	■ Liver	☐ Wind invasion
☐ Wind heat	**Temperature**	
☐ Wind cold	■ Cooling	
☐ Wind damp	☐ Neutral	
☐ Dryness	☐ Warming	

Energetics

Dark leafy greens are nourishing to the Blood and beneficial for the Liver.

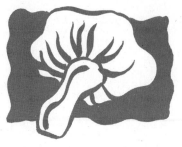

Stout and Tempeh Casserole

This is a dark-flavoured, warming, earthy dish and just the thing for a cold winter's evening. The bitter-sweet flavour of the stout is a perfect complement to the sweet root vegetables and tempeh. It has something of the same satisfaction as a steak and kidney pie.

Preparation time: 20 mins
Cooking time: 80 mins
Serves: 6–8

Ingredients

3 pounds potatoes
Knob of butter
Salt and pepper

12 ounces onion
10 ounces parsnip
1 tablespoon fresh ginger
½ pound celeriac
½ pound swede
6 ounces carrot
6 ounces mushrooms
1 pound tempeh
1 teaspoon ground coriander

¾ pint vegetable stock
1 pint stout
4 teaspoons mustard

Method

Boil the potatoes separately and mash with the butter, salt and pepper.

Meanwhile slice the onions roughly and fry slowly in oil for about 10 minutes. While the onion is cooking, chop all the other vegetables into ½ inch pieces and the tempeh into 1 inch cubes. After 10 minutes add the parsnip and fresh ginger to the onions, stirring occasionally for another 10 minutes. Now add the coriander and all the other vegetables. Stir occasionally for 5 minutes.

Add the stock, stout and mustard, bring to the boil and simmer until the vegetables just start to soften. At this point turn off the heat, transfer to an ovenproof casserole dish, spread the mashed potato over the top of the mixture and put it in the oven. Bake at 400°F/Gas Mark 6 for 40–60 minutes. Serve with dark leafy greens.

Energetics

The casserole method is warming to the body. Tempeh deeply nourishes the Blood and is generally strengthening. The various root vegetables are all sweet and warm with Qi-nourishing actions. The stout is a good Blood tonic. The onion, ginger, coriander and mustard add warmth and movement. Altogether this is a warming recipe which deeply strengthens both Blood and Qi, its primary action, whilst also supporting both Yin and Yang.

Primary actions	Primary influences	Contra-indications
■ Qi ■ Blood	□ Lung	□ Qi def
■ Yin ■ Yang	□ Intestines	□ Blood def
□ Damp	■ Stomach	□ Yin def
□ Phlegm	■ Spleen	□ Yang def
□ Water	□ Heart	□ Damp
□ Qi stagnation	□ Bladder	□ Stagnation
□ Blood stagnation	■ Kidney	□ Heat
□ Heat	■ Gall bladder	□ Cold
■ Cold	□ Liver	□ Wind invasion
□ Wind heat		
□ Wind cold	**Temperature**	
□ Wind damp	□ Cooling	
□ Dryness	□ Neutral	
	■ Warming	

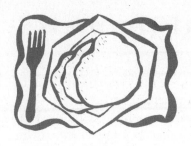

Sweet Potato Patties

Sweet potatoes are delicious just by themselves. They are a perfect ingredient for patties and are excellent with a sauce. Try the recipe for tarator on page 229.

Preparation time: 40 mins
Serves: 6

Ingredients

1 pound sweet potatoes

1 onion
1 egg
1 small knob butter
1 teaspoon dried ginger
2 tablespoons flour
¼ teaspoon cayenne
½ teaspoon nutmeg
Salt and pepper

2 cups coarse oatmeal or breadcrumbs
¼ cup oil

Method

Boil the sweet potato until tender then mash.

Chop the onion very finely, beat the egg and add these to the potatoes together with all the other ingredients and stir in as much oatmeal as is needed to make a stiff mixture and reserve the rest.

Heat the oil in a skillet, make a pile of oatmeal on your chopping board and roll golfball-size pieces of the mixture in the oatmeal to coat. Flatten into patties and fry until browned. Drain off any excess fat and serve warm.

Primary actions	Primary influences	Contra-indications
■ Qi □ Blood	□ Lung	□ Qi def
■ Yin □ Yang	□ Intestines	□ Blood def
□ Damp	□ Stomach	□ Yin def
□ Phlegm	■ Spleen	□ Yang def
□ Water	□ Heart	□ Damp
□ Qi stagnation	□ Bladder	□ Stagnation
□ Blood stagnation	■ Kidney	□ Heat
□ Heat	□ Gall bladder	□ Cold
□ Cold	□ Liver	□ Wind invasion
□ Wind heat	**Temperature**	
□ Wind cold	□ Cooling	
□ Wind damp	□ Neutral	
□ Dryness	■ Warming	

Energetics

Sweet potato nourishes the Yin and the Qi with a strengthening action on the Spleen and Kidney.

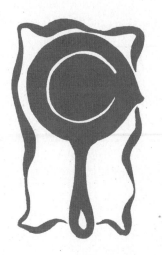

Tartafin

This is a traditional French recipe from Normandy. I have adapted it somewhat by the addition of fennel and thyme to balance the congesting nature of the cheese. Traditionally a strong creamy soft cheese is used but you can experiment with any cheese you like. Tartafin can be a meal by itself. It also goes well with any cooked greens, salad or fish.

Preparation time: 10 mins
Cooking time: 20 mins
Serves: 2

Ingredients

1 pound potatoes
1 small bulb fennel
3 cloves garlic
2 tablespoons olive oil
2 ounces butter
4 ounces cheese
1 teaspoon thyme

Method

Prepare the potatoes and fennel by slicing thinly in rounds. Slice the garlic and fry it gently in the butter and olive oil until you can really smell it. Use a sauté pan or a deep heavy skillet. Do not burn. Add the potatoes and fennel and lay them in the pan. Cover the dish and cook slowly until the potatoes soften. Add slices of cheese on top and sprinkle with thyme. Cook for a few more minutes until the cheese melts.

Energetics

Potatoes are strengthening both to the Qi and the Yin. In combination with the butter and cheese, which also strengthen the Yin, this dish becomes very moistening. Its moist nature is offset by the action of the garlic, fennel and thyme.

Primary actions	Primary influences	Contra-indications
■ Qi □ Blood	■ Lung	□ Qi def
■ Yin □ Yang	□ Intestines	□ Blood def
□ Damp	□ Stomach	□ Yin def
□ Phlegm	□ Spleen	□ Yang def
□ Water	□ Heart	■ Damp
□ Qi stagnation	□ Bladder	□ Stagnation
□ Blood stagnation	■ Kidney	□ Heat
□ Heat	□ Gall bladder	□ Cold
□ Cold	□ Liver	□ Wind invasion
□ Wind heat		
□ Wind cold	**Temperature**	
□ Wind damp	□ Cooling	
■ Dryness	■ Neutral	
	□ Warming	

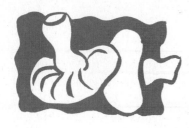

Tofu Mushroom Sauce on Quinoa

The quality of this sauce depends largely on the mushrooms so use open organically grown or wild ones. The blandness of the tofu soaks up the other tastes and creates a creamy consistency similar to a dairy sauce. The sauce can easily be used over any plain vegetables.

Preparation time: 10 mins
Cooking time: 20 mins
Serves: 4

Ingredients	Method
2 cups quinoa 1 teaspoon nori flakes Pinch of sea salt	The quinoa is simply boiled with a pinch of sea salt and a teaspoon of nori flakes. This will take about 20 minutes.
1 onion ½ pound mushrooms ½ tablespoon olive oil ½ tablespoon toasted sesame oil	Chop the onions and mushrooms finely. Sauté the onions for a few minutes in a pan. When they soften add the chopped mushrooms and cook until the mushrooms soften and release their juice.
Half pound tofu 1 cup vegetable stock 1 tablespoon mild miso	Meanwhile blend the tofu, miso and vegetable stock until it turns into a creamy sauce, using as much stock as is needed. Add the tofu cream to the sautéd vegetables and warm thoroughly without boiling (boiling may curdle it).
4 heads broccoli	While the sauce is cooking, steam the broccoli. Serve the broccoli on a bed of quinoa and cover with the sauce.

Primary actions	Primary influences	Contra-indications
■ Qi ■ Blood	☐ Lung	☐ Qi def
■ Yin ☐ Yang	■ Intestines	☐ Blood def
☐ Damp	■ Stomach	☐ Yin def
☐ Phlegm	■ Spleen	☐ Yang def
☐ Water	☐ Heart	☐ Damp
☐ Qi stagnation	☐ Bladder	☐ Stagnation
☐ Blood stagnation	☐ Kidney	☐ Heat
	☐ Gall bladder	☐ Cold
■ Heat	■ Liver	☐ Wind invasion
☐ Cold		
☐ Wind heat	**Temperature**	
☐ Wind cold	■ Cooling	
☐ Wind damp	☐ Neutral	
☐ Dryness	☐ Warming	

Energetics

The combination of tofu, broccoli and quinoa strengthens the Qi and Blood. The mushrooms bring the property of removing Heat and toxins. The overall cooling nature of this meal is slightly offset by the onion.

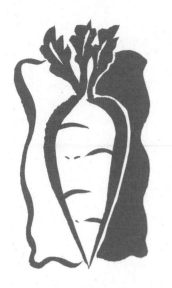

Turkish-style Carrots

This is a simple way with carrots that complements most meals. The sweetness of the carrots is nicely contrasted with the liveliness of the mint and complemented by the rich smoothness of the olive oil and yoghurt. Other root vegetables will also happily swim about in this sauce.

Preparation time: 10 mins
Cooking time: 15 mins
Serves: 4

Ingredients

1 pound carrots
2 tablespoons olive oil
2 tablespoons goat yoghurt
1 clove garlic
Handful chopped mint
Black pepper

Method

Chop the carrots into thick slices and cook very slowly in the oil removing from the heat just before they are completely soft. Turn off the heat and add the yoghurt, crushed garlic and chopped mint. Sprinkle with freshly ground black pepper and serve warm.

Primary actions	Primary influences	Contra-indications
■ Qi ■ Blood	■ Lung	□ Qi def
■ Yin □ Yang	□ Intestines	□ Blood def
□ Damp	□ Stomach	□ Yin def
□ Phlegm	■ Spleen	□ Yang def
□ Water	□ Heart	□ Damp
■ Qi stagnation	□ Bladder	□ Stagnation
□ Blood stagnation	□ Kidney	□ Heat
□ Heat	□ Gall bladder	□ Cold
□ Cold	■ Liver	□ Wind invasion
□ Wind heat	**Temperature**	
□ Wind cold	■ Cooling	
□ Wind damp	□ Neutral	
□ Dryness	□ Warming	

Energetics

Carrots are sweet and nourishing to the Liver, Lung and Spleen. They gently nourish and cleanse the Blood, and nourish both Qi and Yin. The yoghurt adds additional Yin nourishing properties and benefits the Intestines. The mint adds movement and benefits Stagnation.

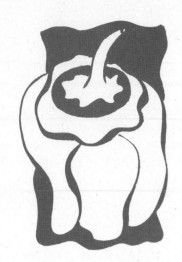

Anchovy Peppers

Anchovies and garlic are delightfully awakening to the taste buds. Sitting inside a red pepper that has slowly and sweetly melted in the oven, they are irresistible.

Preparation time: 10 mins
Cooking time: 45 mins
Serves: 4

Ingredients

3 red peppers
4 tomatoes
6 anchovies
6 cloves garlic
1 teaspoon dried thyme
9 tablespoons olive oil
Black pepper

Method

Slice the peppers lengthways keeping the stalks on but scooping out the seeds and core. Cut the tomatoes into rough chunks and fill each halved pepper. Sprinkle with thyme and lay an anchovy across the top. Thinly slice the cloves of garlic and sprinkle these over the tops. Add a little freshly ground black pepper. Pour 1 $\frac{1}{2}$ tablespoons of olive oil into each halved pepper and bake at 400°F/Gas Mark 6 for 45 minutes or until they are very soft and the peppers are slightly scorched.

Primary actions	Primary influences	Contra-indications
☐ Qi ☐ Blood	■ Lung	☐ Qi def
☐ Yin ■ Yang	☐ Intestines	☐ Blood def
■ Damp	■ Stomach	■ Yin def
☐ Phlegm	☐ Spleen	☐ Yang def
■ Water	☐ Heart	☐ Damp
■ Qi stagnation	☐ Bladder	☐ Stagnation
■ Blood stagnation	☐ Kidney	■ Heat
☐ Heat	☐ Gall bladder	☐ Cold
■ Cold	■ Liver	☐ Wind invasion
☐ Wind heat		
☐ Wind cold	**Temperature**	
☐ Wind damp	☐ Cooling	
☐ Dryness	☐ Neutral	
	■ Warming	

Energetics

This is a warming dish which increases circulation and helps resolve Dampness and Cold. The warming cooking method and the warming and Damp-resolving action of the peppers, anchovies and garlic is balanced by the more cooling action of the tomatoes.

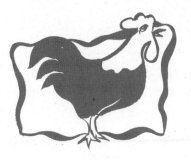

Chicken Marocain

Although it is several years since our French Moroccan friend Catherine cooked this for us, I can still remember it. If I think about it for long enough, I start to salivate. May it make your juices flow too.

Preparation time: 20 mins
Cooking time: 60 mins
Serves: 4–6

Ingredients

2 onions
Handful fresh coriander leaf
½ teaspoon cumin
½ teaspoon paprika
½ teaspoon cinnamon
6 strands saffron

8 pieces skinned chicken (legs or wings)
A little flour
1 tablespoon olive oil
1 tablespoon butter
1 ½ cups chopped tomatoes
1 cup prunes, soaked
Salt and pepper

Method

Roughly chop the onion and fry it in a little olive oil until soft. Add the herbs and spices and fry gently for another minute or two. Put the mixture to one side in a dish.

Dip the chicken pieces in flour and fry in the butter and olive oil mixture on a high flame until browned. This takes about 3 minutes. A wide, deep heavy-bottomed skillet is best. Add the tomatoes and prunes and the onion mixture. Cover the pan and cook slowly for about an hour. Serve with couscous or potatoes and fresh vegetables.

Primary actions	Primary influences	Contra-indications
■ Qi ■ Blood	□ Lung	□ Qi def
■ Yin □ Yang	□ Intestines	□ Blood def
□ Damp	■ Stomach	□ Yin def
□ Phlegm	■ Spleen	□ Yang def
□ Water	□ Heart	■ Damp
□ Qi stagnation	□ Bladder	□ Stagnation
□ Blood stagnation	□ Kidney	□ Heat
■ Heat	□ Gall bladder	□ Cold
□ Cold	■ Liver	□ Wind invasion
□ Wind heat		
□ Wind cold	**Temperature**	
□ Wind damp	□ Cooling	
□ Dryness	□ Neutral	
	■ Warming	

Energetics

Chicken is one of the most effective Qi tonics. It is a mildly warming meat and this property is supported by the herbs and spices. The use of tomatoes and prunes brings a strong moistening and cooling quality, especially useful against Liver Heat. The sweet and sour nature of this recipe means that it will also generate fluids and support the Yin.

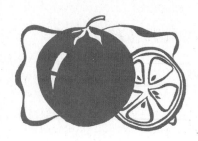

Coconut Lamb

This is a north African way of cooking lamb, very sweet and exotic. You will need only a little to feel very satisfied.

Preparation time: 15 mins
Cooking time: 40 mins
Serves: 4

Ingredients

2 onions
A little olive oil
1 tablespoon fresh coriander
1 teaspoon cumin
Pinch saffron
Salt and pepper
3 carrots
2 tomatoes
1 pound diced lamb
1 cup coconut milk

Method

Roughly chop the onions and fry them in olive oil until soft. Add the herbs and spices and fry gently for another minute or so. Add the carrots, finely sliced, then the tomatoes, then the lamb. Keep turning the mixture for a few minutes. Add the coconut milk, cover the pan and cook slowly for 30-40 minutes. Serve with fresh vegetables.

Primary actions	Primary influences	Contra-indications
■ Qi ■ Blood	☐ Lung	☐ Qi def
■ Yin ■ Yang	☐ Intestines	☐ Blood def
☐ Damp	☐ Stomach	☐ Yin def
☐ Phlegm	■ Spleen	☐ Yang def
☐ Water	■ Heart	■ Damp
☐ Qi stagnation	☐ Bladder	☐ Stagnation
☐ Blood stagnation	■ Kidney	☐ Heat
☐ Heat	☐ Gall bladder	☐ Cold
■ Cold	☐ Liver	☐ Wind invasion
☐ Wind heat	**Temperature**	
☐ Wind cold	☐ Cooling	
☐ Wind damp	☐ Neutral	
☐ Dryness	■ Warming	

Energetics

Lamb is a very warm meat that particularly strengthens the Kidney and Spleen. Coconut warms and strengthens the Heart as well as supplementing the Yin. With the support of the moving and warming action of the herbs and spices, and the counterbalance provided by the tomatoes, this recipe strengthens the Yang of the Heart, Spleen and Kidney; it nourishes Qi and Blood; and it offers support to the Yin.

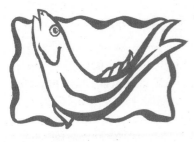

Dill Salmon Bake

I've only cooked this recipe once. It happened spontaneously one evening when I was feeling creative and
wondering how to honour the piece of salmon I had.
Fortunately I was wise enough to write down what I did.
It was unbearably delicious.

Preparation time: 30 mins
Cooking time: 30 mins
Serves: 4

Ingredients

3 pounds potatoes

2 large onions

1 pound salmon
2 glasses white wine
4 teaspoons dill weed
2 ounces butter
Salt
Pepper

Method

Boil the potatoes until about three-quarters cooked.

Meanwhile slice the onions in rings and cook gently in a
little butter for 10 minutes or until they just start to
soften.

Cut the salmon into 1 inch chunks. Put all the ingredients
into a greased ovenproof dish in layers: onions, then
potato, then salmon, then onions and potato again.
Sprinkle with the dill and salt as you build up the layers.
Pour in the white wine and set a few knobs of butter on
top. Sprinkle with freshly ground black pepper, cover and
bake for 25–30 minutes at 400°F/Gas Mark 6.

Primary actions	Primary influences	Contra-indications
■ Qi ■ Blood	■ Lung	□ Qi def
■ Yin ■ Yang	□ Intestines	□ Blood def
□ Damp	■ Stomach	□ Yin def
□ Phlegm	■ Spleen	□ Yang def
□ Water	□ Heart	□ Damp
□ Qi stagnation	□ Bladder	□ Stagnation
□ Blood stagnation	■ Kidney	□ Heat
□ Heat	□ Gall bladder	□ Cold
□ Cold	□ Liver	□ Wind invasion
□ Wind heat		
□ Wind cold	**Temperature**	
□ Wind damp	□ Cooling	
□ Dryness	□ Neutral	
	■ Warming	

Energetics

This is a gently warming dish that will suit all constitutional types. The salmon nourishes the Yin and Blood
whilst also mildly warming the Yang, with assistance
from the wine. The potatoes strengthen the Qi and the
onions warm the body and counteract Phlegm,
Dampness and Stagnation. The dill benefits the digestion.

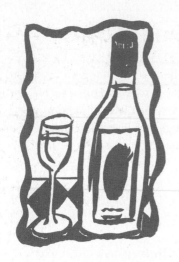

Klefti Lamb

This method of cooking lamb, so the story goes, is modelled on the ways of Greek mountain bandits who developed a technique of tightly sealing their ovens to keep the flavour in and save fuel. If you want to be authentic, use retsina, but any dry white wine will do.

Preparation time: 10 mins
Cooking time: 2 hours
Serves: 2–4

Ingredients

2 large or 4 small lamb chops
Juice of 1 lemon
³/₄ teaspoon salt
2 tablespoons fresh oregano
1 tablespoon fresh rosemary
2 bayleaves
1 glass dry white wine
Black pepper
1 onion
Flour

Method

Preheat the oven to 300°F/Gas Mark 2. Choose an oven-proof dish (earthenware is best) with a tightly fitting lid. Put the lamb in the dish and cover with lemon juice. Sprinkle with the salt, oregano and rosemary and turn so that both sides of the meat are covered. Slice the onion in rings and throw these in. Add the bayleaves, wine and a few twists of freshly ground black pepper. If you like to be authentic, make a dough of flour and water, roll it into a thin 'sausage', moisten the rim of the pot and press the dough onto its rim to create a tight seal. Press the lid on firmly, patch any holes and place it in the oven. Cook for 2 hours or more. When it is done, make a gravy from the juice and serve with plenty of fresh vegetables.

Energetics

Lamb is a hot meat which supports the Yang, especially of the Spleen and Kidney. With the exception of the lemon, all the other ingredients reinforce this warming action.

Primary actions	Primary influences	Contra-indications
■ Qi ■ Blood	□ Lung	□ Qi def
□ Yin ■ Yang	□ Intestines	□ Blood def
□ Damp	■ Stomach	□ Yin def
□ Phlegm	■ Spleen	□ Yang def
□ Water	■ Heart	□ Damp
□ Qi stagnation	□ Bladder	□ Stagnation
□ Blood stagnation	■ Kidney	■ Heat
□ Heat	□ Gall bladder	□ Cold
■ Cold	□ Liver	□ Wind invasion
□ Wind heat		
□ Wind cold	**Temperature**	
□ Wind damp	□ Cooling	
□ Dryness	□ Neutral	
	■ Warming	

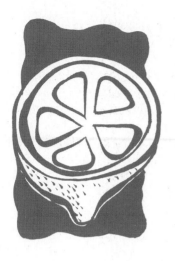

Lemon Chicken Tagine

The tagine is a simple one pot method, popular in northern Africa. Taking only a few minutes to prepare, it enables you to go off and do something else while it sits in the oven. When you come back, a mouth-watering meal awaits you.

Preparation time: 10 mins
Cooking time: 90 mins
Serves: 4–8

Ingredients

4 onions
2 lemons
½ teaspoon cumin
1 teaspoon five spice
A few small pieces cinnamon bark
Pinch saffron
Handful fresh parsley, chopped
Handful fresh coriander, chopped
8 pieces chicken (wings or legs)
Handful green olives

Method

Slice the onions in rings and the lemons into eighths. Lay half of them in an ovenproof dish and sit 4 of the chicken pieces on top. Sprinkle with half the herbs and spices. Repeat the process to make a two-layered dish. Cover the dish and cook in the oven for 1½ hours at 375/Gas Mark 5. Towards the end scatter the olives on top.

Primary actions	Primary influences	Contra-indications
■ Qi ■ Blood	■ Lung	☐ Qi def
☐ Yin ■ Yang	☐ Intestines	☐ Blood def
☐ Damp	■ Stomach	☐ Yin def
☐ Phlegm	■ Spleen	☐ Yang def
☐ Water	☐ Heart	☐ Damp
■ Qi stagnation	☐ Bladder	☐ Stagnation
■ Blood stagnation	☐ Kidney	☐ Heat
☐ Heat	☐ Gall bladder	☐ Cold
■ Cold	☐ Liver	☐ Wind invasion
☐ Wind heat		
☐ Wind cold	**Temperature**	
☐ Wind damp	☐ Cooling	
☐ Dryness	☐ Neutral	
	■ Warming	

Energetics

Chicken warms the body and strengthens the Qi and Blood. The herbs and spices add warmth and movement, as does the onion. The lemon provides a counterbalance and helps the absorption of nutrients from the chicken.

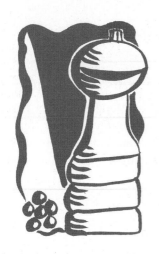

Mackerel Baked in Tea

This is a traditional Cornish method of cooking mackerel to preserve a large catch for several days. It will happily keep for three or four days and actually improves in flavour the day after cooking.

Preparation time: 20 mins
Cooking time: 40 mins
Serves: 2

Ingredients

2 mackerel
2 bayleaves
4 slices lemon
1 teaspoon demerara sugar
½ teaspoon black peppercorns
¼ teaspoon mustard seeds
¼ pint cider vinegar
¼ pint cold tea
Parsley to garnish

Method

Preheat the oven to 350°F/Gas Mark 4. Gut and clean the fish. Lay them in an ovenproof dish and place a bayleaf and two thin slices of lemon inside each one. Sprinkle the sugar, mustard seed and peppercorns over the top then pour on the tea and vinegar. Cover with a lid and bake for about 40 minutes. When cooked, strain out the juice and remove the lemon and bayleaves. Put the fish on a serving plate and garnish with parsley. This dish is eaten cool.

Primary actions	Primary influences	Contra-indications
■ Qi ■ Blood	☐ Lung	☐ Qi def
☐ Yin ☐ Yang	☐ Intestines	☐ Blood def
■ Damp	■ Stomach	☐ Yin def
■ Phlegm	☐ Spleen	☐ Yang def
■ Water	☐ Heart	☐ Damp
☐ Qi stagnation	☐ Bladder	☐ Stagnation
☐ Blood stagnation	☐ Kidney	☐ Heat
	☐ Gall bladder	☐ Cold
☐ Heat	■ Liver	☐ Wind invasion
☐ Cold		
☐ Wind heat	**Temperature**	
☐ Wind cold	☐ Cooling	
☐ Wind damp	■ Neutral	
☐ Dryness	☐ Warming	

Energetics

Mackerel is a sweet fish that strengthens the Qi. It especially strengthens the Stomach and Liver and is effective at drawing Dampness and Water out of the body. The tea has some action against Phlegm in the Lung; the peppercorns are drying and add warmth; the vinegar adds warmth and movement and reinforces the action on the Liver.

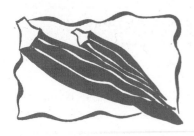

Run Down

Run Down is a Jamaican dish usually served with boiled green bananas and plain dumplings. Any oily fish will do but the lime and the coconut milk give it that authentic Caribbean flavour.

Preparation time: 10 mins
Cooking time: 20 mins
Serves: 6

Ingredients	Method
2 pounds filleted mackerel 3 tablespoons lime juice	Pour the lime juice over the fish and leave to marinate for a while.
3 cups coconut milk 1 large onion 2 cloves garlic 1 jalapeno pepper 1 pound tomatoes 1 teaspoon thyme 1 tablespoon vinegar Salt Pepper	Simmer the coconut milk until it starts to look oily then add all the other finely chopped ingredients. Simmer for a minute or two then pour the mixture over the fish in a large pan, put the lid on and cook for about 10 minutes or until the fish is ready. This dish can also be cooked in the oven or over a barbecue.

Primary actions	Primary influences	Contra-indications
■ Qi ■ Blood	□ Lung	□ Qi def
■ Yin □ Yang	□ Intestines	□ Blood def
□ Damp	■ Stomach	□ Yin def
□ Phlegm	□ Spleen	□ Yang def
□ Water	■ Heart	□ Damp
□ Qi stagnation	□ Bladder	□ Stagnation
□ Blood stagnation	□ Kidney	□ Heat
□ Heat	□ Gall bladder	□ Cold
□ Cold	■ Liver	□ Wind invasion
□ Wind heat		
□ Wind cold	**Temperature**	
□ Wind damp	□ Cooling	
□ Dryness	■ Neutral	
	□ Warming	

Energetics

Mackerel nourishes the Qi and has some influence against Dampness. The coconut is rather more moistening and nourishing to the Yin as well as having an uplifting effect on the Heart. They balance each other well. Lime (or lemon) is useful with all fatty and oily foods, helping to counter Dampness and Stagnation, forming a useful complement to the fish. Most of the other ingredients bring warmth and movement to help the digestion. Overall the soup can be seen as a Yin, Blood and Qi tonic.

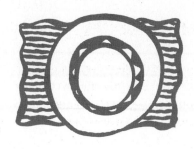

Stir-fried Shrimp on Lettuce

This is a popular Chinese recipe. The crisp lettuce make excellent containers for the strong tasting shrimp and they look very attractive arranged on the plate.

Preparation time: 20 mins
Serves: 4

Ingredients

1 cos/romaine lettuce	
³/₄ pounds shrimp	
1 egg white	
1 tablespoon cornflour	
¹/₄ teaspoon salt	
2 teaspoons fresh ginger	
2 spring onions	
2 tablespoons vegetable oil	
1 teaspoon sesame oil	

Method

Wash and prepare the lettuce, breaking off the whole leaves and putting them to one side.

Clean and chop the shrimp into small pieces, beat the egg white and mix both ingredients together with the cornflour and salt.

Chop the spring onions and ginger finely. Heat the vegetable oil in a large frying pan or wok and throw in the shrimp mixture. Stir for a minute or two then add the ginger and spring onion. Keep stirring and cook for a further two minutes. Add a small splash of water, stir and add the sesame oil before removing from the heat. Heap a portion of the cooked mixture into each lettuce leaf and serve.

Primary actions	Primary influences	Contra-indications
☐ Qi ☐ Blood	■ Lung	☐ Qi def
☐ Yin ■ Yang	☐ Intestines	☐ Blood def
■ Damp	☐ Stomach	☐ Yin def
■ Phlegm	☐ Spleen	☐ Yang def
■ Water	☐ Heart	☐ Damp
☐ Qi stagnation	☐ Bladder	☐ Stagnation
■ Blood stagnation	■ Kidney	■ Heat
☐ Heat	☐ Gall bladder	☐ Cold
■ Cold	■ Liver	☐ Wind invasion
☐ Wind heat	**Temperature**	
☐ Wind cold	☐ Cooling	
☐ Wind damp	☐ Neutral	
☐ Dryness	■ Warming	

Energetics

Shrimp invigorates the Kidney Yang. It is supported in this by the onion and ginger which are both warming. The cool and bitter lettuce provides a counterbalance as well as lessening the chance of reactiveness to the shrimp. Shrimp and lettuce together are reputed to clear skin problems.

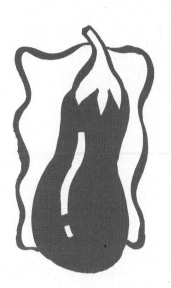

Baba Ghanoush

'Baba Ghanoush' means something like 'daddy spoils you' in Arabic. This is a popular dish in arabic countries where aubergines grow for most of the year. It is a fantastic dip for pieces of raw vegetable or chunks of bread. However you serve it, a dish of olives alongside it is compulsory.

Preparation time: 10 mins
Cooking time: 20 mins
Serves: 4–6

Ingredients

3 aubergines

1 cup light tahini
4 cloves garlic
Juice of 3 lemons
4 tablespoons water
Salt and black pepper to taste
2 tablespoons olive oil
¼ teaspoon paprika
Coriander or parsley to garnish

Method

Cook the aubergines under the grill or in a hot oven and keep turning them until the skin is charred. This takes about 20 minutes. Cut them open, scoop out the insides and mash well.

Combine the tahini, garlic, water and lemon and stir into the pulped aubergine. Add salt and freshly ground black pepper to taste. Serve in a wide dish, pouring the olive oil over the top, sprinkling with paprika and garnishing with chopped parsley or coriander.

Primary actions	Primary influences	Contra-indications
☐ Qi ▨ Blood	☐ Lung	☐ Qi def
▨ Yin ☐ Yang	▨ Intestines	☐ Blood def
☐ Damp	☐ Stomach	☐ Yin def
☐ Phlegm	☐ Spleen	☐ Yang def
☐ Water	☐ Heart	☐ Damp
☐ Qi stagnation	☐ Bladder	☐ Stagnation
▨ Blood stagnation	▨ Kidney	☐ Heat
	☐ Gall bladder	☐ Cold
☐ Heat	▨ Liver	☐ Wind invasion
☐ Cold		
☐ Wind heat	**Temperature**	
☐ Wind cold	☐ Cooling	
☐ Wind damp	▨ Neutral	
☐ Dryness	☐ Warming	

Energetics

Aubergine has the ability to move Stagnant Blood, especially from the Uterus. It also nourishes the Blood. Together with the tahini, which is a rich tonic for the Yin, this makes a deeply nourishing dish for both Blood and Yin. The dampening nature of the tahini is balanced by the lemon and garlic.

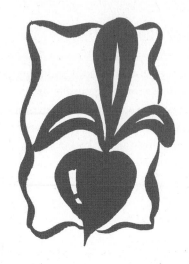

Beetroot and Horseradish Relish

If you have ever had the experience of grating a fresh piece of horseradish you will know its energetics. The horseradish fills the sinus with searing heat, makes the eyes water and wakes up every inch of the lungs' membranes. So, as you might expect, this is a lively relish. The horseradish combines perfectly with the sweetness of the beetroot.

Preparation time: 40 mins
Serves: 4–8

Ingredients

4 beetroot
1 onion
1 teaspoon fresh parsley
4 tablespoons horseradish
¼ cup cider vinegar
1 teaspoon mild honey
Salt

Method

Boil the beetroot and chop or grate very finely. Chop the onion and parsley finely and grate the horseradish or use ready-prepared horseradish from a jar (in which case use a little less cider vinegar). Combine all the ingredients and let them sit for a while, the longer the better, before serving. The relish will keep for a few weeks in a sealed container in the fridge. This recipe will make 2-3 cups.

Primary actions	Primary influences	Contra-indications
☐ Qi ■ Blood	■ Lung	☐ Qi def
☐ Yin ■ Yang	☐ Intestines	☐ Blood def
■ Damp	■ Stomach	■ Yin def
■ Phlegm	☐ Spleen	☐ Yang def
☐ Water	■ Heart	☐ Damp
☐ Qi stagnation	☐ Bladder	☐ Stagnation
■ Blood stagnation	☐ Kidney	■ Heat
☐ Heat	☐ Gall bladder	☐ Cold
■ Cold	■ Liver	☐ Wind invasion
☐ Wind heat		
☐ Wind cold	**Temperature**	
☐ Wind damp	☐ Cooling	
☐ Dryness	☐ Neutral	
	■ Warming	

Energetics

Horseradish is a strong, pungent Yang tonic and Stagnation mover with a special influence on the Lung. Beetroot nourishes the Blood and benefits the Heart and Liver. The onion and cider vinegar are both warming Stagnation movers. So here we have a warming relish which will move the Qi and Blood, break through Stagnation, support the Yang and nourish the Blood.

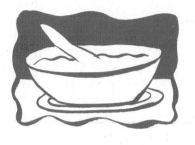

Broad Bean Purée

Dried broad beans are very popular in the Middle East and are known as 'foul' which is an unfortunate translation. Far from being foul tasting these aromatic beans are exciting and mouth-watering. The purée can also be made with fresh broad beans if you want a greener colour and a slightly lighter taste.

Preparation time: 10 mins
Cooking time: 50 mins
Serves: 4–6

Ingredients

¼ pounds dried broad beans
6 bayleaves
Juice and rind of 1 lemon
1 pint water

2 cloves garlic
1 teaspoon aniseed
Handful mint and parsley
1-2 tablespoons olive oil
1 teaspoon nori flakes
Salt and pepper

Method

Presoak the beans, throw away the soaking water and cook until mushy with the bayleaves and lemon rind in a pint of water. When cooked discard the bayleaves and set the mixture aside to cool a little. Mash them if they have not thoroughly disintegrated and soaked up the cooking water.

Crush the aniseed and garlic, chop the herbs finely and add them together with the lemon juice, olive oil, nori flakes, salt and pepper. Serve with bread or crackers.

Primary actions	Primary influences	Contra-indications
☐ Qi ■ Blood	☐ Lung	☐ Qi def
☐ Yin ☐ Yang	☐ Intestines	☐ Blood def
■ Damp	☐ Stomach	☐ Yin def
☐ Phlegm	■ Spleen	☐ Yang def
■ Water	☐ Heart	☐ Damp
☐ Qi stagnation	☐ Bladder	☐ Stagnation
☐ Blood stagnation	■ Kidney	☐ Heat
☐ Heat	☐ Gall bladder	☐ Cold
☐ Cold	☐ Liver	☐ Wind invasion
☐ Wind heat	**Temperature**	
☐ Wind cold	☐ Cooling	
☐ Wind damp	■ Neutral	
☐ Dryness	☐ Warming	

Energetics

The sweet and aromatic broad bean stimulates the action of the Spleen and calms the Stomach. It is effective against Dampness especially when Dampness is combined with Heat. The other ingredients all complement these actions.

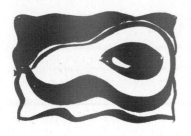

Guacamole

This is a classic Mexican recipe. The avocado acts as a smooth carrier for the sharp and hot flavours of the salsa and the tanginess of the lime. Guacamole can be served in nachos or tortillas; it is equally happy as a dip for crudites, as a side salad or livening up a salad sandwich.

Preparation time: 10 mins
Serves: 4

Ingredients

1 tomato
1 small onion
1 clove garlic
2 ripe avocados
3 tablespoons salsa
Juice of ½ fresh lime
Salt
Pepper
Olive oil

Method

Chop the tomato and onion very small and crush the garlic. Mash the avocado and combine all the ingredients. Leave for a while for the ingredients to blend, covering with a cloth or with a layer of olive oil.

Energetics

Avocados have a cool nature and sweet flavour with a special affinity for the Liver, Lungs and Intestines. They build the Blood and Yin. They are particularly useful as a fat source when the Liver is reactive to other fats. Tomatoes nourish the fluids and a little balancing movement and warmth is brought to this otherwise cool dish by the onion, garlic and salsa spices. The lime assists the Gall Bladder in the breakdown of fat. Overall this dish can be said to nourish the Blood and the Yin although in more severe cases of Yin Deficiency the salsa needs to be very mild.

Primary actions	Primary influences	Contra-indications
☐ Qi ■ Blood	■ Lung	☐ Qi def
■ Yin ☐ Yang	■ Intestines	☐ Blood def
☐ Damp	☐ Stomach	☐ Yin def
☐ Phlegm	☐ Spleen	☐ Yang def
☐ Water	☐ Heart	☐ Damp
☐ Qi stagnation	☐ Bladder	☐ Stagnation
☐ Blood stagnation	☐ Kidney	☐ Heat
☐ Heat	■ Gall bladder	☐ Cold
☐ Cold	■ Liver	☐ Wind invasion
☐ Wind heat	**Temperature**	
☐ Wind cold	☐ Cooling	
☐ Wind damp	■ Neutral	
☐ Dryness	☐ Warming	

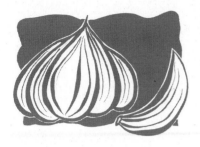

Hummus

This middle eastern classic needs little introduction.

Preparation time: 10 mins
Cooking time: 60 mins
Serves: 4–6

Ingredients

2 cups chickpeas

1–2 lemons
2 cloves garlic, crushed
1 tablespoon tahini
3 tablespoons olive oil
½ teaspoon ground cumin
½ teaspoon salt
Paprika and fresh parsley
to garnish

Method

Soak the chickpeas overnight. Discard the soaking water and cook in enough water to cover the chickpeas by an inch. When the chickpeas are soft, strain and keep the water. Purée the chickpeas adding back as much water as is needed to achieve a creamy but not too runny consistency. Leave the mixture a little rough.

Add the crushed garlic, lemon juice, 1 tablespoon of the olive oil, salt, cumin and tahini. Stir in and add extra lemon and garlic to taste. Turn out the hummus into a serving dish, cover with the remaining olive oil, sprinkle with paprika and garnish with fresh parsley.

Primary actions	Primary influences	Contra-indications
■ Qi ■ Blood	☐ Lung	☐ Qi def
☐ Yin ☐ Yang	☐ Intestines	☐ Blood def
■ Damp	■ Stomach	☐ Yin def
☐ Phlegm	■ Spleen	☐ Yang def
☐ Water	■ Heart	☐ Damp
☐ Qi stagnation	☐ Bladder	☐ Stagnation
☐ Blood stagnation	☐ Kidney	☐ Heat
☐ Heat	☐ Gall bladder	☐ Cold
☐ Cold	☐ Liver	☐ Wind invasion
☐ Wind heat		
☐ Wind cold	**Temperature**	
☐ Wind damp	☐ Cooling	
☐ Dryness	■ Neutral	
	☐ Warming	

Energetics

Chickpeas nourish the Stomach and Heart and are useful against Dampness. In serious conditions of Dampness the tahini can be omitted or reduced. Hummus is easily digested and strengthening to the body.

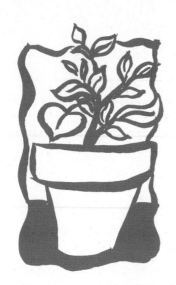

Mediterranean Basil Dip

It is surprising how sweet some foods become when roasted. The garlic and peppers in particular release tremendous sweetness into this dip and the basil, as always, is a delight. It is a magnificent topping on baked potatoes and a good dip for crackers or slipped inside a leaf of crisp cos lettuce.

Preparation time: 15 mins
Cooking time: 25 mins
Serves: 4–8

Ingredients

2 aubergines
2 red peppers
2 green peppers
1 bulb garlic

2 tablespoons olive oil
2 tablespoon red wine vinegar
4 spring onions
1 cup fresh basil
½ teaspoon salt
Black pepper
Paprika

Method

Make a few small slits in the aubergines and place with the peppers on a greased baking tray. Nick the top off the garlic bulb and set it inside a small ovenproof covered pot. Bake the aubergine and peppers at 450°F for 20-30 minutes and set the garlic on the bottom shelf of the oven. Turn the peppers occasionally. Remove when the peppers are blackened.

Let the aubergine and garlic cool and stand the peppers in a paper bag for a few minutes to sweat. Then remove the skin from the peppers, scoop out the flesh of the aubergine and squeeze the pulp out from the garlic skins. Chop the basil and spring onions then combine all the ingredients together. Check for taste when smooth, sprinkle with paprika and decorate with a few basil leaves. Serve at room temperature.

Energetics

Roasting is a very warming method and applying this to such warm foods as garlic and peppers makes this a warming, Yang-strengthening recipe. Many of the ingredients – the aubergine, peppers, garlic, basil, vinegar, black pepper – also have moving properties that makes this a good Stagnation mover for both Qi and Blood. The aubergine is particularly effective at moving Stagnant Blood in the Uterus.

Primary actions	Primary influences	Contra-indications
☐ Qi ☐ Blood	■ Lung	☐ Qi def
☐ Yin ■ Yang	☐ Intestines	☐ Blood def
■ Damp	■ Stomach	☐ Yin def
■ Phlegm	■ Spleen	☐ Yang def
☐ Water	■ Heart	☐ Damp
■ Qi stagnation	☐ Bladder	☐ Stagnation
■ Blood stagnation	☐ Kidney	■ Heat
☐ Heat	☐ Gall bladder	☐ Cold
■ Cold	■ Liver	☐ Wind invasion
☐ Wind heat	**Temperature**	
☐ Wind cold	☐ Cooling	
☐ Wind damp	☐ Neutral	
☐ Dryness	■ Warming	

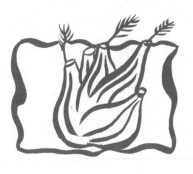

Mixed Vegetable Caponata

Caponata tastes something like a very condensed ratatouille. It is a good way of using seasonal vegetables and you can substitute ingredients freely with this recipe. Serve in small quantities as an accompaniment to fish or vegetable dishes.

Preparation time: 20 mins
Cooking time: 60 mins

Ingredients

2 onions
1 aubergine
1 red pepper
1 green pepper
2 stalks celery
1 bulb fennel
4 ounces string beans
$\frac{1}{2}$ pound mushrooms
2 hot green peppers
1 pound tomatoes
6 cloves garlic
$\frac{1}{2}$ cup olive oil
$\frac{1}{2}$ cup balsamic vinegar
1 cup pitted black olives
2 tablespoons capers
$\frac{1}{2}$ cup fresh basil
$\frac{1}{2}$ cup fresh sorrel
1 teaspoon salt
$\frac{1}{2}$ teaspoon fresh black pepper

Method

Chop all the vegetables very small and put them in a large heavy pot with the olive oil, garlic and vinegar. Do not cover the pot. Cook slowly, stirring occasionally, until most of the fluid has evaporated (about an hour or so). Add the olives, capers, sorrel, basil, salt and pepper. Stir well and cook for another 2-3 minutes. Taste and adjust the seasoning. Serve warm with bread, crackers or as an accompaniment to the main meal. Caponata will keep well in the fridge for a few days.

Energetics

Most of the ingredients in this relish generate movement. Caponata is a good mover of Stagnation and a counter to Dampness. As with all vinegar-based relishes, Caponata stimulates the Liver and benefits the digestion.

Primary actions	Primary influences	Contra-indications
☐ Qi ☐ Blood	☐ Lung	☐ Qi def
☐ Yin ☐ Yang	☐ Intestines	☐ Blood def
■ Damp	☐ Stomach	☐ Yin def
☐ Phlegm	☐ Spleen	☐ Yang def
☐ Water	☐ Heart	☐ Damp
■ Qi stagnation	☐ Bladder	☐ Stagnation
■ Blood stagnation	☐ Kidney	■ Heat
☐ Heat	☐ Gall bladder	☐ Cold
■ Cold	■ Liver	☐ Wind invasion
☐ Wind heat	**Temperature**	
☐ Wind cold	☐ Cooling	
☐ Wind damp	☐ Neutral	
☐ Dryness	■ Warming	

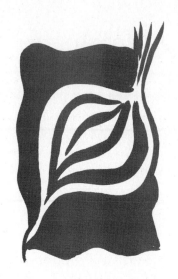

Onion and Mustard Sauce

This is a vibrantly warming sauce suitable for pouring over steamed vegetables or any simple grain.

Preparation time: 5 mins
Cooking time: 20 mins
Serves: 4

Ingredients	Method
2 onions 4 tablespoons olive oil	Chop the onions finely and sauté in the olive oil slowly until they soften and sweeten.
2 ½ tablespoons wheat or spelt flour 2 cups vegetable stock 1 ½ teaspoon tarragon 3 teaspoons mustard	Mix the flour with the stock, stirring in a little at a time until well dissolved. Add the mustard and tarragon then pour it in with the onions. Cook gently, stirring occasionally, until it thickens.

Primary actions	Primary influences	Contra-indications
☐ Qi ☐ Blood	■ Lung	☐ Qi def
☐ Yin ☐ Yang	☐ Intestines	☐ Blood def
■ Damp	☐ Stomach	☐ Yin def
■ Phlegm	☐ Spleen	☐ Yang def
☐ Water	☐ Heart	☐ Damp
■ Qi stagnation	☐ Bladder	☐ Stagnation
☐ Blood stagnation	☐ Kidney	☐ Heat
☐ Heat	☐ Gall bladder	☐ Cold
■ Cold	☐ Liver	☐ Wind invasion
☐ Wind heat	**Temperature**	
■ Wind cold	☐ Cooling	
■ Wind damp	☐ Neutral	
☐ Dryness	■ Warming	

Energetics

The mustard, tarragon and onions generate movement and warmth. This is an ideal sauce for supporting the digestive fire and for conditions of Cold, Damp and Stagnation.

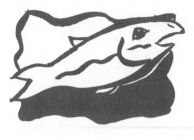

Pauper's Dip

This delicious recipe was given to me by Riverford Farm Shop, our local and magnificent suppliers of organic meat, fruit and vegetables. Apparently it is modelled on a recipe for 'poor man's caviar' – quite cheap to make but expensive tasting.

Preparation time: 10 mins
Cooking time: 20 mins
Serves: 10

Ingredients

2 pounds aubergines
1 pound smoked mackerel
½ pound curd cheese
½ pound yoghurt
4 tablespoons olive oil
2 cloves garlic
Juice of 2 lemons
3 ounces parsley
2 ounces salt
1 ounce black pepper

Method

Roast the aubergine for 20 minutes or so in a hot oven, until the flesh is soft. Scoop it out into a bowl. Crush the garlic, finely chop the parsley and add these to the bowl together with all the other ingredients. Mash the ingredients together with a fork. Serve on bread or crackers.

Primary actions	Primary influences	Contra-indications
■ Qi ■ Blood	■ Lung	□ Qi def
■ Yin □ Yang	□ Intestines	□ Blood def
□ Damp	■ Stomach	□ Yin def
□ Phlegm	■ Spleen	□ Yang def
□ Water	□ Heart	■ Damp
□ Qi stagnation	□ Bladder	□ Stagnation
□ Blood stagnation	□ Kidney	□ Heat
	□ Gall bladder	□ Cold
□ Heat	■ Liver	□ Wind invasion
□ Cold		
□ Wind heat	**Temperature**	
□ Wind cold	■ Cooling	
□ Wind damp	□ Neutral	
□ Dryness	□ Warming	

Energetics

This is a highly nutritious recipe, nourishing the Qi, Blood and Yin. The aubergines nourish and move the Blood; the mackerel strengthens the Qi and counters the dampening nature of the Yin-strengthening cheese and yoghurt; the parsley brings additional nourishment to the Blood.

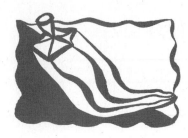

Roasted Pepper and Avocado Dip

This recipe blends together hot and cool tastes. It is a smooth, silky, beautifully coloured dip with a perky undertaste. The dip can be served as an accompaniment to many meals, used in salad dressing or in sandwiches or even as filling for a baked potato.

Preparation time: 10 mins
Cooking time: 30 mins
Serves: 4

Ingredients

1 red pepper
1 green pepper
1 red chilli pepper
¹/₂ avocado
3 cloves garlic
3 tablespoons fresh coriander leaf
Juice of ¹/₂ lime
¹/₄ cup olive oil
¹/₂ teaspoon salt
1 heaped tablespoon capers

Method

Roast the peppers in a hot oven (450°F/Gas Mark 8) removing them when almost burned (about 30 minutes). Let the peppers sweat for a while in a covered dish or paper bag and when they are cool remove their skins as best you can. Scrape out the seeds from both kinds of pepper. Now blend together all the ingredients except the capers which are turned in once the dip is made. This recipe will make about two cups.

Primary actions	Primary influences	Contra-indications
☐ Qi ■ Blood	☐ Lung	☐ Qi def
☐ Yin ☐ Yang	☐ Intestines	☐ Blood def
☐ Damp	■ Stomach	☐ Yin def
☐ Phlegm	☐ Spleen	☐ Yang def
☐ Water	☐ Heart	☐ Damp
■ Qi stagnation	☐ Bladder	☐ Stagnation
■ Blood stagnation	☐ Kidney	☐ Heat
☐ Heat	☐ Gall bladder	☐ Cold
☐ Cold	■ Liver	☐ Wind invasion
☐ Wind heat	**Temperature**	
☐ Wind cold	☐ Cooling	
☐ Wind damp	☐ Neutral	
☐ Dryness	■ Warming	

Energetics

Avocados are a cool tonic for the Blood and Yin with a moistening action on the Lungs and Intestines. They also pacify and smooth the action of the Liver. The peppers and garlic on the other hand stimulate circulation and Yang energy. They are supported in this by the gentler action of the coriander. Lime is very beneficial for the Liver and helps with the digestion of the rich avocado. The extreme action of the hottest ingredients is well balanced by the avocado's soothing and moistening action. This relish is especially helpful in cases of Liver Qi Stagnation.

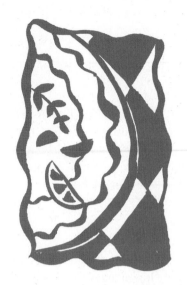

Tarator (Tahini Sauce)

This simple sauce is delicious over vegetables. It also works well over homemade vegetable burgers and rissoles. Try it with the sweet potato patties recipe on page 206.

Preparation time: 10 mins
Serves: 4

Ingredients

1 cup tahini
1 cup water
3–5 cloves garlic
¼ teaspoon cumin
½ teaspoon paprika
1 teaspoon sea salt
Juice of 4 lemons
1 cup chopped parsley

Method

Pour the tahini into a jug and slowly stir in the water using a fork. Crush the garlic and add this with the salt, cumin and paprika. Add the lemon, stirring until well blended, then add the chopped parsley.

Primary actions	Primary influences	Contra-indications
☐ Qi ■ Blood	☐ Lung	☐ Qi def
■ Yin ☐ Yang	☐ Intestines	☐ Blood def
☐ Damp	☐ Stomach	☐ Yin def
☐ Phlegm	☐ Spleen	☐ Yang def
☐ Water	☐ Heart	■ Damp
☐ Qi stagnation	☐ Bladder	☐ Stagnation
☐ Blood stagnation	■ Kidney	☐ Heat
☐ Heat	☐ Gall bladder	☐ Cold
☐ Cold	■ Liver	☐ Wind invasion
☐ Wind heat	**Temperature**	
☐ Wind cold	☐ Cooling	
☐ Wind damp	■ Neutral	
☐ Dryness	☐ Warming	

Energetics

Tahini is a rich source of nourishment, supplementing the Yin and benefiting the Kidney and Liver. Both the lemon and the garlic have a strong anti-mucus action which reduces the dampening effect of the tahini. From a western perspective, lemon increases the absorption of minerals from the tahini. The parsley brings additional nourishment to the Blood and has a strengthening effect on the Kidney.

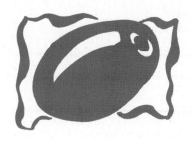

Vegetarian Tapenade

A tapenade is a dip or spread infused with garlic. This is a French recipe with a distinctly Mediterranean feel. This tapenade is strongly flavoured with olives, garlic and capers and given an interesting texture by the pinenuts. It is excellent on toast, ricecakes or oatcakes.

Preparation time: 10 mins
Serves: 4–6

Ingredients

2 tablespoons chives
1 ½ cups parsley
1 cup pinenuts
1 ½ cups pitted black olives
2 tablespoons capers
2 cloves garlic
1–2 tablespoons lemon juice
3 tablespoons olive oil
½ teaspoon thyme
Black pepper

Method

Crush the pinenuts and finely chop the parsley and chives. Combine all the other ingredients and mash or blend fairly coarsely. Then fold in the parsley, chives and pinenuts. It can be served immediately or allowed to infuse for a while. It will keep for a few days in the fridge. Anchovies (about 6-8) can replace the pinenuts for a more traditional recipe.

Primary actions	Primary influences	Contra-indications
☐ Qi ■ Blood	■ Lung	☐ Qi def
■ Yin ☐ Yang	■ Intestines	☐ Blood def
■ Damp	■ Stomach	☐ Yin def
■ Phlegm	☐ Spleen	☐ Yang def
☐ Water	☐ Heart	☐ Damp
■ Qi stagnation	☐ Bladder	☐ Stagnation
☐ Blood stagnation	■ Kidney	☐ Heat
☐ Heat	☐ Gall bladder	☐ Cold
☐ Cold	■ Liver	☐ Wind invasion
☐ Wind heat		
☐ Wind cold	**Temperature**	
☐ Wind damp	☐ Cooling	
☐ Dryness	■ Neutral	
	☐ Warming	

Energetics

This tapenade combines nourishment to the Yin and the Blood with Qi moving qualities. Pinenuts nourish the Yin and lubricate the Intestines, parsley nourishes the Blood and nourishes the Kidney, whilst the capers, thyme and black pepper add warmth, movement and some action against Dampness. Olives are known for their detoxifying properties and their beneficial affect on the Lung and Liver.

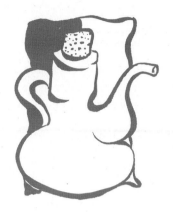

Zogghiu

Zogghiu is a Sicilian dialect word from the Palermo region meaning to add oil to food. This particular version of pesto is good with fish or white meat. You can also make a more textured version by adding pine kernels or walnuts.

Preparation time: 15 mins
Serves: 4

Ingredients

1 cup fresh parsley
1 cup fresh mint
4 cloves garlic
³/₄ cup olive oil
1 ¹/₂ tablespoon white wine vinegar
Salt

Method

Grind the herbs and garlic together in a mortar and pestle until they form a paste. Slowly whip in the olive oil and vinegar adding salt to taste. This will make about 3/4 of a cup. To make a more textured sauce, add some lightly toasted pine kernels, ground to a rough meal.

Primary actions	Primary influences	Contra-indications
■ Qi ■ Blood	■ Lung	□ Qi def
□ Yin □ Yang	□ Intestines	□ Blood def
□ Damp	□ Stomach	□ Yin def
□ Phlegm	□ Spleen	□ Yang def
□ Water	□ Heart	□ Damp
■ Qi stagnation	□ Bladder	□ Stagnation
■ Blood stagnation	■ Kidney	□ Heat
□ Heat	□ Gall bladder	□ Cold
□ Cold	■ Liver	□ Wind invasion
□ Wind heat		
□ Wind cold	**Temperature**	
□ Wind damp	□ Cooling	
□ Dryness	■ Neutral	
	□ Warming	

Energetics

Parsley is a Blood tonic and a useful tonic for the Kidney Qi. The olive oil base is soothing and nourishing to the Liver and the pungent garlic, vinegar and mint bring movement to balance the oil's richness.

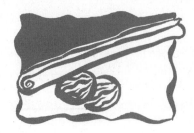

Baharat

Baharat is a middle eastern spice mixture traditionally used to flavour meat and fish. It is also very tasty sprinkled over vegetables. This is a very hot condiment so go gently with it.

Preparation time: 10 mins

Ingredients

1 teaspoon cloves
1 teaspoon coriander seeds
3 cardamom pods
1 teaspoon black peppercorns
1 teaspoon ground cinnamon
1 teaspoon ground nutmeg
½ teaspoon chilli powder
1 teaspoon paprika

Method

Grind the whole ingredients using a pestle and mortar then work in the other ingredients. The mixture will keep for a long time but will become less strong after a while.

Primary actions	Primary influences	Contra-indications
☐ Qi ☐ Blood	☐ Lung	☐ Qi def
☐ Yin ■ Yang	☐ Intestines	☐ Blood def
■ Damp	■ Stomach	■ Yin def
☐ Phlegm	☐ Spleen	☐ Yang def
☐ Water	☐ Heart	☐ Damp
■ Qi stagnation	☐ Bladder	☐ Stagnation
■ Blood stagnation	■ Kidney	■ Heat
☐ Heat	☐ Gall bladder	☐ Cold
■ Cold	☐ Liver	☐ Wind invasion
☐ Wind heat		
■ Wind cold	**Temperature**	
☐ Wind damp	☐ Cooling	
☐ Dryness	☐ Neutral	
	■ Warming	

Energetics

All these spices are warming and effective at moving Stagnation and Cold. Baharat will increase the digestibility of rich food such as meat, stimulating and warming the digestion. It is a useful condiment for Yang Deficiency but should not be overused.

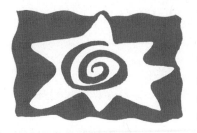

Dukkah

This is the perfect condiment to sprinkle over root vegetables, guaranteed to ping the tastebuds awake. I especially like it over mashed swede. It will also flavour salads and rice dishes.

Preparation time: 15 mins

Ingredients

½ pound sesame seeds
4 ounces coriander seeds
4 ounces hazelnuts
2 ounces cumin
1 teaspoon salt
¼ teaspoon freshly ground black pepper

Method

Dry roast each ingredient separately then grind everything together in a pestle and mortar. Be careful not to create a paste, especially if using mechanical means. This is a dry condiment for sprinkling.

Primary actions	Primary influences	Contra-indications
■ Qi ☐ Blood	☐ Lung	☐ Qi def
■ Yin ☐ Yang	☐ Intestines	☐ Blood def
☐ Damp	■ Stomach	☐ Yin def
☐ Phlegm	☐ Spleen	☐ Yang def
☐ Water	☐ Heart	☐ Damp
■ Qi stagnation	☐ Bladder	☐ Stagnation
☐ Blood stagnation	■ Kidney	☐ Heat
☐ Heat	☐ Gall bladder	☐ Cold
☐ Cold	■ Liver	☐ Wind invasion
☐ Wind heat	**Temperature**	
☐ Wind cold	☐ Cooling	
☐ Wind damp	☐ Neutral	
☐ Dryness	■ Warming	

Energetics

Sesame seeds and hazelnuts provide rich nourishment for the Yin. The inclusion of cumin and coriander provides mild warmth and enough movement to avoid congestion. This mixture stimulates the Qi, nourishes the Yin and is useful where there is some Stagnation.

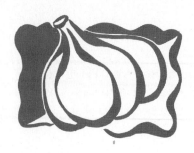

Garlic and Walnut Dressing

This is a rich dressing suitable for any green salad. It also tastes good on new potatoes, on beansprouts or on rice salad.

Preparation time: 5 mins
Serves: 6

Ingredients

½ cup walnuts
4 cloves garlic
1 tablespoon fresh parsley
6 tablespoons olive oil
1 teaspoon salt
3 tablespoons cider vinegar

Method

Crush the nuts with a rolling pin or back of a wooden spoon. Chop and crush the garlic and finely chop the parsley. Combine the ingredients and leave to stand before use. The dressing can also be blended with a whizzer.

Primary actions	Primary influences	Contra-indications
☐ Qi ■ Blood	■ Lung	☐ Qi def
☐ Yin ■ Yang	☐ Intestines	☐ Blood def
☐ Damp	☐ Stomach	☐ Yin def
■ Phlegm	☐ Spleen	☐ Yang def
☐ Water	☐ Heart	☐ Damp
■ Qi stagnation	☐ Bladder	☐ Stagnation
■ Blood stagnation	■ Kidney	☐ Heat
☐ Heat	■ Gall bladder	☐ Cold
■ Cold	■ Liver	☐ Wind invasion
☐ Wind heat		
☐ Wind cold	**Temperature**	
☐ Wind damp	☐ Cooling	
☐ Dryness	☐ Neutral	
	■ Warming	

Energetics

This is a Yang strengthening dressing, nourishing to the Kidney and Lung. Walnuts and parsley are traditional tonics for the Kidney. Garlic warms and opens the Lung and both garlic and walnuts have a strong action against Phlegm.

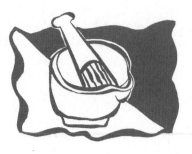

Gomasio

The smell of freshly prepared gomasio is hard to resist. It is also very simple to make. Try using it instead of plain salt at the dinner table.

Preparation time: 10 mins

Ingredients

20 parts sesame seeds
1 part sea salt

Method

Dry roast the ingredients in a skillet until the aromas are released then grind together with a pestle and mortar or use a whizzer.

Primary actions	Primary influences	Contra-indications
☐ Qi ☐ Blood	☐ Lung	☐ Qi def
■ Yin ☐ Yang	☐ Intestines	☐ Blood def
☐ Damp	☐ Stomach	☐ Yin def
☐ Phlegm	☐ Spleen	☐ Yang def
☐ Water	☐ Heart	☐ Damp
☐ Qi stagnation	☐ Bladder	☐ Stagnation
☐ Blood stagnation	■ Kidney	☐ Heat
☐ Heat	☐ Gall bladder	☐ Cold
☐ Cold	■ Liver	☐ Wind invasion
☐ Wind heat	**Temperature**	
☐ Wind cold	☐ Cooling	
☐ Wind damp	■ Neutral	
☐ Dryness	☐ Warming	

Energetics

This is a Yin nourishing condiment whose action is directed by the salt towards the Kidney.

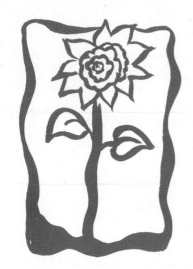

Shoyu Roasted Seeds

These toasted seeds are always popular. They are a delightful snack and can be sprinkled over salads, plain vegetables or grains.

Preparation time: 10 mins

Ingredients

1 cup sunflower seeds	
½ cup pumpkin seeds	

2 tablespoons soya sauce

Method

Heat the sunflower seeds in a heavy skillet over a medium flame for about 5 minutes. Add the pumpkin seeds and continue dry roasting until they begin to brown and the first seeds begin to pop.

Pour the soya sauce over them and turn quickly so that they are all coated. Keep roasting and turning the seeds for a few minutes until the soya sauce is well absorbed.

Primary actions	Primary influences	Contra-indications
■ Qi □ Blood	□ Lung	□ Qi def
□ Yin □ Yang	■ Intestines	□ Blood def
□ Damp	□ Stomach	□ Yin def
□ Phlegm	■ Spleen	□ Yang def
□ Water	□ Heart	□ Damp
□ Qi stagnation	■ Bladder	□ Stagnation
□ Blood stagnation	■ Kidney	□ Heat
□ Heat	□ Gall bladder	□ Cold
□ Cold	□ Liver	□ Wind invasion
□ Wind heat		
□ Wind cold	**Temperature**	
□ Wind damp	□ Cooling	
□ Dryness	■ Neutral	
	□ Warming	

Energetics

These seeds help strengthen the Qi and support the Spleen and Kidney. The soya sauce draws the action down into the Intestines and lower Jiao.

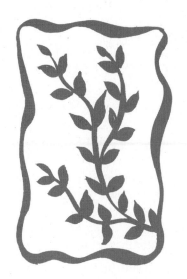

Zaatar

This dry mixture of sesame seeds, salt and herbs is popular in the Middle East and is traditionally served with bread and olive oil. Break off a hunk of bread, dip it in the oil and then into the dry herbs. The explosion of taste in the mouth is an evocative experience. The mixture is excellent sprinkled on salads or over cooked vegetables. The secret is to use freshly dried herbs no more than a year old.

Preparation time: 5 mins

Ingredients

½ teaspoon thyme
1 teaspoon sumac
3 teaspoons sesame seeds
¼ teaspoon sea salt

Method

Dry roast and grind together the sesame seeds and salt. Add the thyme and sumac, grind a little more and mix well. Keep it in a well sealed jar.

Primary actions
☐ Qi ☐ Blood
■ Yin ☐ Yang
■ Damp
■ Phlegm
☐ Water
■ Qi stagnation
☐ Blood stagnation
☐ Heat
☐ Cold
☐ Wind heat
☐ Wind cold
☐ Wind damp
☐ Dryness

Primary influences
■ Lung
☐ Intestines
☐ Stomach
☐ Spleen
☐ Heart
■ Bladder
■ Kidney
☐ Gall bladder
☐ Liver

Temperature
■ Cooling
☐ Neutral
☐ Warming

Contra-indications
☐ Qi def
☐ Blood def
☐ Yin def
☐ Yang def
☐ Damp
☐ Stagnation
☐ Heat
☐ Cold
☐ Wind invasion

Energetics

Sumac is an astringent herb that tones the Kidney Qi and counters Dampness in the Bladder. Sesame seeds nourish the Kidney Yin and the salt directs the action of the mixture downwards. Thyme stimulates the Qi, especially in the Lung and acts against Phlegm. The mixture is slightly cooling.

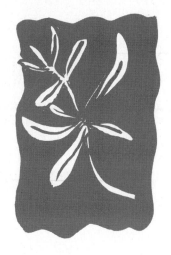

Castagnaccio (Sweet Chestnut Bread)

Castagnaccio is a traditional Tuscan recipe with many local variations. I first encountered this bread when someone pulled it out of her lunchbox in a class I was teaching. One nibble and I was nobbled, as they say. So sweet and enticing. After several failed attempts to reproduce it myself, she sent the recipe just as I was finishing this book. You will probably have to find an Italian delicatessen to buy chestnut flour but it's worth the effort. Because chestnut flour spoils easily, it is normally only available for a few months after harvest in September.

Preparation time: 10 mins
Cooking time: 40 mins
Makes one loaf

Ingredients

3 cups chestnut flour
1 cup water
4 tablespoons olive oil
Pinch of salt

Handful pine kernels
Handful raisins (optional)
Generous sprig fresh rosemary

Method

Preheat the oven to 350°F/Gas Mark 4 and oil a shallow 12 inch baking dish with a generous amount of olive oil. Meanwhile mix together the flour, salt, olive oil and water. Add the water gradually, stirring well to avoid lumps. Stop adding water when you have achieved a thick pouring consistency.

Stir in the pine kernels and some fresh rosemary leaves. Add the raisins if desired. Spread the batter in the tin and garnish with plenty of rosemary. Bake for 40 minutes or until deep cracks appear on the surface. Allow to cool before cutting into wedges.

Energetics

Chestnut is a sweet and warming nut. It strengthens the Yang of the Kidney and Spleen and gently moves the circulation of the Blood. The addition of pine kernels and raisins makes this a fairly comprehensive recipe, nourishing the Yin, Blood and Qi as well as supporting the Yang.

Primary actions	Primary influences	Contra-indications
■ Qi ■ Blood	□ Lung	□ Qi def
■ Yin ■ Yang	□ Intestines	□ Blood def
□ Damp	■ Stomach	□ Yin def
□ Phlegm	■ Spleen	□ Yang def
□ Water	□ Heart	□ Damp
□ Qi stagnation	□ Bladder	□ Stagnation
■ Blood stagnation	■ Kidney	□ Heat
□ Heat	□ Gall bladder	□ Cold
□ Cold	■ Liver	□ Wind invasion
□ Wind heat		
□ Wind cold	**Temperature**	
□ Wind damp	□ Cooling	
□ Dryness	□ Neutral	
	■ Warming	

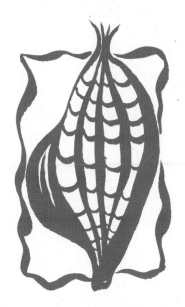

Journey Bread

Sometimes called 'journey bread' or 'johnny cakes', corn bread is one of the easiest breads to make. It is light and more like a cake in texture.

Preparation time: 5 mins
Cooking time: 30 mins
Makes one loaf

Ingredients

1 1/2 cups cornmeal
3/4 cup wheat/spelt flour
4 teaspoons baking powder
1/2 cup sesame seeds
1/2 cup crushed walnuts
1 teaspoon salt
2 eggs
1 1/4 cups soya milk
1/4 cup sunflower oil
1 tablespoon maple syrup

Method

Mix together all the dry ingredients in a bowl. Beat the eggs and milk together. Stir these into the dry mixture along with the oil and maple syrup. The mixture should be quite wet. Grease one large or two small bread tins and fill to two thirds. Bake at 400°F/Gas Mark 6 for about 30 minutes. Test with a knife to ensure that it is cooked all the way through.

Primary actions	Primary influences	Contra-indications
■ Qi ■ Blood	□ Lung	□ Qi def
■ Yin □ Yang	□ Intestines	□ Blood def
□ Damp	■ Stomach	□ Yin def
□ Phlegm	■ Spleen	□ Yang def
□ Water	□ Heart	□ Damp
□ Qi stagnation	□ Bladder	□ Stagnation
□ Blood stagnation	■ Kidney	□ Heat
□ Heat	□ Gall bladder	□ Cold
□ Cold	□ Liver	□ Wind invasion
□ Wind heat		
□ Wind cold	**Temperature**	
□ Wind damp	□ Cooling	
□ Dryness	■ Neutral	
	□ Warming	

Energetics

Grains are basically nourishing to the Blood and Qi. The use of sesame seeds, spelt flour and the addition of eggs increases the nourishment to the Yin whilst the walnuts support both Yin and Yang.

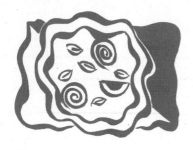

Polenta Pizza

Polenta makes an unusual and effective base for a pizza. A quick spell in a very hot oven hardens it sufficiently to hold the pizza topping. The topping can be varied according to taste from the usual array of olives, mushroom, anchovy, onion and tomato to perhaps more adventurous toppings such as smoked tofu, leeks or asparagus tips. For those trying to avoid wheat or yeast, this is an excellent and tasty alternative.

Preparation time: 15 mins
Cooking time: 75 mins
Serves: 6

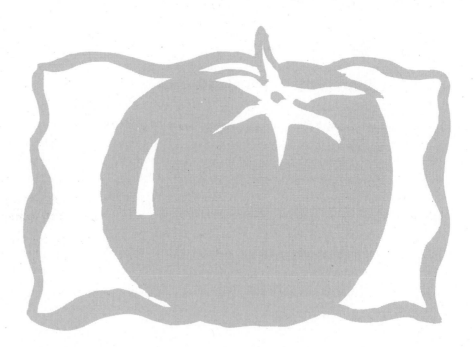

Primary actions	Primary influences	Contra-indications
■ Qi ■ Blood	□ Lung	□ Qi def
□ Yin □ Yang	□ Intestines	□ Blood def
□ Damp	■ Stomach	□ Yin def
□ Phlegm	□ Spleen	□ Yang def
□ Water	■ Heart	□ Damp
□ Qi stagnation	□ Bladder	□ Stagnation
□ Blood stagnation	■ Kidney	□ Heat
□ Heat	□ Gall bladder	□ Cold
□ Cold	□ Liver	□ Wind invasion
□ Wind heat		
□ Wind cold	**Temperature**	
□ Wind damp	□ Cooling	
□ Dryness	■ Neutral	
	□ Warming	

Energetics

Corn is nourishing to the Kidney, Stomach and Heart. It is also mildly diuretic. It provides a good counterbalance to the moistening action of the tomatoes. The rich nourishment of the cheese is balanced by the decongesting action of the onion, pepper and garlic. This is a well balanced and broadly nourishing meal.

Ingredients	Method
3 cups cornmeal 5 cups water 2 teaspoons salt	To make the polenta, put 2 cups of the cornmeal in a heavy-bottomed pot and slowly add the water. Stir carefully to avoid lumps. Add the salt and cook on a medium heat for 20-30 minutes. Stir often, especially towards the end. When the polenta stiffens and pulls away from the side of the pan, it is cooked. Now stir in the other cup of cornmeal or as much as is needed to make a very stiff mixture. Press the polenta firmly into a large greased baking tray (14 inches diameter or thereabouts). The polenta should be about a half inch thick. Bake in a very hot oven (450°F/Gas Mark 8) for about 20 minutes or until the surface feels crusty.
6 tomatoes 2 large onions 1 small green pepper 4 cloves garlic 6 ounces olives 6 artichoke hearts, quartered 2 handfuls fresh basil	Meanwhile roughly chop the onions, pepper and tomatoes. Fry the onions gently until they start to soften, then add the other ingredients and cook for 3-4 minutes adding the basil at the last minute.
2–3 cups grated cheese Black pepper	Take the polenta base out of the oven, spoon the topping evenly over the surface and cover with grated cheese. Return to the oven at 375°F/Gas Mark 5 and bake for a further 20 minutes or until the cheese is melted. Serve with a green salad and sprinkle with fresh black pepper.

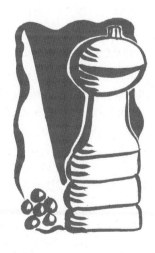

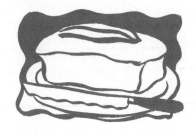

Soda Bread

If making yeasted bread seems too laborious, soda bread is a good place to start. It is easy to make and delicious.

Preparation time: 10 mins
Cooking time: 40 mins
Serves: 4

Ingredients

1 pound spelt flour
1 teaspoon salt
2 teaspoons bicarbonate of soda
2 teaspoons cream of tartar
2 ounces butter or vegetable oil
½ pint buttermilk or plain yoghurt

Method

Sift the flour, salt and raising agents into a bowl and mix well. Rub in the fat and gradually add the buttermilk to make a soft dough. (If it is too sticky add more flour). Knead the dough briefly and shape it into a dome 6-8 inches across. Cut a deep cross into the top and bake on a greased baking tray at 425°F/Gas Mark 7 for about 30 minutes. Break or cut into wedges and serve. If you find the bread is too crumbly an egg can be added.

Primary actions	Primary influences	Contra-indications
■ Qi ■ Blood	□ Lung	□ Qi def
■ Yin □ Yang	□ Intestines	□ Blood def
□ Damp	□ Stomach	□ Yin def
□ Phlegm	■ Spleen	□ Yang def
□ Water	■ Heart	□ Damp
□ Qi stagnation	□ Bladder	□ Stagnation
□ Blood stagnation	□ Kidney	□ Heat
	□ Gall bladder	□ Cold
□ Heat	□ Liver	□ Wind invasion
□ Cold		
□ Wind heat	**Temperature**	
□ Wind cold	□ Cooling	
□ Wind damp	■ Neutral	
□ Dryness	□ Warming	

Energetics

This is a moist bread that nourishes the Yin without being too dampening. Spelt is a mildly warm grain with a generally higher nutritional value than its relative, wheat. Though high in gluten, it is frequently tolerated by those with celiac disease and is less likely to provoke the formation of mucus. The buttermilk or yoghurt add to this bread's Yin nourishing value.

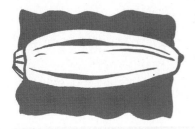

Sweet Bread

This is a very moist bread, more like a cake. Although it keeps well for a couple of days, try eating it fresh from the oven for a real treat.

Preparation time: 15 mins
Cooking time: 30 mins
Makes one loaf

Ingredients

3 large eggs
½ cup safflower oil
½ teaspoon vanilla
3 tablespoons yoghurt
1 teaspoon maple syrup
1 cup grated carrot
½ cup grated courgette
Grated rind of 1 orange

1 ½ cups rice flour
1 level teaspoon baking soda
1 level teaspoon baking powder
1 tablespoon ground almonds
¼ teaspoon cinnamon

Method

Lightly beat the eggs and combine with the oil, vanilla, yoghurt, maple syrup, carrot, courgette and orange rind.

Mix all the dry ingredients together in another bowl, making sure the baking powder and bicarbonate are well distributed.

Mix the dry and wet ingredients together and stir lightly. Pour the mixture into a bread tin and bake at 350°F/Gas Mark 4 for 40 minutes or so.

Primary actions	Primary influences	Contra-indications
■ Qi ■ Blood	☐ Lung	☐ Qi def
☐ Yin ☐ Yang	☐ Intestines	☐ Blood def
☐ Damp	■ Stomach	☐ Yin def
☐ Phlegm	■ Spleen	☐ Yang def
☐ Water	☐ Heart	☐ Damp
☐ Qi stagnation	☐ Bladder	☐ Stagnation
☐ Blood stagnation	☐ Kidney	☐ Heat
☐ Heat	☐ Gall bladder	☐ Cold
☐ Cold	☐ Liver	☐ Wind invasion
☐ Wind heat		
☐ Wind cold	**Temperature**	
☐ Wind damp	☐ Cooling	
☐ Dryness	■ Neutral	
	☐ Warming	

Energetics

This bread nourishes the Blood and Qi and is easily digested.

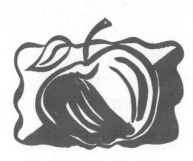

Apple and Chestnut Tart

Preparation time: 45 mins
Serves: 6–8

Apple and chestnut are the bisexuals of the world of cooking, at home both in savoury and sweet dishes. They are perfect companions in this tart. Both the apple and lemon bite nicely through the thick textured chestnut. Enjoy.

Ingredients

One 9 inch pastry case
1 pound chestnut purée
Peel of one lemon
1 teaspoon cinnamon
1 tablespoon date syrup

1 large cooking apple
½ cup flaked almonds
Juice of one lemon
½ teaspoon cinnamon
1 tablespoon brown sugar

Method

Boil and purée the chestnuts or use tinned purée. Grate the lemon peel, and add it to the purée together with one teaspoon of cinnamon and the date syrup. Press the mixture into the pastry case.

Cover the surface with thinly sliced apple and the flaked almonds. Pour the lemon juice over the top, sprinkle with a mixture of the sugar and the remaining cinnamon and bake at 400°F/Gas Mark 6 for about 20-30 minutes.

Primary actions	Primary influences	Contra-indications
■ Qi ■ Blood	■ Lung	□ Qi def
■ Yin ■ Yang	□ Intestines	□ Blood def
□ Damp	■ Stomach	□ Yin def
□ Phlegm	■ Spleen	□ Yang def
□ Water	■ Heart	□ Damp
■ Qi stagnation	□ Bladder	□ Stagnation
■ Blood stagnation	■ Kidney	□ Heat
□ Heat	□ Gall bladder	□ Cold
□ Cold	□ Liver	□ Wind invasion
□ Wind heat		
□ Wind cold	**Temperature**	
□ Wind damp	□ Cooling	
□ Dryness	■ Neutral	
	□ Warming	

Energetics

Chestnuts strengthen the Yang and benefit the Kidney, Stomach and Spleen. The apple nourishes the Yin of the Heart, Lung and Stomach. They are supported respectively by the cinnamon and lemon.

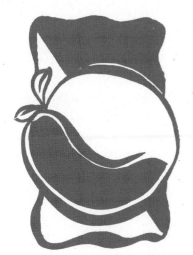

Apricot Whatnot

This dessert will send your family wild with excitement. The sweetness of these fruits melts into the body like sunshine. It's an ideal dish for a winter's day when fresh summer fruits are out of season.

Preparation time: 5 mins
Cooking time: 15 mins
Serves: 4

Ingredients

1 cup dried apricots
½ cup dried dates
1 cup yoghurt

Method

Soak the dates and apricots overnight or for an hour before cooking. Stew them until soft, then purée. Combine with yoghurt. Serve warm and make enough for second helpings.

Primary actions	Primary influences	Contra-indications
■ Qi ■ Blood	■ Lung	☐ Qi def
■ Yin ☐ Yang	■ Intestines	☐ Blood def
☐ Damp	☐ Stomach	☐ Yin def
☐ Phlegm	■ Spleen	☐ Yang def
☐ Water	☐ Heart	☐ Damp
☐ Qi stagnation	☐ Bladder	☐ Stagnation
☐ Blood stagnation	☐ Kidney	☐ Heat
☐ Heat	☐ Gall bladder	☐ Cold
☐ Cold	■ Liver	☐ Wind invasion
☐ Wind heat		
☐ Wind cold	**Temperature**	
☐ Wind damp	☐ Cooling	
■ Dryness	■ Neutral	
	☐ Warming	

Energetics

Apricots strengthen the Blood and moisten the Lung. In their dried form they are gently warming. Dates nourish both Qi and Blood, also with a mildly warming action and a strengthening effect on the Liver and Spleen. Yoghurt is cooling, moistening and nourishes the Lung, Intestines and Stomach. This simple dish provides a tonic for the Blood, Qi and Yin.

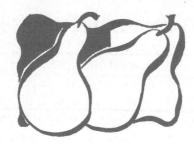

Baked Pears with Juniper

This recipe was inspired by an idea in Nigel Slater's 'The Thirty Minute Cook'. Choose pears that are smallish and properly ripe. This is a perfect dish for the autumn, 'season of mists and mellow fruitfulness'. It goes well with a few seasonal nuts.

Preparation time: 10 mins
Cooking time: 30 mins
Serves: 4

Ingredients

8 small ripe pears
6 tablespoons apple juice concentrate
1 tablespoon lemon juice
½ teaspoon crushed coriander seeds
8 juniper berries, crushed
Honey
Yoghurt
Flaked almonds

Method

Halve the pears and place them in a covered dish. Pour the apple juice concentrate and lemon over them and sprinkle with the crushed coriander seeds and juniper. Bake at 400°F/Gas Mark 6 for about 30 minutes. Serve with honey, yoghurt and a sprinkle of toasted flaked almonds.

Primary actions	Primary influences	Contra-indications
☐ Qi ☐ Blood	■ Lung	☐ Qi def
■ Yin ☐ Yang	☐ Intestines	☐ Blood def
☐ Damp	■ Stomach	☐ Yin def
☐ Phlegm	☐ Spleen	☐ Yang def
☐ Water	☐ Heart	☐ Damp
☐ Qi stagnation	☐ Bladder	☐ Stagnation
☐ Blood stagnation	☐ Kidney	☐ Heat
■ Heat	☐ Gall bladder	☐ Cold
☐ Cold	☐ Liver	☐ Wind invasion
☐ Wind heat	**Temperature**	
☐ Wind cold	■ Cooling	
☐ Wind damp	☐ Neutral	
☐ Dryness	☐ Warming	

Energetics

Pears moisten the Lung and nourish the Yin which is the main action of this dish. The juniper slightly offsets the coolness of the pears, as does the baking method. The apple juice concentrate and lemon support the action of the pears. The yoghurt is also moistening, cool and nourishing to the Yin.

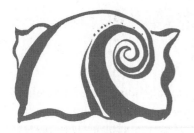

Coconut Macaroons

Coconut macaroons are very sexy food. Pull them out of your repertoire for a very special occasion.

Preparation time: 15 mins
Cooking time: 30 mins
Makes 24

Ingredients

¹/₄ cup almonds
4 egg whites
¹/₄ teaspoon cream of tartar
¹/₂ teaspoon baking powder

³/₄ cup maple syrup
Generous splash rosewater
3 cups dessicated coconut

Method

Blanch the almonds then grind them to a coarse meal. Beat the eggwhites with the cream of tartar until they begin to stiffen then add the baking powder.

In another bowl combine the ground almonds with all the other ingredients. Fold in the eggwhites. Spoon the mixture onto a greased baking tray, one tablespoon per macaroon loosely shaped into rounds. Bake for 30 minutes at 300°F/Gas Mark 2. Remove from the tray while still warm.

Primary actions	Primary influences	Contra-indications
■ Qi ☐ Blood	■ Lung	☐ Qi def
☐ Yin ☐ Yang	☐ Intestines	☐ Blood def
☐ Damp	☐ Stomach	☐ Yin def
☐ Phlegm	☐ Spleen	☐ Yang def
☐ Water	■ Heart	■ Damp
☐ Qi stagnation	☐ Bladder	☐ Stagnation
☐ Blood stagnation	☐ Kidney	☐ Heat
☐ Heat	☐ Gall bladder	☐ Cold
☐ Cold	☐ Liver	☐ Wind invasion
☐ Wind heat	**Temperature**	
☐ Wind cold	☐ Cooling	
☐ Wind damp	■ Neutral	
☐ Dryness	☐ Warming	

Energetics

Coconut tends to warm and nourish the Heart and this sweet treat will uplift the spirit. The eggwhites and almonds nourish the Lung. As with all very sweet foods, a little will be beneficial but too much will overwhelm the Spleen and undo its benefits.

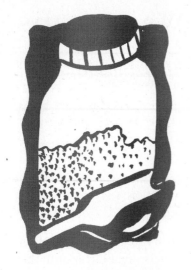

Date and Walnut Flapjack

My grandmother used to make me a date and walnut loaf that no other cake has ever bettered. Unfortunately I don't have her recipe, but here is another near perfect combination: walnuts, dates and oats. These flapjacks will satisfy even someone whose grandmother spoiled them like mine did.

Preparation time: 40 mins
Serves: 8

Ingredients

6 ounces walnuts
8 ounces dates
A little hot water
1 handful sesame seeds
1 cup sunflower oil
2 eggs, beaten
2 tablespoons molasses
1 tablespoon cinnamon
1 teaspoon ginger
20 ounces oatflakes

Method

Crush the walnuts and chop the dates finely. Add a small amount of hot water to the dates, leave for a few minutes then mash until the dates dissolve a little. Add the molasses, crushed walnuts, sesame seeds, oil, spices and eggs. Stir well. Gradually add the oats until the mixture is thick and moist. Push it into a shallow baking tray and bake at 400°F/Gas Mark 6 for about half an hour. Cut when still warm.

Primary actions	Primary influences	Contra-indications
■ Qi ■ Blood	■ Lung	☐ Qi def
■ Yin ■ Yang	■ Intestines	☐ Blood def
☐ Damp	■ Stomach	☐ Yin def
☐ Phlegm	■ Spleen	☐ Yang def
☐ Water	■ Heart	☐ Damp
☐ Qi stagnation	☐ Bladder	☐ Stagnation
☐ Blood stagnation	■ Kidney	☐ Heat
☐ Heat	☐ Gall bladder	☐ Cold
■ Cold	■ Liver	☐ Wind invasion
☐ Wind heat		
☐ Wind cold	**Temperature**	
☐ Wind damp	☐ Cooling	
☐ Dryness	☐ Neutral	
	■ Warming	

Energetics

The combination of walnuts, dates, sesame seeds, eggs, molasses and oats is nourishing to most aspects of our system: the Yin, Yang, Blood and Qi. Its moistening action is partially moderated by the drying and warming action of the spices. Because of its richness, too much will be dampening. This is a warming energy tonic that will support the whole system.

Marmalade Slice

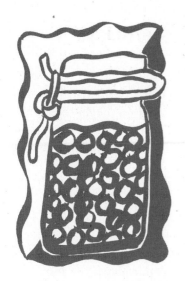

Marmalade's lively, zesty taste deserves more than routine appearances on toast at breakfast. In this recipe marmalade brings the flapjack sharply alive in the mouth and it's hard not to reach for that second piece.

Preparation time: 10 mins
Cooking time: 30 mins
Serves: 4–6

Ingredients

3 cups oatflakes
½ cup dessicated coconut
2 teaspoons dry ginger

½ cup saffflower oil
1 egg

6–8 ounces sugar-free marmalade

Method

Pour the oats, coconut and ginger into a bowl. Rub the mixture firmly through your hands a few times to crumble the oats a little more.

Beat the egg then gently stir in the oil. Add the egg and oil mixture to the dry ingredients stirring it in well. Grease a 7 inch baking tray, spoon in half the mixture and press down firmly.

Spread the marmalade evenly over the surface then cover with the remaining mixture. Press down firmly. Bake at 400°F/Gas Mark 6 for about 30 minutes or until very lightly browned. Leave to cool before slicing.

Primary actions	Primary influences	Contra-indications
■ Qi ■ Blood	■ Lung	☐ Qi def
☐ Yin ☐ Yang	☐ Intestines	☐ Blood def
☐ Damp	☐ Stomach	☐ Yin def
☐ Phlegm	■ Spleen	☐ Yang def
☐ Water	☐ Heart	☐ Damp
■ Qi stagnation	☐ Bladder	☐ Stagnation
☐ Blood stagnation	☐ Kidney	☐ Heat
☐ Heat	☐ Gall bladder	☐ Cold
■ Cold	☐ Liver	☐ Wind invasion
☐ Wind heat	**Temperature**	
☐ Wind cold	☐ Cooling	
☐ Wind damp	☐ Neutral	
☐ Dryness	■ Warming	

Energetics

Oats are a gently warming grain, strengthening to the Qi and Blood. The marmalade is a strong mover of Stagnation and, provided it is sugar-free, a reducer of Phlegm. The oats and marmalade complement each other: the tendency of oats to be a little heavy is countered by the action of the marmalade. Nevertheless, the overall richness of this recipe makes it unsuitable for serious conditions of Phlegm and Dampness.

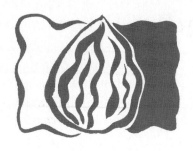

Molasses Cookies

These are very rich cookies reminiscent of christmas pudding. They are dark coloured, sweet and enlivened by the tang of the citrus peel. They are adapted from a recipe originally found in Ed Brown's 'Tassajara Bread Book' which has the honour of being the first recipe book I ever bought.

Preparation time: 20 mins
Cooking time: 25 mins
Serves: 6–8

Ingredients

1 ½ cups molasses
3 tablespoons butter
1 tablespoon baking powder
3 cups spelt flour

½ cup chopped almonds
2 tablespoons fresh lemon peel
2 tablespoon fresh orange peel
3 teaspoons cinnamon
½ teaspoon cardamom
¼ teaspoon cloves

Method

Heat the molasses slowly in a pan with the butter. When the butter is melted and blended with the molasses, remove from the heat and add the baking powder and about half the flour, stirring well.

Turn in all the other ingredients, then add more flour until the mixture becomes stiff and sticky. The amount of flour used depends on its absorbency. Press the mixture to a depth of just under half an inch into a greased tray. Bake at 350°F/Gas Mark 4 for about 20-25 minutes and remove from the tray while still warm. Cut into about two dozen squares. The bars should be chewy rather than crisp.

Primary actions	Primary influences	Contra-indications
■ Qi ■ Blood	■ Lung	☐ Qi def
☐ Yin ☐ Yang	☐ Intestines	☐ Blood def
☐ Damp	☐ Stomach	☐ Yin def
☐ Phlegm	■ Spleen	☐ Yang def
☐ Water	■ Heart	■ Damp
☐ Qi stagnation	☐ Bladder	☐ Stagnation
☐ Blood stagnation	☐ Kidney	☐ Heat
	☐ Gall bladder	☐ Cold
☐ Heat	☐ Liver	☐ Wind invasion
☐ Cold		
☐ Wind heat	**Temperature**	
☐ Wind cold	☐ Cooling	
☐ Wind damp	☐ Neutral	
☐ Dryness	■ Warming	

Energetics

The molasses, spelt and butter make a moist combination that nourishes the Blood and Qi and uplifts the Heart. The richness is balanced by the drying and moving properties of the various spices and powerful Stagnation-moving properties of the citrus peel.

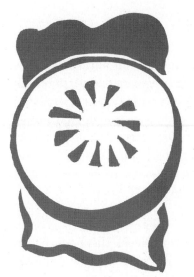

Peppered Fruit Salad

The first mouthful of this dessert is always a surprise. The contrast between the fruit and the pepper is very exciting.

Preparation time: 15 mins
Cooking time: 45 mins
Serves: 4–6

Ingredients

3 kiwi fruit
3 peaches
Juice of 2 lemons
4 tablespoons date syrup
1 teaspoon szechuan peppercorns
½ teaspoon coriander seeds
½ pound strawberries

Method

Halve the kiwi and peaches, removing the peach stones. Set them face down in a shallow ovenproof dish. Pour the lemon juice and date syrup over the fruit. Crush the coriander seeds and peppercorns and sprinkle them over the top. Cover the dish and bake at 325°F/Gas mark 3 for 45 minutes. When the dish is cooked, set aside to cool a little. Add the strawberries, quartered, and turn them in the syrup. Serve as they are or with plain yoghurt.

Energetics

Fruits, combining sweet and sour flavours in their flesh, are generally moisture-generating, cooling and nourishing to the Yin. However, peach is a somewhat warm fruit and the baking method and the addition of peppercorns and coriander makes this less cooling than most fruit dishes, quite well tolerated by most people with cool constitutions. The subtle balance of cool and moistening fruit with warm and drying spices is an unusual example of a dish which harmonises Yin and Yang.

Primary actions	Primary influences	Contra-indications
☐ Qi ■ Blood	☐ Lung	☐ Qi def
■ Yin ☐ Yang	☐ Intestines	☐ Blood def
☐ Damp	■ Stomach	☐ Yin def
☐ Phlegm	☐ Spleen	☐ Yang def
☐ Water	■ Heart	☐ Damp
☐ Qi stagnation	☐ Bladder	☐ Stagnation
☐ Blood stagnation	■ Kidney	☐ Heat
☐ Heat	☐ Gall bladder	☐ Cold
☐ Cold	■ Liver	☐ Wind invasion
☐ Wind heat		
☐ Wind cold	**Temperature**	
☐ Wind damp	☐ Cooling	
☐ Dryness	■ Neutral	
	☐ Warming	

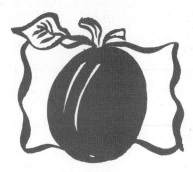

Plum Fool

The plum season is very short and for only a few weeks of the year the local greengrocers seem to overflow with their sweet heady scent. Even the wasps go crazy. So many ripe plums all at once and what to do? A fruit fool makes a refreshing dish at any time of day and it is very easy to make. I use sweet yellow plums for this recipe but any ripe and tasty plum will do. This recipe will send an excited ripple round the dinner table.

Preparation time: 10 mins
Cooking time: 20 mins
Serves: 4

Ingredients

1 pound plums or gooseberries
1 teaspoon fennel seeds
$1/2$ teaspoon dried ginger
4 tablespoons concentrated apple juice

Method

Stone and halve the plums and cook them gently in a covered pan with the spices. After about 20 minutes remove them from the heat, mash or purée. Add the apple juice concentrate, combining well. Plum fool can be served warm or cool and with a swirl of yoghurt if desired.

Primary actions	Primary influences	Contra-indications
☐ Qi ■ Blood	☐ Lung	☐ Qi def
■ Yin ☐ Yang	☐ Intestines	☐ Blood def
☐ Damp	■ Stomach	☐ Yin def
☐ Phlegm	☐ Spleen	☐ Yang def
☐ Water	☐ Heart	☐ Damp
■ Qi stagnation	☐ Bladder	☐ Stagnation
☐ Blood stagnation	☐ Kidney	☐ Heat
■ Heat	☐ Gall bladder	☐ Cold
☐ Cold	■ Liver	☐ Wind invasion
☐ Wind heat		
☐ Wind cold	**Temperature**	
☐ Wind damp	■ Cooling	
☐ Dryness	☐ Neutral	
	☐ Warming	

Energetics

Plums are cooling and strengthening to the Liver. They are an excellent remedy for Liver Heat and helpful for Stagnation in the Intestines. The spices provide a counterpoint to this dish's coolness. Gooseberries may be substituted for the plums as they have similar energetic properties.

Sesame Treats

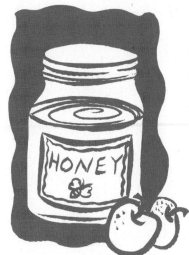

This is a very rich snack, like halva. Try these marble-sized treats with a cup of dark grain coffee or cup of tea.

Preparation time: 20 mins
Serves: 6

Ingredients

2 cups sesame seeds
2 tablespoons melted butter
¼ cup honey
1 tablespoon sesame oil
1 teaspoon vanilla extract
½ teaspoon cinnamon

Method

Dry roast the sesame seeds until their aroma is strong, but do not burn. Grind them as finely as possible then stir in all the other ingredients and press together. Let it cool and harden then wet the hands and shape the mixture into balls the size of marbles. They are ready to serve.

Primary actions	Primary influences	Contra-indications
■ Qi □ Blood	□ Lung	□ Qi def
■ Yin □ Yang	□ Intestines	□ Blood def
□ Damp	□ Stomach	□ Yin def
□ Phlegm	□ Spleen	□ Yang def
□ Water	■ Heart	■ Damp
□ Qi stagnation	□ Bladder	□ Stagnation
□ Blood stagnation	■ Kidney	□ Heat
□ Heat	■ Gall bladder	□ Cold
□ Cold	■ Liver	□ Wind invasion
□ Wind heat		
□ Wind cold	**Temperature**	
□ Wind damp	□ Cooling	
■ Dryness	■ Neutral	
	□ Warming	

Energetics

The sesame seeds strengthen the Yin and the honey is a sweet tonic for the Qi. The fat increases the moistening quality of the 'halva'. The cinnamon provides a counterpoint with its warming and drying energy. As this snack is so nutritious it needs to be eaten in small doses otherwise it will be too dampening.

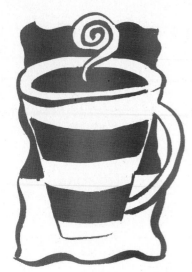

Aniseed, Fennel and Caraway Tea

This simple tea freshens and enlivens the mouth. It is best drunk after a meal as an aid to digestion. A few teaspoons of this tea can also be given to babies to relieve colic.

Preparation time: 5 mins
Makes 3 cups

Ingredients

1 teaspoon aniseed
1 teaspoon caraway
1 teaspoon fennel

Method

Simply put the seeds in a teapot and pour on boiling water. If you like it a little stronger, simmer the seeds in a pot for about 5 minutes.

Primary actions	Primary influences	Contra-indications
☐ Qi ☐ Blood	■ Lung	☐ Qi def
☐ Yin ☐ Yang	☐ Intestines	☐ Blood def
■ Damp	☐ Stomach	☐ Yin def
■ Phlegm	■ Spleen	☐ Yang def
☐ Water	☐ Heart	☐ Damp
■ Qi stagnation	■ Bladder	☐ Stagnation
☐ Blood stagnation	■ Kidney	☐ Heat
☐ Heat	☐ Gall bladder	☐ Cold
■ Cold	☐ Liver	☐ Wind invasion
☐ Wind heat		
☐ Wind cold	**Temperature**	
☐ Wind damp	☐ Cooling	
☐ Dryness	☐ Neutral	
	■ Warming	

Energetics

These are all warming spices that generate movement and help relieve digestive Stagnation. The tea counters Dampness and promotes Qi circulation.

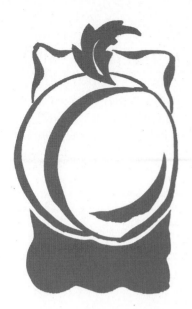

Apricot and Nettle Wine

Tonic wines are wonderful. What better excuse to sit back in the evening with a glass of wine knowing that your pleasure is also your medicine.

Preparation time: 20 mins
3 weeks to mature

Ingredients

1 bottle red wine
1 pint fresh nettles
24 dried apricots

Method

You will need a large clean glass jar or bottle, a little bigger than your wine bottle, with a good screw-top lid or cork. Sterilise it by rinsing with cold water and heating it in the oven for about 20 minutes. Pick the nettles fresh and push them into the jar, packing them down gently to make room for a few more. The exact quantity is not important. Put the dried apricots on top (the unsulphured variety are best) and pour in a cheap bottle of red wine, filling to near the brim. Seal and leave the bottle in a dark cupboard at room temperature for three weeks. Drink a glass each day as a tonic. The nettles can go into the compost heap afterwards but the boozy fruits taste delicious.

Energetics

Apricots and nettles are both excellent Blood tonics. Infused in wine, their properties are easily carried into the body. The red grapes from which the wine is made are also Blood-nourishing and the alcohol makes this a warming drink.

Primary actions	Primary influences	Contra-indications
☐ Qi ■ Blood	■ Lung	☐ Qi def
☐ Yin ☐ Yang	☐ Intestines	☐ Blood def
☐ Damp	☐ Stomach	☐ Yin def
☐ Phlegm	■ Spleen	☐ Yang def
☐ Water	■ Heart	☐ Damp
■ Qi stagnation	■ Bladder	☐ Stagnation
■ Blood stagnation	■ Kidney	■ Heat
☐ Heat	☐ Gall bladder	☐ Cold
■ Cold	■ Liver	☐ Wind invasion
☐ Wind heat		
☐ Wind cold	**Temperature**	
☐ Wind damp	☐ Cooling	
☐ Dryness	☐ Neutral	
	■ Warming	

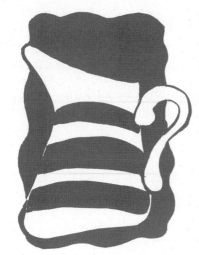

Barley Water

Some people swear that barley water is the secret of their good health and it is rumoured that the Queen of England drinks it daily. It can be a refreshing summer drink as well as a strengthening and soothing drink during convalescence.

Preparation time: 1 hour
Makes 3 cups

Ingredients

2 ounces barley
2 pints water
Lemon juice
Pinch salt

Method

Gently dry roast the barley, add the water and bring to a rolling boil for about 15 minutes. Then simmer for 30-45 minutes or until the barley is soft and disintegrating. Strain and add a twist of lemon juice. It can be drunk 'neat' or diluted a little. Barley malt can be added for sweetness.

Primary actions	Primary influences	Contra-indications
■ Qi ■ Blood	□ Lung	□ Qi def
□ Yin □ Yang	■ Intestines	□ Blood def
■ Damp	■ Stomach	□ Yin def
□ Phlegm	■ Spleen	□ Yang def
■ Water	□ Heart	□ Damp
□ Qi stagnation	□ Bladder	□ Stagnation
□ Blood stagnation	□ Kidney	□ Heat
■ Heat	■ Gall bladder	□ Cold
□ Cold	■ Liver	□ Wind invasion
□ Wind heat		
□ Wind cold	**Temperature**	
□ Wind damp	■ Cooling	
□ Dryness	□ Neutral	
	□ Warming	

Energetics

Barley water is a traditional remedy for all conditions of Damp Heat, especially when it is focused in the genitourinary system or the Liver. It will also soothe the Intestines, strengthen the Spleen and cool the Blood.

Chai

This version of chai is not the caustic throat-stripper served on every street corner in India. Instead here is a blended tea that will enliven, delight and refresh. Try it at breakfast for an uplifting start to the day.

Preparation time: 15 mins
Makes 4 cups

Ingredients

1 tablespoon cinnamon bark
1 tablespoon cardamom pods
1 tablespoon dried orange peel
½ tablespoon fresh ginger
½ teaspoon coriander seeds
⅓ teaspoon black peppercorns
5 cloves
2 whole star anise
½ teaspoon black tea leaves
(optional)
1 ½ pints water

Method

Simmer all the ingredients together for 15 minutes with the lid off so that the liquid reduces slightly. A few black tea leaves can also be added. Serve sweetened with honey. A little warmed milk can be added when serving, if desired.

Energetics

Chai stimulates the circulation, warms the body and expels Cold. It also stimulates digestion and supports the Kidney Yang.

Primary actions	Primary influences	Contra-indications
☐ Qi ☐ Blood	■ Lung	☐ Qi def
☐ Yin ■ Yang	☐ Intestines	☐ Blood def
■ Damp	■ Stomach	■ Yin def
■ Phlegm	■ Spleen	☐ Yang def
☐ Water	☐ Heart	☐ Damp
■ Qi stagnation	☐ Bladder	☐ Stagnation
■ Blood stagnation	■ Kidney	■ Heat
☐ Heat	☐ Gall bladder	☐ Cold
■ Cold	☐ Liver	☐ Wind invasion
☐ Wind heat		
☐ Wind cold	**Temperature**	
☐ Wind damp	☐ Cooling	
☐ Dryness	☐ Neutral	
	■ Warming	

Ease Digestion Tea

This is a pleasant, light after-dinner tea. If you have access to fresh herbs, use twice the amount. Fennel can also be substituted for the aniseed.

Preparation time: 5 mins
Makes 3 cups

Ingredients

1 teaspoon basil
1 teaspoon peppermint
1 teaspoon aniseed

Method

Infuse all ingredients in a teapot for 5 minutes.

Primary actions	Primary influences	Contra-indications
☐ Qi ☐ Blood	■ Lung	☐ Qi def
☐ Yin ☐ Yang	☐ Intestines	☐ Blood def
■ Damp	■ Stomach	☐ Yin def
■ Phlegm	■ Spleen	☐ Yang def
☐ Water	☐ Heart	☐ Damp
■ Qi stagnation	☐ Bladder	☐ Stagnation
☐ Blood stagnation	☐ Kidney	☐ Heat
☐ Heat	☐ Gall bladder	☐ Cold
☐ Cold	☐ Liver	☐ Wind invasion
☐ Wind heat	**Temperature**	
☐ Wind cold	☐ Cooling	
☐ Wind damp	■ Neutral	
☐ Dryness	☐ Warming	

Energetics

All three herbs counter nausea and indigestion, or rebellious Stomach Qi as it is known in Chinese medicine. This tea will also stimulate the Lung, resolve Phlegm and clear the sinuses.

Hom

This is a very satisfying and soothing drink highly treasured in the Ayurvedic tradition. It is best drunk as a meal by itself or as an in-between meals snack. It can be drunk in the evening to promote good sleep.

Preparation time: 10 mins
Serves: 2

Ingredients

20–30 almonds
2 cups milk
1 teaspoon honey
6 cardamom pods, lightly crushed
Good pinch fresh black pepper

Method

The almonds are best if soaked for 36 hours, then the skins rub off easily and the almonds have begun to release more of their goodness. (If you are in a rush, simply blanch and peel the almonds). Heat the milk gently with the spices and simmer for a few minutes, then bring to a quick boil and remove from heat. Strain out the cardamom pods. Blend with the almonds and honey in a whizzer and serve warm.

Primary actions	Primary influences	Contra-indications
■ Qi ■ Blood	■ Lung	□ Qi def
■ Yin □ Yang	■ Intestines	□ Blood def
□ Damp	□ Stomach	□ Yin def
□ Phlegm	□ Spleen	□ Yang def
□ Water	□ Heart	■ Damp
□ Qi stagnation	□ Bladder	□ Stagnation
□ Blood stagnation	□ Kidney	□ Heat
	□ Gall bladder	□ Cold
□ Heat	□ Liver	□ Wind invasion
□ Cold		
□ Wind heat	**Temperature**	
□ Wind cold	□ Cooling	
□ Wind damp	■ Neutral	
■ Dryness	□ Warming	

Energetics

Almonds strengthen the Qi of the Lung and help in the transformation of Phlegm. Milk is a general Qi tonic with a special affinity for the Lung. Together they provide a strong Lung Qi and Yin tonic. Both almonds and milk will also lubricate the Intestines. The moisture-generating nature of the milk is moderated by the spices which counteract Dampness and by heating which improves its digestibility. However, Hom is not recommended for Damp conditions or when there is diarrhoea.

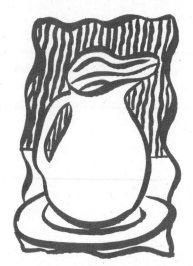

Lassi

Lassi is a simple and quick drink from India that serves as a nutritious snack. This is a sweet version but salted lassi is also very popular. Lassi is probably the ancestor of the modern 'smoothie'.

Preparation time: 1 min

Ingredients

1 part plain yoghurt
3 parts water
A few drops rose essence
Honey to sweeten

Method

The ingredients are simply combined and beaten until blended. There is plenty of scope for experimenting with different additions such as mint or various ground spices.

(To make smoothies simply reduce the water to one part, omit the rose essence and add one part fruit. Any soft fruit will do and bananas make an especially good base. Here too is plenty of scope for experiment.)

Energetics

Yoghurt is cooling and nourishing for the Yin and Qi. It is also beneficial for the Intestines.

Primary actions	Primary influences	Contra-indications
■ Qi □ Blood	■ Lung	□ Qi def
■ Yin □ Yang	■ Intestines	□ Blood def
□ Damp	□ Stomach	□ Yin def
□ Phlegm	□ Spleen	■ Yang def
□ Water	□ Heart	■ Damp
□ Qi stagnation	□ Bladder	□ Stagnation
□ Blood stagnation	□ Kidney	□ Heat
	□ Gall bladder	■ Cold
■ Heat	□ Liver	□ Wind invasion
□ Cold		
□ Wind heat	**Temperature**	
□ Wind cold	■ Cooling	
□ Wind damp	□ Neutral	
■ Dryness	□ Warming	

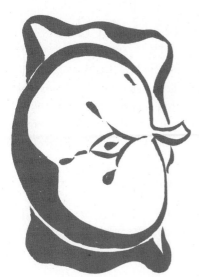

Summer Cooler

This is a cooling, refreshing tea, perfect for a hot summer's day. It is also helpful during feverish illnesses.

Preparation time: 5 mins
Makes 4 cups

Ingredients

1 teaspoon peppermint
2 teaspoons rosehip
1 tablespoon concentrated apple juice
One pint water
Lemon juice to taste

Method

Pour boiling water over the herbs and brew for 5 minutes. Pour in the concentrated apple juice just before serving and add lemon juice to taste.

Energetics

This is a simple cooling drink for hot conditions. It will cool an overheated Stomach or Liver and is ideal for conditions of Summer Heat.

Primary actions	Primary influences	Contra-indications
☐ Qi ☐ Blood	■ Lung	☐ Qi def
☐ Yin ☐ Yang	☐ Intestines	☐ Blood def
☐ Damp	☐ Stomach	☐ Yin def
☐ Phlegm	☐ Spleen	☐ Yang def
■ Water	☐ Heart	☐ Damp
☐ Qi stagnation	■ Bladder	☐ Stagnation
☐ Blood stagnation	■ Kidney	☐ Heat
■ Heat	☐ Gall bladder	■ Cold
☐ Cold	■ Liver	☐ Wind invasion
☐ Wind heat		
☐ Wind cold	**Temperature**	
☐ Wind damp	■ Cooling	
☐ Dryness	☐ Neutral	
	☐ Warming	

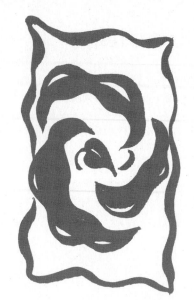

Tea for Wind Cold

You may well be raising your eyebrows at this tea and rightly so: it is not for the faint-hearted. But when you feel shivery, cold and know that you are going down with a cold or flu, this tea is may yet save the day. Make several strong cups, drink up and then crawl under the bedclothes to sweat it out.

Preparation time: 10 mins
Makes 2 cups

Ingredients

2 teaspoons fresh ginger
1 teaspoon cinnamon bark
1 clove garlic
1 spring onion
¹/₄ teaspoon cayenne pepper
2 cups water

Method

Simmer the ginger and cinnamon for 10 minutes, adding the chopped spring onion, garlic and cayenne pepper just before the end. Sweeten with a little honey if desired.

Primary actions	Primary influences	Contra-indications
☐ Qi ☐ Blood	■ Lung	☐ Qi def
☐ Yin ■ Yang	☐ Intestines	☐ Blood def
☐ Damp	☐ Stomach	☐ Yin def
☐ Phlegm	☐ Spleen	☐ Yang def
☐ Water	☐ Heart	☐ Damp
☐ Qi stagnation	☐ Bladder	☐ Stagnation
☐ Blood stagnation	■ Kidney	☐ Heat
☐ Heat	☐ Gall bladder	☐ Cold
☐ Cold	☐ Liver	☐ Wind invasion
☐ Wind heat		
■ Wind cold	**Temperature**	
■ Wind damp	☐ Cooling	
☐ Dryness	☐ Neutral	
	■ Warming	

Energetics

These are very heating herbs which drive Cold out of the body and 'release the exterior'. Pungent and heating, they are the perfect match for invasions of Wind Cold.

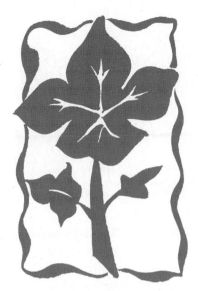

Tea for Wind Heat

Definitely the tea for the feverish beginnings of flu or colds. It has the added bonus of being very pleasant.

Preparation time: 5 mins
Makes 3 cups

Ingredients

1 teaspoon peppermint
1 teaspoon elderflower
1 teaspoon yarrow
3 cups water

Method

Pour boiling water over the leaves and leave to steep for 5 minutes.

Primary actions	Primary influences	Contra-indications
☐ Qi ☐ Blood	■ Lung	☐ Qi def
☐ Yin ☐ Yang	☐ Intestines	☐ Blood def
☐ Damp	☐ Stomach	☐ Yin def
☐ Phlegm	☐ Spleen	☐ Yang def
☐ Water	☐ Heart	☐ Damp
☐ Qi stagnation	☐ Bladder	☐ Stagnation
☐ Blood stagnation	☐ Kidney	☐ Heat
☐ Heat	☐ Gall bladder	☐ Cold
☐ Cold	☐ Liver	☐ Wind invasion
■ Wind heat		
☐ Wind cold	**Temperature**	
■ Wind damp	■ Cooling	
☐ Dryness	☐ Neutral	
	☐ Warming	

Energetics

This tea 'releases the exterior', allowing invading pathogens to leave the body. The pungent flavour of the herbs pushes the invaders away and stops them from penetrating more deeply. This is a classic tea for the onset of colds or flu manifesting with hot symptoms.

How to Create a Self-Healing Recipe

Cooking according to one's own condition can be a fun and creative process. To engage with food, bringing attention and creativity into this central aspect of life, is itself an act of healing. To open to the delight of good food and to celebrate its miracles helps us open to life itself.

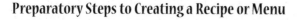

This book is as much about encouraging you to create your own delicious recipes as it is about providing them ready-made. The basic principles that underlie the recipes chosen for this book are explained here to help you in your own personal healing journey.

Self-healing requires action, practice and consistency – actually preparing and applying a remedy provides a lot more healing impetus than almost any amount of reading

Dylana Accola and Peter Yates, *Back to Balance*

Preparatory Steps to Creating a Recipe or Menu

Step One. The first part of this book helps the reader to understand the various patterns defined by traditional Chinese medicine. To create personal recipes it is important first to understand one's condition and the general approach to eating that best supports healing. These principles include the general eating style that is most appropriate and the various temperatures, flavours and types of food that are helpful. The first step is therefore to read about and determine the particular condition, then to assimilate the essential principles.

For example, when working with a condition of Spleen Qi Deficiency, the important principles are the use of well-prepared foods, mostly cooked, which are easy on the digestion. Soups, stews and casseroles are helpful methods whereas raw and cold foods are to be favoured less. Food needs to be mostly sweet in flavour and slightly warm with support from aromatic and mildly pungent flavours. A grain and vegetable based diet is ideal with the use of foods high in complex carbohydrates such as yams and root vegetables.

(As this book is not designed as a diagnostic aid and if you are not already familiar with traditional Chinese medicine, I recommend that you visit a qualified practitioner to understand the patterns that you are working with in your life at this time. Even as an experienced practitioner, I value and use the perceptions of other practitioners to help me see more clearly the landscape of my own being.)

Step Two. The second step is to become familiar with the natures of various foods: their temperatures, flavours and actions. These have been touched on briefly in this book and are listed on the wallchart (available from Meridian Press) and in its companion manual 'Helping Ourselves'. Foods can be selected from these sources to form a basis for individual recipes. As you become more attuned to the energetics of food, you will develop a body-knowing about a food's properties which will help you sense the properties of foods not listed in the current literature on food energetics.

Step Three. Once the range of appropriate foods and cooking methods has been established, the creative process of recipe-making can begin. The condition in question indicates the overall direction the diet needs to take. However, this is a question of merely tilting the balance in one favoured direction, not the pursuit of one direction at the expense of everything else. A recipe can be supported by several ingredients that tilt the meal in the same direction but that direction also needs to be moderated, held in dynamic balance by the inclusion of some foods and flavours with counterbalancing properties.

For example, lamb may be chosen as a main ingredient to generate warmth and support the Yang of the body. It may be roasted (to enhance the warming quality) with rosemary (a Yang strengthening herb), and accompanied by several warming root vegetables. To create a dynamic balance, this meal can be served with a light green salad which is cool and Damp-resolving or with apple sauce which is also cool. The overall balance – one main direction moderated by a smaller amount of foods that have opposite actions – is more effective and safer than the total exclusion of all opposite-natured foods.

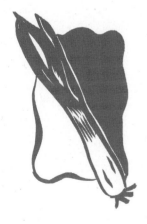

Step Four. It is important to remember that there is no one label which successfully describes the totality of one's needs. It is possible to express several different, even conflicting, patterns at the same time. For example, a person may express signs of Yang Deficiency concurrently with signs of Yin Deficiency. When the patterns appear complex it is better to meet them with simplicity rather than try to match them in their complexity. A simple wholefood diet with a wide variety of organic vegetables, fruits and a moderate amount of good quality protein (a common sense approach to food) will benefit almost any condition. It is far more important that we relax and enjoy our food than it is to cleverly concoct sophisticated recipes to heal our every ill. When the patterns appear complex it is often time to simplify and listen gently to what our bodies are saying.

Complex patterns may also demand that we prioritise. Which pattern is the deepest? Sometimes, when Yin and Yang Deficiency co-exist, we can address the more pronounced of the two patterns and the other may also begin to resolve. If, for example, Yin Deficiency is the deeper pattern, a Yin strengthening diet will provide better quality 'fuel' which in turn enables the Yang to be stronger. In the reverse case, a Yang supportive diet will increase digestive efficiency and so enable the Yin to be better nourished.

The decision of what to support also depends on a person's relative strength. When, for example, there is Spleen Qi Deficiency and chronic Dampness we must assess how much direct reduction of the Dampness a person's system can tolerate. A balanced decision is made about supporting the strength of the Spleen on the one hand and reducing Dampness on the other. The overuse of Damp-resolving foods or herbs may be too much for a person when they are weak.

To make this example more concrete we can imagine two people each presenting with Dampness. The first person is robust and energetic with a huge appetite for food and for life. She presents with Dampness that comes from overconsumption of rich food and beer. The second person is exhausted with a post-viral illness. His Dampness is the result of the body's inability to transform even the more modest diet he is eating. In the first case more emphasis can be given to Damp-resolving foods and a restricted diet. In the second more emphasis needs to be given to strengthening the body to increase its ability to transform food into nourishment.

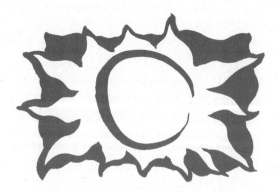

A step by step example:

'Spleen Yang Deficiency'

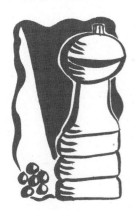

- This three word diagnostic label indicates a need to nourish Deficiency, strengthen the Yang and support the Spleen. Deficiency is nourished through the use of sweet foods; the Yang is strengthened through the use of warming cooking methods and warm-natured foods with some use of the pungent flavour; the Spleen is supported through eating easily-digested, sweet-flavoured foods with help from aromatic and pungent flavours. We also know that cold or chilled foods may worsen the condition and that bitter and sour flavours will tend to move the diet in the opposite direction. Knowing these things, the kinds of foods and cooking methods become clear. The ingredients chosen need to be mostly warming in temperature as do the cooking methods. Casseroles and stews would be good choices. Grains and root vegetables offer good support to the Spleen. Warm foods and some pungent flavours strengthen the Yang.

- Create a list of foods which are both warming and supportive of the Spleen. These include oats, chicken, squash, sweet rice, sweet potato, date, chestnut, aniseed, caraway, ginger, garlic and molasses. Also note the various foods which have a reputation for strengthening the Yang such as cinnamon, lamb, rosemary, trout, walnut, shrimp. These will be given an important place in the creation of a recipe or menu.

- Now devise recipes around some of these ingredients, e.g., chicken stewed with sweet potato, ginger and garlic; or porridge flavoured with molasses and sprinkled with walnuts; or chestnuts roasted with rosemary. This is the time to let creativity soar. These recipes can be balanced by the inclusion of a few opposite-flavoured foods, e.g., lemon can be added to a chicken stew. Various complementary or balancing dishes can be chosen as accompaniments, e.g., the chicken stew can be supported by rice cooked with aromatic and warming spices and balanced by the inclusion of a few button mushrooms which are cool in nature.

The principles are not complicated. The central ingredient of the recipe can be:

(1) supported by foods of similar properties

(2) complemented by foods of harmonious properties

(3) balanced by foods of opposite properties.

For example:

Pumpkin and Chestnut Soup
for Spleen Yang Deficiency

Pumpkin five parts

Potato one part

Carrot one part

Onion one part

Chestnut two parts

Cinnamon

Pepper

Lemon

The main ingredient, pumpkin, is sweet and warm. It supports the Spleen and helps resolve Dampness. It is supported in this action by the chestnut which is also sweet and warm and additionally has the complementary action of strengthening the Yang. The potato and carrot lend support by strengthening the Spleen Qi and the carrot has a complementary action of strengthening Blood. The onion brings movement, a complementary action to counteract Stagnation. The cinnamon and black pepper reinforce the Yang-strengthening effect. A twist of lemon in each bowl as the soup is served provides a counterbalance.

Each recipe in the recipe section of this book has a similar description of its actions. It is a simple matter to substitute various ingredients either because they are not to hand or because you want to tilt the recipe in a particular direction. Again I encourage you to be creative and have fun with cooking. The final judgment of whether a recipe works or not is in the body's response to it. Use your own body as a kind of 'tuning fork' to feel the resonance of each meal that you create. My sincere hope is that this book will awaken a lasting habit of listening to your own body-knowing.

> **Each person carries his own doctor inside him....we are at our best when we give the doctor who resides within each patient a chance to go to work**
>
> **Albert Schweizer**

Part Four
Leftovers

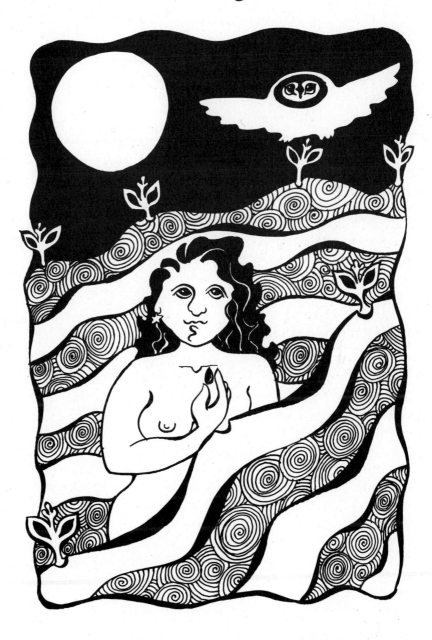

There is such a thing as
food and such a thing as
poison. But the damage
done by those who pass
off poison as food is far
less than that done by
those who generation
after generation convince
people that food is poison

Paul Goodman

Coffee and Tea

Coffee is interesting energetically. Though it initially releases heat very fast and efficiently into the system, it is quickly spent. Its effect is to liberate heat without giving the means to generate more. Ultimately coffee appears to rob us of heat, leaving us cold inside. It opens the door to the furnace rather than stokes the furnace itself. It may be a question of quantity: a little behaves in much the same way as a Yang tonic, a lot is Cold medicine which weakens the Yang.

Coffee is not without benefits. It does stimulate the digestive system, helps to break down Stagnation and Dampness, and activates the brain. It also stimulates bowel movement and diuresis. A little coffee will benefit the person who is Stagnant, Damp or Yang Deficient. Those who are Yin or Blood Deficient should be very careful with it. 'Coffee is cold and dry,' says Hajji Khalifat writing in Turkey in 1635, 'for its heat is a strange heat with no effect.....By its dryness coffee repels sleep. To those of a moist temperament it is highly suited'.

Like alcohol, coffee has been the target of many prohibition movements. Charles II tried unsuccessfully to ban it in England; in the seventeenth century women led a movement against 'the excessive use of that drying and enfeebling liquor that does so enfeeble our men'; it was even banned in Turkey around the same time. As a recreational, mood-altering drug it has a long history and probably is better recognised for this special status. Perhaps we should declare it sacred, reserve it for special occasions and drink each cup with reverence!

In small quantities tea is a great digestive stimulant and helps in the breakdown of Dampness and Phlegm. It refreshes the spirit and helps move Stagnation. Energetically, tea is cool so is less suitable for Cold people and generally is less suitable for Deficient conditions. In the large quantities and strength that we drink it today tea tends to be weakening, especially to the Kidney and Bladder Qi, and too much strong tea can actually cause Phlegm. It weakens through the chronic overstimulation of the nervous system. It tends to make the kidneys hard and contracted, leaches some vitamins and minerals and blocks the absorption of protein on its journey through the body.

Cool/Deficient types will find that mixing warming spices such as cardamom and cinnamon with their black tea will somewhat counteract its cooling effect as well as increase its Damp-resolving properties. Generally the larger the leaf, the less damaging the tea; cheap commercial tea which releases its brown colour almost instantly is the most suspect. Green teas and the various twig teas have a much better benefit/damage ratio.

Stimulants are generally tolerated better during the morning which is seen as the Yang part of the day, suited to greater stimulus and energy release. It is also worth noting that women are more vulnerable to the negative effects of coffee than men, and its consumption should be carefully regulated whenever there are malign developments in the breasts and reproductive organs.

Alcohol

Alcohol has a time-honoured place in the celebration of human life. Books about health often discourage the use of alcohol because of the potentially life-threatening nature of alcohol abuse. But just like tea and coffee, when treated with respect, alcohol can be an enjoyable and beneficial part of a healthy lifestyle.

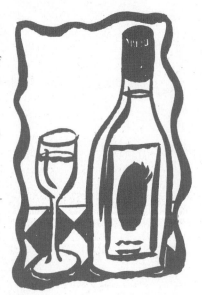

Energetically, alcohol is warm, becoming warmer the more concentrated it is. Beer is the coolest, wine somewhere in the middle and spirits at the top end. Beer's flavour is bitter and sweet and generally we can say that the more the bitter flavour predominates the less Dampening the beer will be. Darker beers have somewhat more nutritional value and can nourish the Blood. Overconsumption of beer tends to overwhelm the Spleen and Kidneys and create a mixed pattern of Heat and Cold in the body (the alcohol creates pockets of Heat, the sheer volume of fluid douses the fire of the lower body). As beer is very Dampening it is best restricted by those with Damp constitutions or conditions. Seasonally, it is better drunk in summer as it can be too cooling during the winter.

Drink a glass of wine after your soup and you steal a rouble from your doctor

Russian proverb

Wine is energetically warm, red wine being warmer than white. Its flavour includes sweet, sour and bitter. An occasional glass of wine for many people is a relaxant, helping to move Stagnation and stimulate the circulation of Blood and Qi. It is a helpful accompaniment to heavy meals. Mulled with spices it can be an effective remover of Cold from the body; infused with medicinal herbs, wine serves as an excellent carrier of the herbs' tonic effect. Red wine is also mildly nourishing to the Blood. In cooking, wine can add heat to a dish.

Spirits are to be handled with more caution. They are potent Stagnation movers but easily become toxic to the body. Overconsumption will stress the Liver and lead to the accumulation of Heat.

How much is too much? This really depends on the strength of a person's constitution and their lifestyle. A strong person leading an active life can tolerate more than a weaker person, and some people can not tolerate alcohol at all.

Sugar

In traditional cultures sugar or intensely sweet foods were reserved for times of significant celebration as were most intoxicants. In today's western culture, addicted to 'feelgood' sensations, sugar ('the great white death') has become our most popular drug, finding its way into almost everyone's diet. The constant sugar high on which our culture lives overlies our avoidance of deeper

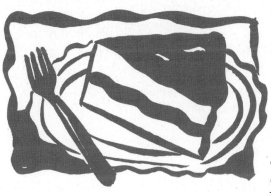

feelings, our cultural diseases of niceness, sentimentality and other forms of removal from the raw experience of life. Sugar is used as a substitute for love and satisfaction, a filler of voids with its corollary of the 'sugar blues'.

From a western point of view, sugar overstimulates the pancreas and exhausts the adrenals, leaches some minerals (specifically, upsetting the phosphorus/calcium balance causing excretion of calcium supplies) and upsets the protein/carbohydrate balance. Its overconsumption is a major cause of immune weakness and allergy. In Chinese medicine we describe this as overwhelming the Spleen and draining the Kidney. Overuse of sugar will also weaken the Blood and tend to produce both Heat and Dampness. It is a powerful substance which can easily destabilise, creating swings in energy and moods.

Because sugar is so pervasive in our diets it is not something we can avoid without adopting quite extreme and restrictive practices. In my view the best we can do is become more aware of what the body experiences with intake of sugar, and only eat as much as we know can be tolerated. The place for sugar seems to me to be times of celebration. There is also a role for sugar as a carrier of the effects of certain medicines. In cookery, sugar is sometimes used to harmonise other flavours.

White sugar is one of the great dietary disasters of our age, far too sweet and too sudden for the body to handle in more than the smallest quantity. To be weaned away from white sugar the palate needs to be reeducated to enjoy the darker sugars and molasses, the date and malt extracts, honey and so on, which are nutritionally more acceptable. But whatever the source, too much condensed sweetness is overwhelming to the Spleen and is the root of many physical and psychic disorders.

Some helpful ways to regulate sugar intake:

- Presoaking foods and using longer, slow-cooking methods will release more of a food's natural sweetness.

- Well-chewed food will also release more of its sweetness.

- Eating adequate amounts of complex carbohydrates will ensure more sustained release of sugars into the bloodstream.

- The inclusion of more dark greens and bitter foods will reduce sweet cravings and replenish some of the leached nutrients.

- Drinking a glass of water when craving sugar will often significantly reduce the hankering for something sweet. Often sugar cravings are actually a sign of dehydration.

- Establishing regular eating habits can also help regulate sugar craving with sweet treats made from natural unsugared ingredients on standby for those important moments when something sweet is the perfect thing.

One day a mother brought her young son to see Mahatma Ghandi and asked if he would please tell her child to stop eating sugar. 'Come back in a week,' said Ghandi. Puzzled, she went away and came back a week later as asked. Then Ghandi did what the woman had originally asked and advised the young boy to stop eating sugar. Afterwards, the woman asked him why he had delayed. 'Oh,' he answered, 'first I had to give up sugar.'

Dairy

Dairy foods are a rich source of nourishment although far more problematic for the human digestive system than most other foods. Dairy will not suit everybody, and in some cases it is best avoided altogether. However, given that it occupies such a prominent place in the western diet it is worth looking at certain considerations here.

About 20% of Caucasian people and 80% of Asian and Black people are lactose intolerant. The enzymes present in the human body in its early years sometimes stop being produced in early childhood. Lactose intolerance shows initially as digestive disturbance such as diarrhoea, flatulence and cramping. Later it may be the cause of many Damp conditions and cause major obstruction and difficulty in the whole body. There may be allergic reactions to milk with chronic inflammation of the lungs' mucus membranes, runny nose, sore throat and ear infections.

Despite its reputation as a source of calcium and its recommendation as preventative for osteoporosis, milk's high protein content and its disproportionate phosphorus/calcium ratio makes it at best a dubious source. Milk is more likely to increase the rate at which calcium is excreted from the body, overtaxing the kidneys. Statistically the countries with the highest milk consumption (the USA and Scandinavia) have the highest osteoporosis rates in the world[40].

If the system is overburdened by milk it will store those products it can't eliminate. Milk is frequently the cause of calcium deposits in the kidneys, leading to kidney stones, especially when fortified milk is consumed. Women's reproductive organs are also highly vulnerable and dairy consumption is frequently linked to cysts, to various kinds of obstruction of the menstrual cycle and to infertility. In Chinese medicine this is described as the build-up of Dampness or Phlegm.

The fat content of milk has recently been targeted as a cause for concern. However, cow's milk has less fat than human breast milk and the removal of fat to make low-fat milk is probably misguided.

Removing the fat imbalances the food and increases the chances of adverse reactions in the body. When the level of fat is reduced the level of protein is relatively increased which in turn overtaxes the kidneys. The butterfat in milk is actually necessary to properly digest its protein content. Other practices such as pasteurisation, homogenisation and heat treatment further damage the milk and make it less digestible. Under no circumstances should low-fat or fortified milk be given to young children and babies.

Contamination is also an issue. The presence of antibiotics and growth hormones in milk may further increase the likelihood of reactions and some of the more obscene practices of modern farming, such as feeding other animal parts to cattle, has already resulted in death and maiming. Organophosphates used to treat warble fly in cattle may also impact the human nervous system.

With these considerations in mind, what is the best approach to dairy consumption in a western diet? The good news is that naturally soured dairy products such as yoghurt, kefir or buttermilk are more easily digested by most people as are moderate amounts of raw milk. Despite dairy's Dampening nature it does have a useful place. For the Yin Deficient and Dry constitution it is especially helpful and it is useful in convalescence from debilitating, Yin-depleting illness such as tuberculosis.

- Favour certified raw organic whole milk over other kinds. This has the added advantage of avoiding the consumption of lactation-promoting hormones, accumulated pesticide residues, antibiotics, mucus and other unsavoury ingredients commonly found in commercial cow's milk. Cancer-inducing viruses have also been found[41] and dairy farmers, interestingly, have the highest rate of leukemia of any occupational group.

- Use naturally fermented or soured milk products, especially in cases of lactose intolerance.

- Favour goat or sheep products if there is a tendency towards Dampness.

- Use dairy more for conditions of Blood, Qi and Yin Deficiency and less for Yang Deficient, Damp or Stagnant conditions.

- Reduce or avoid dairy when the Spleen Qi is weak and there is a tendency for mucus to accumulate in the Lung.

- If pasteurised milk is used, it is best brought to the boil then cooled slightly to be drunk warm. Cardamom, ginger, garlic and honey are beneficial added ingredients. Heating milk with a slice of raw onion in the bottom of the pan will also reduce its Dampening effects.

- Combine dairy with decongesting foods such as vegetables and fruit.

- Avoid combining dairy with meat as this is excessively Dampening.

- Avoid homogenised milk altogether as it leads to increased fatty deposits in the arteries.

- If using soya milk as an alternative, note that whereas dairy enters the Lung channel, soya milk goes to the Spleen and is somewhat less Dampening. However, in excess, soya milk will also produce Phlegm.

Vegetarianism

To be or not to be a vegetarian? I would like to rephrase that question as 'what proportion of meat in the diet can be considered healthy?' and I would like to set the question in the context of both personal and planetary health. So what are the considerations?

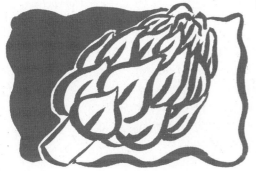

From the viewpoint of Gaia it appears to be a natural law that many animals eat other animals. This is part of the natural ecology that maintains balance. There is much debate about whether humans were originally vegetarians but the reality is that now most cultures are omnivorous. The question is whether we eat within the laws of ecology or whether we choose to disrespect them. When the planet is pushed into oversupporting meat production, the price is starvation in poorer parts of the planet.

Quite clearly our western meat-eating habits cause vast distortions of the planet's ecology. Most agricultural land in the USA is used to produce food for livestock and it is estimated that if Americans alone reduced their national meat intake by 10% enough grain could be saved to feed 60 million people. From my early experiences as a farmer I know that some land is hard to grow crops on and best used for sheep grazing and that the raising of livestock can complement the growth of grains, vegetables and fruits.

From the viewpoint of personal health some of the following considerations are helpful. First, note that the protein content of human breast milk is 5%. This alone suggests that our anxieties about receiving sufficient protein may be unnecessary. From a nutritional point of view proteins are most easily and effectively assimilated when they comprise about 10% of any meal.

In western terms, two major considerations regarding protein consumption are the oxygen balance, and the acid/alkaline balance. Oxygen accomplishes many of the tasks assigned to Qi in the body and it provides most (perhaps 90%) of the metabolic energy. Within our diets the most oxygen-rich foods are vegetables, sprouts, fruits, grains, nuts and seeds. The lowest levels of oxygen are found in meat and fats. Nutrients are more concentrated in denser foods. From the point of view of oxygen availability it would seem that a relatively small proportion of our food should consist of meat and fat.

In terms of acid and alkaline, the body maintains a pH level of around 7.4 despite our attempts to sabotage it! This is because a few points either way will result in death. In order to support the body in maintaining its pH balance we need to eat a generally alkalising diet. Acid-forming foods are defined by their mineral composition, not whether or not they taste acidic. Lemons, for example, are alkalising. Meat, dairy, sugar and most proteins are acid forming, although yoghurt and raw milk are slightly alkalising. Soya beans, tofu, Kidney beans, aduki beans, almonds, brazils, green corn and millet are exceptions to this tendency. Coffee is also acid-forming. So again we see that meat is best moderated by high intake of typically 'vegetarian' food.

Modern western nutritionists encourage a very low intake of meat and dairy because of the potentially negative impact they have on our health. From the oriental point of view, meat and dairy are highly respected as nutritious foods and it is for this reason that they are generally eaten in small quantities. Meat is seen as 'healthy' provided it is eaten in proportion. An overconsumption of meat results in the accumulation of Dampness and often Heat. An

I do not ask devotees not to eat meat. If meat suits someone's body, helping it to be strong, then eating it is not wrong. In general, if something suits your body, then you should eat it. To be spiritual it is not necessary to destroy all desire. The fulfilment of those desires that strengthen you and make others happy is good. Which desires should be fulfilled varies from person to person

Mother Meera

often-quoted 'ballpark' figure for meat consumption is two ounces of meat eaten three times a week.

We must add to this picture the problem of toxic accumulation from modern industrial farming practices. Unless it is organically reared, all meat adds a toxic burden to the body that is the price of its nutritional value. This is especially true of beef, pork and chicken. When the animals are intensively reared by inhumane methods, such as calves are for veal, there is also a psychic burden which we receive through the meat. Lamb, venison and game are likely to be less toxic.

For many people, opening their awareness to receive the pain of the animal reared for meat is unbearable and they turn to vegetarianism. Others continue to eat meat in the spirit of reverence and thanks. Many rarely give it a thought and yet remain relatively healthy. My own view is that meat eaten with awareness, from a place of informed choice, is a perfectly healthy practice and for some people a very necessary one. Having spent eighteen years of my own life as a vegetarian in a gesture to rebalance a world gone crazy, I also know that a vegetarian diet supported me well enough. There is clearly no 'right' or 'wrong' position here.

For those who choose vegetarianism as their dietary path I would like to add one or two words of advice: without the quick fix of meat it is important to give more attention to balancing the diet and including good quality vegetable protein. The system will also be more clean on a good vegetarian diet. This means that imbalance will be registered more easily. Vegetarians are therefore advised to be especially careful with sugar and caffeine which meat eaters will tolerate more easily. In fact, there is often a tendency to binge on sugar and starch to compensate for the lack of animal fats and protein. For those new to nutritional ideas there are many excellent books available on the vegetarian diet and I recommend becoming as informed as possible.

Lastly, vegetarianism is best supported by spiritual belief, a trust that all necessary nourishment is available through our relationship with the divine. When we investigate our beliefs as vegetarians, we often find places of denial, places in the psyche that crave meat, that repress meat-eating as part of a more deep suppression of the life force. I encourage the exploration of these places so that ultimately one might embrace a more full and life-

From what I've seen, vegetarianism works best when accompanied by a deeply felt spiritual commitment. When spirit and emotion support a diet devoid of animal products (or with dairy only), our bodies seem perfectly able to extract and transform all the nutrients they need for maintenance and repair from plant products. Vegetarianism does not appear to have equally positive effects when embarked upon solely for 'sensible' reasons of health; if passion and emotion are not involved, we seem to be less efficient at processing vegetable matter, and symptoms of insufficiency may result after a number of years. Moreover, if the diet doesn't work, intellectual reasoning or ideology may at times block our awareness of the signals given out by our body indicating distress or discomfort

Annemarie Colbin,
Food and Healing

affirming vegetarian practice. It is my experience that those whose vegetarianism is supported by positive life-affirming beliefs rather than guilt and denial, or even the retreat from pain, generally maintain full vitality. When vegetarianism is ensnared in righteous anger or suppression of instinct, it is rarely supportive of full vitality. A healthy vegetarianism is rooted in the practice of listening to the body and mediating with the realities of today's world.

Raw Food

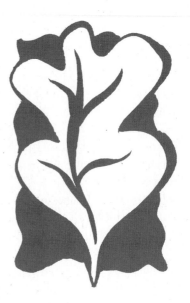

Cooking is a kind of alchemy. Through the use of fire and the skilful mixing of herbs and spices, food is made ready to be transformed into nourishment within our bodies. Although to the purist, cooking may seem an unnatural act unique to the human being, generations of experience have established that cooking food liberates its potential for nourishment more effectively than eating it raw.

To cook or not to cook is a debate that persists so it is worth considering it briefly here. Raw food is essentially cool, cleansing and slightly more sour than when it is cooked. It is very effective at purging excess Heat from the body and cleansing the Liver. In these days of high toxicity raw food is finding a stronger place in our eating patterns once again. The important consideration is who benefits from raw food.

Those prone to Heat and toxicity benefit from raw food, at least until the patterns of Heat and toxicity are resolved. Everyone can to some extent benefit from the inclusion of some raw food provided it is well chewed. Those tending towards Deficiency and Cold, however, should be careful as too much raw food will worsen their condition. It is not possible to say how much is acceptable as this will vary from person to person and will also depend on climate and season. Spring and summer are generally times when raw food is more easily tolerated.

It is not a question of raw food being good or bad in itself. Raw food is wonderful: it is simply a question of how much and for whom. Although Chinese cooking makes little use of raw food, this is in part because of the danger of parasites and considerations of hygiene and it is always a mistake to try to import one culture's eating habits into another without adapting them for climate and tradition. My own view is that everyone can benefit from a little raw food and that it would be a sad loss not to enjoy the taste of a fresh apple or fresh herbs and leaves.

Pregnancy

The ten lunar months of pregnancy are clearly a special time in a woman's life. Despite the multitude of dietary advice offered regarding the nutrients which will be needed to ensure a healthy pregnancy, the best approach, where possible, is to maintain a sensible, healthy diet and to trust the body wisdom that is intensified during this time. Supplements are helpful in some cases, but not necessary if the diet is good and the woman is reasonably well.

Some special considerations may be helpful:

'Eating for Two'. To overeat during pregnancy is a mistake, especially if this means eating more quick-fix carbohydrates. It is natural to eat more, but quality is far more important than quantity. In particular it is important to eat more dark green vegetables and good quality protein sources. In the later stages of pregnancy it may be easier to eat several smaller meals during the day to help bridge any drops in sugar level.

It is natural for the energy of the Spleen, Kidney and Liver to be slightly lower than usual during pregnancy. Their energy is being drawn on to nourish the developing child. Whilst it is important to maintain their strength, it is not usually advisable to over-tonify as this may result in rejection of the foetus/embryo. For this reason heavy supplementation is not usually advised.

Pregnancy is also a time when the mother detoxifies more strongly than at other times. Drastic changes to the diet may result in too much toxicity being released at once so all dietary change should be gradual, ideally beginning before conception. Avoidance of toxins will occur instinctively in the mother and needs to be honoured. It is helpful to review such things as air quality, water purity and chemicals generally entering the diet. Sudden exposure of the developing child to toxins, e.g., through a spell of heavy alco-

hol consumption, can be as damaging as lower level, more chronic exposure, so consistent moderation is the best approach.

Following the principles of minimal intervention will obviously lead to avoidance of the use of antibiotics, aspirin, antacids or any other drugs that may be used during pregnancy. Many of these drugs are energetically Cold in nature and may damage the developing child. Cold foods are also to be treated with caution during pregnancy. Caffeinated drinks, sugar, alcohol, saturated fat and recreational or medicinal drugs are all best kept to a minimum. Exposure to extremes of cold, or of heat (such as sauna) are generally to be avoided where possible.

Other kinds of intervention such as scans and electrical monitoring or invasive tests are often unnecessary, and being well-informed and supported by a strong advocate is advisable. Even in techniques as apparently non-invasive as ultrasound, the baby has been shown to move away from the sound waves, suggesting that this procedure is disturbing, at least.

Birth is a time when the mother has another opportunity to detoxify and this is a natural part of the process. During the immediate postpartum stage the cleansing process is supported by keeping to a simple and nourishing diet for a few days. Only when this cleansing process is complete is it advisable to begin the strengthening process to replace the loss of Blood and Qi. Tonifying herbs and a more strengthening diet are begun as soon as the cleansing is complete, to nourish the mother through breast-feeding and the work of motherhood.

Chicken soup is a classic tonic for the immediate postpartum period, fortified with some ginger and the Blood-strengthening herb Dong Quai. During the postpartum period a nursing mother's needs change again. It is normal and healthy to eat more than usual.

There are a few things to avoid during pregnancy and through the lactating period. All foods consumed by the mother will be passed through to some degree to the child. It is therefore best to keep strong stimulants and alcohol to a minimum. Excessive dairy consumption by the mother is a common cause of colic in babies and excessive consumption of oranges sometimes causes hyperactivity. Otherwise it is best to simply eat widely, generously and to enjoy the food.

Alfalfa is one of the most useful postpartum foods as it encourages the production of quality breast milk and increases its flow. A few herbs are also useful: aloe vera has external applications for postnatal conditions such as torn perineum or labia, for haemorrhoids and vaginal yeast infections (as well as being useful for nappy rash!). Internally it is a useful general tonic and it soothes the digestive tract. Like alfalfa, fennel is a helpful tea for increasing the quality and amount of breast milk as well as being helpful for colic. Raspberry leaf is used before and after childbirth to tone the uterus.

An effective postpartum bath can be made from simmering equal parts of uva ursi, shepherd's purse, comfrey root and garlic for a half hour or so. This speeds healing remarkably. Internally a tea of raspberry leaf, shepherd's purse, licorice root, comfrey and false unicorn root is reputed to be a fairly comprehensive healer.

There is not the space in this book to advise more fully on pregnancy and childbirth. Fortunately there are many good books available now, a few of which are listed in the bibliography.

Babies and Children

Children's dietary needs are somewhat different from those of adults. At birth their digestive system is immature, specially geared to digest breast milk and not ready to try out anything else. Generally, a child will let you know when he or she is ready to try out solid foods. When this time comes it is best to keep the foods simple and to introduce foods one at a time and slowly.

At first, simple well-cooked baby rice or oats are usually best, followed by the gradual introduction of cooked and pureed vegetables such as carrot. Carrot is especially useful as it is easy to digest and it also strengthens the Spleen. It is better to choose foods which are not too Cold energetically, as the healthy development of the digestive system depends on its ability to generate warmth. Fruits, which are generally cooling, are best cooked initially and Cold fruits such as bananas or oranges are best avoided at this early stage. Starchy root vegetables are generally well received by most babies, but vegetables of the onion or cabbage family often prove indigestible and tomatoes may cause adverse reactions. When a child's digestion is upset by a food, it is best to withdraw that food for a few weeks and try again later.

If babies are kept to this simple diet for long enough, their digestion will gradually strengthen, enabling them to move on to more complex foods, and they will avoid food Stagnation which is the cause of much early illness. It is often said that almost all childhood diseases of the first six or seven years begin either as emotional distress or as a form of food Stagnation leading to the accumulation of Phlegm. This accumulation of Phlegm leads to many of the familiar childhood illnesses such as respiratory infection, nasal congestion, ear infection, diarrhoea and allergic reactions.

Amongst well-meaning parents it sometimes happens that damage is done by feeding the baby whole foods too early. The harsh bran of whole grains and the roughage of root vegetable or fruit skins can be too scouring for the intestines. It is also worth noting that too much fruit and the use of raw foods will tend to cool and weaken the digestion.

A few more guidelines may be helpful:

· For the first two years at least, food should be well cooked and initially pureed or well mashed. It should also be quite simple.

· Strong flavours are best kept until the digestive system is more mature.

· Refined sweeteners obviously are best avoided and fruit or vegetable juices are best diluted.

· All food is best served warm or at room temperature.

· Flours cause mucus to accumulate and may cause allergic reactions, so are best avoided for the first two years.

· The onion family may be too strong and should be used attentively, watching for any discomfort.

· Honey may be toxic to children under eighteen months.

· Salt is best introduced after the child is a year old.

· Egg white is best avoided for the first year, though egg yolk may be introduced sooner.

Otherwise, common sense is probably the best guide, avoiding the use of sugar and sweeteners, processed foods and chemicals as far as possible. Worrying doesn't help the child so, speaking as a parent myself, I believe that the home we provide and the love and support we give make up for most gaps in the child's diet. Creating a happy relationship with food is a good preparation for adult life, more important than getting stuck on the small details. And despite the well-informed preparations of any parent, a child has a will of its own and will make its own choices about food.

It takes seven years to fully develop the digestive system and for children to reach an awareness of their emotions as separate from themselves. During the first two years in particular, when the digestive system is very immature, it is common for the digestion to be overstrained leading to 'accumulation disorder', a backlog of undigested foods that overwhelms the Spleen and leads to obstruction of the system by Heat and Dampness. To support the Spleen, it is best not to have too many foods combined in one meal. It is also best not to overstimulate a child during and immediately after meal times so that sufficient energy remains available to the Stomach for digestion.

At two years old a child goes through significant transitions, developing a stronger sense of its individuality and testing out its will. Passing feverish illnesses are common as this is a 'hot' phase of development. Children are naturally more 'yang' than most adults and overheating is therefore more common. A decline in appetite is also common around this time. Avoiding sugar and other sweeteners is important as is keeping the relationship with food fun, creative and low on stress.

During the first seven years children are also more susceptible to the emotions of the adults around them and will easily pick up on a parent's feelings, whether these feelings are out in the open or not. By the age of seven most of the patterns of adult life have been prepared. If an enjoyable and relaxed relationship with food has been established during this time then the child is well set up for the future.

Even when good habits have been established in early childhood, adolescence can still be a difficult time nutritionally. Most teenagers, through both peer culture and their high demand for energy, will gravitate towards sugar and erratic eating patterns. Maintaining a high intake of complex carbohydrates in the shape of grains and legumes will help to balance this, as will a higher intake of protein. The demand for vitamins and minerals is also higher so keeping plenty of fruit available and offering teenagers high nutrient foods such as 'smoothies'(see recipe for 'lassi') enriched with fruit, wheatgerm, nuts and brewers yeast is helpful. Young girls have a higher need for iron and will benefit from iron-rich foods such as molasses.

If teenagers cannot be persuaded to look after themselves nutritionally, then it may be worthwhile considering supplements. A food-derived general vitamin and mineral formula would be appropriate. So would chlorella which is the best tolerated of all the various 'green' foods. Otherwise the best parents can do is lead by example, be gentle and creative with advice and, the biggest test of all, relax.

Slimming and Obesity

The slimming industry is big business. This is not surprising in a western culture which is undeniably overweight. However, the slimming industry is more successful at making money than at helping people slim. New products and new diets come and go with varying degrees of success and failure but obesity doesn't go away. In fact, obesity is on the increase in the western world, and in countries which adopt a western way of life. Something, clearly, is awry.

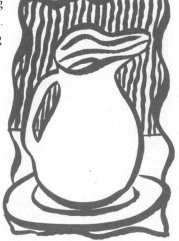

From the viewpoint of Chinese medicine, accumulated fat is the accumulation of Phlegm and Dampness. The transformation of Dampness, as we have seen, is dependent on the strength of the Spleen and the body's Yang. The causes of Spleen weakness and weakness of the Yang are not just about overeating (although this certainly doesn't help) but also about poor food choices and lifestyle habits.

Obesity will not be overcome by starvation diets (which further weaken the Spleen), nor by the consumption of Cold or purgative foods (which further weaken the Yang), but by a diet which nourishes and protects these functions. In other words, unless the Spleen and the Yang are strengthened, weight will always be put back on no matter how well the diet has been adhered to.

The implication of this is that overweight people need to nourish themselves rather than starve or punish themselves in order to regulate obesity. This means eating warm, cooked foods, plenty of vegetables, soups and stews, a little meat and low-fat protein, whole grains and legumes, flavoured with gentle warm-energy pungent herbs and spices that support the digestive fire. Naturally, sugar and saturated fat and refined starch need to be reduced as much as possible, but if over-restrictive, ultra-low calorie, Cold-energy diets are followed, the craving for just those foods will simply increase.

A high vegetable, whole food diet of warm cooked meals will not make anyone fat. Nor will it leave a person feeling chronically hungry. Despite the calorie-counting obsession of the slimming world, losing or gaining weight is not ultimately about calories: it is about fire and internal strength. Nor is maintaining a healthy body weight just about what a person eats. Exercise is vital for strengthening the metabolism and our ability to transform the food we eat. Adequate levels of exercise will actually reduce appetite in most people and put them more in touch with their body's true needs.

If I could offer one piece of advice to those who truly suffer from being overweight, it would be to throw away the diet books, commit to eating the best quality organic wholefood diet and get that body moving. I do not mean to dismiss the genuine difficulty of living in an overweight body. The suffering can be deep. However, I also see immense suffering in the guilt, anxiety and self-hatred that the dieting culture fosters. The steps I have suggested above are intended to reduce some of this suffering.

Deeper at work in the psyche there are often powerful messages about the body that any amount of dieting will not shift. Fashionable magazines are adorned with body images verging on the anorexic; religious teaching frequently reviles the flesh; and natural bodily functions are frequently shamed throughout western culture. Often painful feelings from childhood or earlier experience lie buried in folds of fat and there is a desire to keep them there.

Once responsibility for our own well-being has been accepted and all the sensible measures to regulate weight have been adopted, loving acceptance of the body is the key to the transformation of suffering. It may not be possible to achieve or return to 'perfect' weight. However, if what has been achieved is greater ease and comfort with our own bodies, then perhaps that is enough.

As human beings we need a certain amount of gratification, and if we don't get it in quality we tend to make up for it in quantity

Dr. Dean Ornish

Fasting

Fasting is not commonly practised within Chinese medicine but it does have a time-honoured place in Qi Gong tradition. It has become quite common in the West, perhaps as a reaction to our overconsuming lifestyle and the tendency to accumulate toxins. It therefore seems useful to include a few paragraphs here at the end of this book.

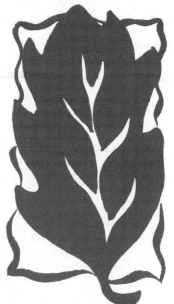

Perhaps the most useful regular fast that we all do is that between supper and next morning's breakfast. The digestive system needs periods of rest, both overnight and between meals. So the habit of continual snacking is seen in Chinese medicine as exhausting to the Spleen. The physical need for more long-term fasting arises when the digestive system needs rest and the body needs encouragement to expel toxins. It may also arise in certain illnesses that affect the digestive system.

There are many ways to fast. What they have in common is a simplification of what we take into our bodies. A water-only fast is suitable for those with a strong constitution. It is best accompanied by extra rest (perhaps during all those hours saved on cooking, eating and washing up!) and the entry and exit from the fast need to be gradual. On entry it is best to prepare the body by eating a cleansing diet for a few days so that the colon is not congested and the body is not shocked by a sudden withdrawal from food. Exit needs also to be gradual, eating only small amounts at first of easily-digested food.

A rice fast will also cleanse the body whilst offering a more continuous energy supply. This simple fast of brown wholegrain rice will gently cleanse the colon, reduce stress throughout the system and remove toxins gradually from the liver. It is a useful fast for those of a more Deficient constitution or for the winter months. A little olive oil and lemon juice can be poured over the rice if desired. Fruit and juice fasts are more cooling, suitable for Hot conditions or hot climates.

It is not generally a good idea to fast when pregnant or breastfeeding or when very weak. The following conditions should also be cause for care and possibly supervision if considering a fast: underweight, weak heart, low blood pressure, diabetes, peptic ulcers and mental illness. Fasting is also more demanding in cold weather. Fasts of more than three or five days may also be best with some supervision. Healing crises often occur during periods of fasting but uncomfortable reactions that persist for more than a day or two should be carefully monitored.

The potential benefits of fasting are great. Waste products can be eliminated from the cells, fat can be converted to energy and toxins are commonly released from the colon, bladder, kidneys, lungs, sinuses and skin. In Chinese medicine terms, Dampness and Heat in particular are resolved by fasting and patterns of Stagnation can also be addressed by this method. In other words, it is conditions of an Excess, congested kind that are most successfully addressed by fasting.

> **Fasting is the opposite of addiction. All addiction numbs us, while fasting leaves us emotionally naked**
>
> Dr Kabir Helminski

Finally, fasting is about more than physical elimination. The most benefit can be had if the fast is accompanied by plenty of rest and good use of the time to withdraw from 'doing' mode into a more reflective and contained way of being. The practice of fasting can be a mental, emotional and spiritual practice. Most people experience greater clarity and inner peace, and renewed energy to deal with what is truly important in life. Fasting brings us to explore more closely our hungers, and by emptying out at the physical level we also have the opportunity to quieten our busy-ness and become more open and receptive to the deeper nature of our experience of this life.

Microwave Ovens

Microwave cookery is significantly different from other methods in that food is heated from the inside outwards. There is no transfer of heat from an external source to the food. Instead, heat is generated by friction between the molecules. Contrary to popular belief, there is considerable destruction of a food's nutritional value during the process of microwave cooking.

Whereas in conventional methods the cell walls of foods will remain intact, the reversal of polarity caused by microwave cookery has been shown to rupture the cell wall and induce destructive changes in the molecular structure of nutrients[42]. Other significant tests show that microwaved breast milk loses much of its immunological properties through microwave heating[43] and that microwaved food causes measurable changes in the blood, indicative of a pathogenic process beginning, similar to those found in the early stages of cancer[44].

It is my own observation that many people who regularly use microwave ovens to cook their food develop or reinforce conditions of Blood Deficiency and that these conditions do not shift until the use of microwaves is reduced. Occasional consumption of microwaved food is unlikely to hurt anybody: its effects are more cumulative and appear to involve lowered immunity and detrimental changes in blood composition.

Anecdotal evidence, reported by anthroposophist A. Bohmert, suggests that microwaved water loses its ability to bring grain to germination[45]. This suggests that the energetic structure of water (and therefore all foods) is harmed by intense exposure to microwave radiation. Because of its military applications, results of research into the effects of microwave radiation tends to be restricted. Until further research has been carried out, I suggest that microwave ovens be treated with extreme caution.

Genetic Engineering [46]

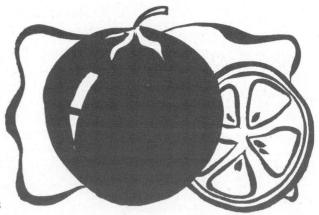

Genetic engineering involves taking genes from one species and inserting them into another in an attempt to reproduce a desired trait. This could mean, for example, selecting a gene which leads to the production of a chemical with antifreeze properties from an arctic fish (such as the flounder), and splicing it into a tomato or strawberry. Natural barriers normally prevent gene transfers of this kind. It is now possible for scientists to cross food plants with genes taken from bacteria, viruses, insects, animals or even humans.

It has been suggested that genetic engineering is simply 'the latest in a 'seamless' continuum of biotechnologies practised by human beings since the dawn of civilisation, from bread and wine-making, to selective breeding.' Although it is true that the food crops we are eating today bear little resemblance to the wild plants from which they originated, there are clear differences between genetic engineering and traditional breeding. In traditional forms of breeding, variety has been achieved through selection from the multitude of genetic traits already existing within a species' gene pool. A rose can be crossed with a different kind of rose, but a rose will never cross with a potato. In nature, genetic diversity is created within certain limits.

There are a number of techniques in the genetic engineer's toolkit. A biochemical process is used to cut the strings of DNA in different places and select the required genes. These genes are usually then inserted into circular pieces of DNA (plasmids) found in bacteria. Because the bacteria reproduce rapidly, within a short time thousands of identical copies (clones) can be made of the 'new' gene. Two principal methods can then be used to insert a 'new' gene into the DNA of a plant that is to be engineered.

1) A 'ferry' is made with a piece of genetic material taken from a virus or a bacterium. This is used to infect the plant and in doing so smuggle the 'new' gene into the plant's own DNA. A bacterium called Agrobacterium tumefaciens (which causes gall formation in plants) is commonly used for this purpose.

2) The genes are coated onto large numbers of tiny pellets made of gold or tungsten, which are fired with a special gun into a layer of cells taken from the recipient plant. Some of these pellets may pass through the nucleus of a cell and deposit their package of genes, which in certain cases may be integrated into the cell's own DNA.

Because the techniques used to transfer genes have an extremely low success rate, the scientists need to be able to find out which of the cells have taken up the new DNA. So, before the gene is transferred, a 'marker gene' is attached, which codes for resistance to an antibiotic. Plant cells which have been engineered are then grown in a medium containing this antibiotic, and the only ones able to survive are those which have taken up the the 'new' genes with the antibiotic-resistant marker attached. These cells are then cultured and grown into mature plants.

As it is not possible to insert a new gene with any accuracy, the gene transfer may also disrupt the tightly controlled network of

DNA in an organism. Current understanding of the way in which genes are regulated is extremely limited, and any change to the DNA of an organism at any point may well have knock-on effects that are impossible to predict or control. The new gene could, for example, alter chemical reactions within the cell or disturb cell functions. This could lead to instability, the creation of new toxins or allergens, and changes in nutritional value.

The food and biotech industries argue that it would be discriminatory to enforce mandatory labelling of GE food, and suggest that this would constitute an illegal trade barrier. Mandatory labelling could mean that not only would consumers be able to boycott GE products, but also that segregation would need to be introduced, potentially making GE food uneconomical for the food industry. There is clearly an issue of civil liberty here: without thorough segregation and labelling, people are unable to exercise free choice.

Labelling of GE food is essential in order to be able to trace any health problems that may arise. In Europe, at the time of this writing, GE soya is present in about 60% of all processed food in forms such as vegetable oil, soya flour, lecithin and soya protein; GE maize can be found in about 50% of processed foods as corn, corn starch, cornflour and corn syrup; and GE enzymes are used widely throughout the food industry. Over 90% of these ingredients are excluded from the current labelling legislation. The only certain way to avoid GE food is to eat organic produce.

The biotech industry is dominated by a handful of multinational corporations which hold interests in food, additives, pharmaceuticals, and chemicals. These corporations are beginning to hold monopolies in the global market for genetically engineered products. This is being facilitated through international free-trade agreements, patenting rights, and a systematic process of acquisitions and mergers. These mergers incorporate seed companies, biotechnology companies and other related interests.

Biotech companies are trying to persuade the public that genetic engineering will reduce the use of damaging herbicides, yet these same companies are actually increasing production capacity for the herbicides themselves and requesting permits for higher residues of these chemicals in GE food. Until now, most of the research by biotech companies has focused on making crops resistant to their own 'broad-spectrum' herbicides. This means that a

Numerous studies show that when more primitive populations begin to consume a western diet, they start dying of heart attacks and cancer. But the main difference between what they're eating and what we're eating is not meat or fats, but whole foods. The culprit appears to be the large-scale adulterating or dismembering of everything we put in our mouths

The Better Diet Book

field can be covered with chemicals and everything will die except for the resistant crop.

International free-trade agreements favour the interest of multi-national corporations and make it difficult for any country to refuse a new product or technology even if they have concerns about its effect on health or the environment. Rather than feed the world, the biotech industry threatens the diversity of truly sustainable farming practices; it has the potential to increase poverty in agricultural communities and drive small farmers from the land; and it will increase the flow of resources from Third World countries to corporations in the industrialised nations.

There is growing evidence that genetic engineering poses new threats to ecosystems. Once released, the new living organisms made by genetic engineering are able to interact with other forms of life, reproduce, transfer their characteristics and mutate in response to environmental influences. They can never be recalled or contained. Any mistakes or undesirable consequences are likely to be passed on to all future generations of life. Resistant weeds and crop pests seem likely to emerge[47], biodiversity could be threatened, new viruses could be created and farmlands may soon become devoid of wildlife[48]. With the planned release of so many GE organisms, and with so little understanding of the way they will interact with the wider environment, it is unsurprising that some of the scenarios imagined are truly nightmarish.

From the viewpoint of Chinese medicine, to intervene at the genetic level is to tamper with the essence (Jing). The Jing is responsible for our proper growth and development and is considered to be a treasure, to be conserved and protected. Damage to the Jing through the unpredictable effects of genetic engineering could result in such consequences as compromised immunity, growth abnormalities and hormonal dysfunction.

In Devon, where I live, public resistance to irresponsible genetic engineering is strong: large-scale public education, court actions against the biotech companies and civil disobedience including the uprooting of trial crops. Positive, empowering actions include the exercise of consumer power by refusing to buy genetically engineered products, by supporting organic growers, pressuring retailers and government agencies, and by becoming educated. I am personally hopeful that the force of public resistance to the short-sighted, power-motivated misuse of science will not only stop it in its tracks, but also add new force to the growing movement towards sustainable, organic and humane agriculture.

For further information see Useful Addresses at the end of this book.

The Energetic Actions of Vitamins, Minerals and Common Drugs

The interpretation of the energetic actions of vitamins, minerals and common drugs listed below is derived mostly from the thoughtful work of Bob Flaws[49] and Dr. Stephen Gascoigne[50] . It is included because of the rising popularity of supplements and the widespread use of western medications. In order to use supplements within the framework of traditional Chinese medicine, an understanding of their energetics is clearly useful. It is also useful in diagnosis to establish whether supplements or medicinal drugs are contributing in any way to a particular condition.

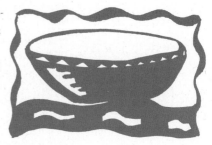

Vitamins

Very broadly speaking, the actions of most vitamins are to tonify and regulate Blood and Qi.

Vitamin A: main action is to tonify and cool the Blood with additional benefit to the bones and eyes

B vitamins: the general action of B vitamins on the nervous system is described in Chinese medicine as easing Liver Qi Constraint/Stagnation. Most B vitamins also nourish the Blood. B6 and Choline help pacify internal Wind; B5 and B6 clear Damp Heat from the Liver and Gall Bladder

Vitamin C: cools Heat and is therefore useful during infection

Vitamin D: may be seen as a Kidney tonic, strengthening the Jing and the bones

Vitamin E: supports the Kidney Yang and nourishes Liver Blood

> If you take a vitamin A pill in the morning, you may be spending the rest of the afternoon looking for the rest of the carrot
>
> AnneMarie Colbin

Vitamin K: has an astringent effect on bleeding. Affects the Intestines and helps contain Lung Qi

Bioflavonoids: clear Heat, especially Liver Heat, and ease Blood Stagnation

Beta-carotene: moves the Qi, clearing Qi Stagnation and reducing Heat

Minerals

Minerals tend to be tonifying to the Yin and strengthening to the Kidney. Some also nourish the Liver. Many nourish sinews and bones, and minerals may generally be seen as supporting the deep structures and processes of the body. They are important to proper growth, development and fertility.

Calcium: strengthens the Yin and the Bones and is generally calming to the Shen

Chromium: tonifies Qi and Blood and strengthens the Spleen

Cobalt: tonifies Qi and Blood

Copper: drains Dampness and Damp Heat, strengthens the Spleen

Fluorine: tonifies the Kidney and the Yin, and is therefore important to the bones and teeth

Iodine: clears Heat, especially from the Liver

Iron: nourishing to the Yin and Blood, cools and disperses blood and is generally cooling to the body

Magnesium: supports the Yin and calms the Shen

Manganese: nourishes both Yin and Jing

Molybdenum: tonifies Blood and Yin and is generally cooling, especially to the Blood

Phosphorus: strengthens the Yin and Jing of the Kidney

Potassium: helps to leach Water and Dampness from the system, is generally cooling and helps clear Damp Heat from the Liver/Gall Bladder

Selenium: nourishes Yin, secures the Jing and calms the Shen

Silica and **Silicon**: general Kidney tonics especially strengthening to the bones

Sodium: strengthening to the Kidney and Liver, softening accumulations (an action of the salty flavour)

Sulphur: Nourishes the Liver and both cools and strengthens the Blood

Zinc: benefits the Jing, Blood and bones

Common Drugs

Western medical drugs can sometimes confuse a traditional Chinese diagnosis. An understanding of their energetics can be helpful in assessing the causes of imbalance.

Anti-Parkinsonian drugs: a hot drug affecting the Liver and Heart

Antibiotics (except sulphonamides): Cold and Damp drugs affecting the Lung, Intestines and Spleen

Antidepressants: hot drugs affecting the Heart and Liver

Antifungals: hot drugs affecting the Spleen and Liver

Aspirin: a warm, dispersing drug affecting the Lung and the Blood

AZT: a hot drug affecting the Liver and Kidney

Betablockers: cold drugs affecting all the Yin Organs

Bronchodilators: warm, dispersing drugs affecting the Lung

Cancer chemotherapy: a hot treatment affecting the Liver

Codeine: a hot drug affecting the Heart, Lung and Large Intestine

Corticosteroids: hot drugs affecting the Lung, Spleen and Kidney

Digoxin: a warm drug affecting the Heart and Kidney

Diuretics: cold drugs affecting the Kidney

For good health we
need a love potion.
No amount of herbs,
pills, injections and
ointments will help
us unless we are kind
to ourselves, to others,
to animals and plants.
Pills must be coated
with compassion;
then they will be
truly effective

Romio Shresta

Female sex hormones: cold drugs affecting the Kidney, Liver, Heart and Spleen

Insulin: a cold drug affecting the Spleen, Lung and Kidney

Nitrates: hot drugs affecting the Heart and Liver

Non-steroidal anti-inflammatories: warm, dispersing drugs affecting the Kidney and Liver

Sulphasalazinine: a warm, dispersing drug affecting the Lung

Sulphonamide: a warm, dispersing drug affecting the Lung and Kidney

Tranquillisers: cold drugs affecting the Heart and Liver

Long-term use of recreational drugs generally damages the Yin and Essence. Most people who are addicted to either alcohol or drugs develop patterns of Liver and Kidney Yin Deficiency. This may be as much the product of a malnourished lifestyle as the influence of the drugs themselves. Over time, patterns of Qi and Yang Deficiency are also likely to emerge. A Yin-nourishing diet, with the support of broad-based mineral and vitamin supplements, is usually the best course of dietary action.

Footnotes

1 See glossary. The Chinese medical term for acupoint is 'qi xue' meaning 'qi hole' or 'qi chamber'. The same term (xue) is used in geomancy to refer to harmonious sites in the landscape which would be selected for burial sites. At these sites the forces of heaven and earth are seen as balanced.

2 The term 'bodymind' is used several times in this book to indicate the inseparable nature of body and mind, a principle that underlies any holistic vision of health.

3 Throughout this book, words which have a specific meaning within Chinese medicine are capitalised. When the same word is used in lower case, this indicates that the common western meaning applies.

4 This story can be found in Esquival, Laura. *Like Water for Chocolate.* Black Swan, 1998 edition.

5 Myss, Carolyn. *Energy Anatomy*, audiotapes. Sounds True, 1996.

6 Edwards, D. 'Your Healthy House'. *What Doctors Don't Tell You*, volume 10, no. 1 (1999).

7 Qi Gong is a self-development practice originating in China. Unlike the aerobic exercise practices of the West, Qi Gong emphasises relaxed attention and conservation of energy. Despite its generally gentle approach, Qi Gong can help a person attain high levels of physical fitness, good health and mental, emotional and spiritual clarity. The practice of Qi Gong is considered by many to be the root of all Chinese medicine.

8 Giono, Jean. *The Man Who Planted Trees.* Chelsea Green, 1985.

9 Walker, Brian (trans.). *Hua Hu Ching*, attributed to Lao Tsu. Harper, 1992, p 106.

10 The meditative practice of 'circulating the Light' is the subject of many oral and written teachings. The following extract is taken from the esoteric Chinese text *The Secret of the Golden Flower*: 'The light is not in the body alone, nor is it only outside the body. Mountains and rivers and the great earth are lit by the sun and moon; all that is light. Therefore it is not only within the body. Understanding and clarity, perception and enlightenment, and all movements (of the spirit) are likewise this light; therefore it is not just something outside the body. The lightflower of heaven and earth fills all the ten thousand spaces.

But also the lightflower of the individual body passes through heaven and covers the earth. Therefore, as soon as the light is circulating, heaven and earth, mountains and rivers, are all circulating with it at the same time.'

The notion of light within the human body is used in W.G. Sutherland's *Contributions to the Science of Osteopathy*. The information that photons are actually produced and circulate within the human body comes from the craniosacral therapy training at the Karuna Institute in Devon, England but I have been unable to trace the original source. The emission of infra-red light from bone, which is perhaps related to this phenomenon, is reported in Becker, Robert. *The Body Electric*. Quill/William Morrow, 1985, pp.128-131.

11   Reported in the *Journal of Chinese Medicine* May 1998. The original research was carried out at the Carnegie Mellon University in Pittsburgh.

12   The theory of meridian development is discussed at length in: Matsumoto, Kiiko and Birch, Stephen. *Hara Diagnosis: Reflections on the Sea*. Paradigm Publications, 1988.

13   See: Bensoussan, Alan. *The Vital Meridian*. Churchill Livingstone 1991. This is a fascinating review of Chinese and western research into the nature of meridians and the mechanisms of acupuncture.

14   Qi Gong is the ancient art of cultivating the subtle energy, or Qi. It is widely practised in China and is becoming increasingly popular in the West. The vast variety of styles can be broadly divided into spiritual, health, martial, medical and paranormal paths of development. See the Recommended Reading section for useful books and addresses.

15   Mast cells are present in most body tissues and are an important part of the immune system. They are particularly involved in allergic response, releasing substances such as histamine into the tissue.

16   In a fascinating experiment, people were tested after receiving healing. All participants showed significant increase in their Spleen energy after healing, suggesting that healing energy is also received via the Spleen. These experiments were carried out by Dr. Motayama and Sandra Hill and reported in: Hill, Sandra. *Reclaiming the Wisdom of the Body*. Constable, 1997.

17   Only a few acupuncturists or Chinese herbalists support the view that the Large Intestine has a major role in immunity. However, it is the common experience of Shiatsu practitioners and some Japanese acupuncturists that the Large Intestine meridian shows up weak when immunity is low and that treatment of the meridian can improve immunity. For a discussion of this issue see: Flaws, Bob. *Scatology and the Gate of Life*. Blue Poppy Press.

18 Bach, E. *Heal Thyself* . C.W. Daniel Company Ltd,1931.

19 A Dutch study reported in *The Journal of Traditional Chinese Medicine* (May 1996) suggests that the consumption of flavonoids, which are found in fruit and vegetables as well as black tea, green tea and red wine, offer protection against heart disease.

20 From: Walker, Brian (trans.). *Hua Hu Ching*. Harper, 1992. This book is sometimes attributed to Lao Tsu but not verified as his work.

21 Zhang Zai (AD 1020-1077), quoted with several other writers exploring this idea by Giovanni Maciocia in: Maciocia, Giovanni. *The Foundations of Chinese Medicine*. Churchill Livingstone, 1989, pp 36-37.

22 The classic text *Simple Questions* ch.23 describes the five 'exhaustions' as follows: 'Excessive use of the eyes injures the Blood (Heart); excessive lying down injures Qi (Lung); excessive sitting injures the muscles (Spleen); excessive standing injures the bones (Kidney); excessive exercise injures the sinews (Liver).'

23 The impact of lifestyle and emotions on the physical body are discussed in the *Simple Questions*. More modern discussion of the relationship between emotional tendencies and the life of the physical body within traditional Chinese medicine can be found in: Seem, Mark. *Bodymind Energetics*. Thorsons, 1987; Requena, Yves. *Character and Health*. Paradigm, 1989; and Diamond, John. *Life Energy and the Emotions*. Edengrove Editions 1997.

24 Although ginseng is easily available over the counter, I suggest that it is better to consult a trained practitioner before using it. Some ginseng can be too heating for certain people.

25 A syndrome is a pattern of disharmony in the bodymind which is diagnosed by the presence of related signs and symptoms. 'Signs and symptoms' must be understood in a much wider sense than is normally meant in the West. A pattern of disharmony can be seen in many aspects of physical function, appearance and emotion. These may include such widely different things as changes in urine, the presence or absence of thirst, vague sensations of heat in the afternoon, irritability, dreaming or changes in facial colour. Signs and symptoms range from the gross and physical to the slight and subtle and reflect Chinese medicine's holistic view of the inter-related nature of all phenomena.

26 Jeffers, Susan. *Feel the Fear and Do It Anyway*. Rider, 1991.

27 William Shakespeare, *Henry V*, Act III Scene I.

28 'The hundred diseases develop from wind': *Su Wen* section 12 chapter 42.

29 The use of the sweet flavour to strengthen the body is a very Chinese concept. In the west, bitter and aromatic flavours have traditionally been used to strengthen the system. It is here that care is needed when importing the medicine of one culture into another. Bitter and aromatic tonics clear out Dampness, stimulate sluggish digestive systems and decongest the Liver (appropriate for a western culture consuming relatively large amounts of meat and alcohol and prone to over-nutrition); sweet tonics nourish the Spleen (suitable for a culture such as China where meat consumption has been traditionally low, grain consumption is high and under-nutrition is common). For this reason it is important to respect the experience of our own culture and not to reach out undiscriminatingly for sweet-flavoured foods at the expense of bitter and aromatic flavours. I am indebted for this insight to an interview with Jeremy Ross published in *The Empty Vessel*, Fall 1998.

30 'Cleansing' is not a concept much talked about in Chinese medicine but is more common to western naturopathy. The Judao-Christian tradition at the root of western culture views the body as essentially dirty and this deeply embodied belief underlies a system of natural medicine which emphasises toxicity as the major cause of disease. This book seeks to translate the concepts of Chinese medicine into a western context and the concept of cleansing is so fundamental to traditional western medicine that I have simply let it be. In terms of Chinese medicine, cleansing may be taken to mean cooling/stimulating Liver function/easing Qi Stagnation/decongesting Blood.

31 Jim Garvey (Garvey, Jim. *The Five Phases of Food*. Well-being Books, 1983) postulates another analysis of food cravings. Basing his idea on the five constituents of cells (carbohydrates, proteins, water, fats and electrolytes), he suggests that craving for carbohydrates indicates Spleen weakness, protein craving indicates Lung weakness, water/fluid craving indicates Kidney weakness, fat craving indicates Liver weakness and craving for stimulants (electrolytes) indicates Heart weakness.

32 Tiquia, Rey. *Traditional Chinese Medicine*. Choice Books, 1996.

33 Mayer, Anne-Marie. 'Historical changes in the mineral content of fruits and vegetables'. *British Food Journal* Volume 99 no. 6, (1997): pp.207–211. This report documents statistically significant reductions in seven out of the eight minerals commonly analysed in food (Na, K, Ca, Mg, P, Fe, Cu, Zn) over the last 50 years in Britain based on figures produced by the Ministry of Agriculture, Fisheries and Food.

34 In the US, the organic food market is currently the fastest growing segment of the grocery industry and a similar trend can be found in Europe. Obtaining organic/naturally grown food is becoming easier

and some suggestions for finding suppliers are included at the end of this book.

35 *Annual Report of the Working Party on Pesticide Residues*. 1993 & 1994. A discussion of this report can be found in *Ethical Consumer* magazine Issue 40 (March/April 1996).

36 Data provided by the Environmental Working Group , tel: (001) 202-667-6982; e-mail: www.ewg.org

37 Chinese medicine is sometimes described in the language of the Five Elements (Earth, Metal, Water, Wood and Fire). Sometimes translated as 'phases', the elements are processes and qualities in nature which can also be seen at work in the human being. According to Giovanni Maciocia 'It could be said that the theory of the five elements, and its application to medicine, marks the beginning of what one might call 'scientific' medicine and a departure from shamanism.' (Maciocia, Giovanni. *The Foundations of Chinese Medicine*. Churchill Livingstone, 1989, p.16).

38 Ehmke, Karen & Jim. *Food For Life*. Whole Health Institute, 1989.

39 The descriptions of the energetic properties of herbs and spices given throughout this book are normally, but not always, in accord with the traditions of Chinese medicine. From time to time, functions ascribed to the herb by traditional western herbalism are reinterpreted as Chinese energetic functions. This is not a question of right or wrong but rather a question of 'marriage', an expression of the fertile meeting of two traditions. Hawthorn, for example, is cited as a herb which nourishes Heart Yin; this is because its use in the west is to nourish the heart muscle and to treat essential hypertension. In Chinese medicine it is used primarily to move food Stagnation and Blood Stagnation. Readers are referred to Peter Holmes' book *The Energetics of Western Herbs* from which I drew most of the instances where such cross-over occurs.

40 *Clin Ortho Related Res*, 152 ;35, (1980), quoted in What Doctors Don't Tell You Vol. 5 no. 1.

41 *Medical World News*, 16 May (1969) reports that cancer-inducing viruses which are resistant to being killed by pasteurisation have been recovered from supermarket supplies.

42 Schrumpf, E./Charley, H. : 'Texture of broccoli and carrots cooked by microwave energy'. *Journal of Food Science*, no. 40, (1975).

43 Quan, R et al. : 'Effects of microwave radiation on anti-infective factors in human milk'. *Pediatrics*, no. 89 (4), (1992).

44 Hertel, H.: 'Are microwave ovens a source of danger?' *Journal of Natural Science* vol. 1 no. 2 (1998).

45 ibid.

46 I am grateful to genetic campaigner Luke Anderson who supplied the information and much of the text for this section.

47 'Probably the greatest threat from genetically altered crops is the insertion of modified virus and insect virus genes into crops. It has been shown in the laboratory that genetic recombination will create highly virulent new viruses from such constructions. Certainly the widely used cauliflower mosaic virus is a potentially dangerous gene. It is a pararetrovirus which means that it multiplies by making DNA from RNA messages. It is very similar to the Hepatitis B virus and related to HIV. Modified viruses could cause famine by destroying crops or cause human and animal diseases of tremendous power.' Dr. Joseph Cummins, Professor Emeritus of Genetics at the University of Western Ontario.

48 'The ability to clear fields of all weeds using powerful herbicides which can be sprayed onto GE herbicide-resistant crops will result in farmlands devoid of wildlife and spell disaster for millions of already declining birds and plants.' Graham Wynne, Chief Executive of the RSPB (Royal Society for the Protection of Birds).

49 These brief descriptions of the energetic actions of vitamins and minerals are mostly taken from the pioneering work of Bob Flaws in his book *Something Old, Something New; Essays on the TCM Description of Western Herbs, Pharmaceuticals, Vitamins and Minerals.* The actions of vitamins, minerals and amino acids are discussed more extensively in this book and in his more recent *The Dao of Healthy Eating* and I am grateful to Bob Flaws for his permission to refer to his descriptions in this book. Please refer to either of Bob Flaws' books for a fuller exploration.

50 This information was kindly provided for me by Dr. Stephen Gascoigne and can be found in Volume Two of his excellent resource book: Gascoigne, Stephen. *The Manual of Conventional Medicine for Alternative Practitioners.* Jigme Press, 1994.

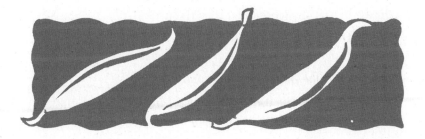

Bibliography

Acupuncture in the Treatment of Children. Julian Scott. Eastern Press, 1991 edition

Arisal of the Clear. Bob Flaws. Blue Poppy Press, 1991

Ayurvedic Cookbook, The. Amadea Morningstar. Lotus Press, 1990

Back to Balance – A Holistic Self-Help Guide to Eastern Remedies. Dylana Accolla with Peter Yates. Kodansha International, 1996

Barefoot Doctor's Manual. Revolutionary Health Committee of Hunan Province. Routledge and Kegan Paul. 1978

Between Heaven and Earth. Harriet Beinfield and Efrem Korngold. Ballantine Books, 1991

Body Electric, The. Robert Becker and Gary Selden. Quill/William Morrow, 1985

Bodymind Energetics – Toward a Dynamic Model of Health. Mark Seem. Thorsons Publishing Group, 1988

Book of Jook, The – Chinese Medicinal Porridges. Bob Flaws. Blue Poppy Press, 1995

Bulletins of the Institute for Traditional Medicine. Institute of Traditional Medicine. 1992-1995

Character and Health. Yves Requena. Paradigm Publications, 1989

Chemistry of Herb Energetics. Christopher Hobbs. Extracted from Michael Tierra's *Planetary Herbology*. Lotus Press, 1988

Chinese Dietary Therapy. Liu Jilin ed.. Churchill Livingstone, 1995

Chinese Foods for Longevity. Henry Lu. Sterling Publishing, 1990

Chinese Herbal Medicine. John Hicks. Thorsons, 1997

Chinese Herbal Medicine. Daniel Reed. Thorsons, 1987

Chinese Medicated Diet. ed. Zhang Enqin. Publishing House of Shanghai College of Traditional Chinese Medicine, 1990

Chinese Medicine. Angela Hicks. Thorsons, 1996

Chinese Medicine, The Web that has no Weaver. Ted Kaptchuk. Rider, 1985

Chinese System of Food Cures. Henry Lu. Sterling Publishing, 1986

Chinese System of Natural Cures. Henry Lu. Sterling Publishing, 1994

Doctor's Manual of Chinese Food Cures and Western Nutrition Volumes 1 and 2. Henry Lu. Academy of Oriental Heritage, 1993 edition

Eating Your Way To Health – Dietotherapy in Traditional Chinese Medicine. Cai Jingfeng. Foreign Languages Press, Beijing, 1988

Energetics of Western Herbs Volumes 1 and 2. Peter Holmes. NatTrop Publishing, 1993 edition

Five Phases of Food. John Garvey. Well-being Books, 1983

Food and Healing. Annemarie Colbin. Ballantine, 1986

Food for Life. Jim and Karen Ehmke and Larry Krantz. Whole Health Institute, 1991

Foundations of Chinese Medicine. Giovanni Maciocia. Churchill Livingstone, 1989

Fruit as Medicine. Dai Yin-fang & Liu Cheng-jun. Rams Skull Press, 1986

Hara Diagnosis: Reflections on the Sea. Kiiko Matsumoto and Stephen Birch. Paradigm Publications, 1988

Healing Cuisine of China, The. Zhuo Zhao & George Ellis. Healing Arts Press, 1998

Healing With Whole Foods. Paul Pitchford. North Atlantic Books, 1993

Herbs of Life. Lesley Tierra. The Crossing Press, 1992

Hua Hu Ching – The Unknown Teachings of Lao Tzu. Brian Walker. Harper, 1994

Keeping Your Child Healthy with Chinese Medicine. Bob Flaws. Blue Poppy Press, 1996

Kitchen Pharmacy, A Book of Healing Remedies for Everyone. Rose Elliot and Carlo De Paoli. Quill William Morrow, 1992

Life Energy and the Emotions. John Diamond. Edengrove Editions, 1997

Manual of Conventional Medicine for Alternative Practitioners. Stephen Gascoigne. Jigme Press, 1994

May All Be Fed – Diet for a New World. John Robbins. William Morrow, 1992

Natural Medicine for Children. Julian Scott. Gaia Books, 1996

Prince Wen Hui's Cook. Bob Flaws. Paradigm Publications, 1993

Publications of Jiangsu Science and Technology Publishing House.
(Yin Shi Zhi Liao Zhi Nan)

Reclaiming the Wisdom of the Body – A Personal Guide to Chinese Medicine. Sandra Hill. Constable, 1997

Secret of the Golden Flower, The. Translated by Richard Wilhelm. Routledge & Kegan Paul, 1962

Secret Treatise of the Spiritual Orchid, The. Claude Larre and Elisabeth Rochat de la Vallee. Monkey Press 1992

Simple Path to Health, The, – A Guide to Oriental Nutrition & Well-being. Kim Le. Rudra Press, 1996

Staying Healthy with Nutrition. Elson Haas. Celestial Arts, 1992

Tao of Health, Sex and Longevity, The. Daniel Reid. Simon & Schuster, 1989

Tao of Natural Breathing, The. Dennis Lewis. Mountain Wind Publishing, 1997

Tao of Nutrition, The. Maoshing Ni. Shrine of the Eternal Breath of Tao, 1987

Traditional Chinese Medicine. Rey Tiquia. Choice, 1996

Traditional Foods Are Your Best Medicine. Ronald Schmid. Healing Arts Press, 1987

Vegetables as Medicine. Chang Chao-liang, Cao Qing-rong and Li Bao-zhen. Rams Skull Press, 1989

Vital Meridian, The, – A Modern Exploration of Acupuncture. Alan Bensoussan. Churchill Livingstone, 1991

Way to Good Health with Chinese Herbs. Hong-Yen Hsu. Oriental Healing Arts Institute, 1982

What Doctors Don't Tell You. Monthly bulletins

Yellow Emperor's Classic of Internal Medicine. Translated by Ilza Veith. University of California Press, 1992

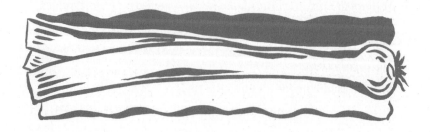

Further Reading

Recipe Books

Cooking with Stones. Stones Print 0 9514076 0 0

A vibrantly alive book containing some of the best vegetarian cookery available in England. Stones restaurant is magically situated alongside the ancient stone circle of Avebury, Wiltshire.

Sundays at Moosewood. The Moosewood Collective. Fireside 0 671 67990 2

Recipes from all over the world lovingly compiled, as served in the famous Moosewood Restaurant. A huge feast of a book.

Healing Foods Cookbook. Jane Sen. Thorsons 0 7225 3322 5

Extraordinarily simple and elegant recipes from the Bristol Cancer Centre and the best food photography I have ever seen.

Kitchen Pharmacy. Rose Elliot and Carlo de Pauli. Quill 0 688 12111 X

A cookbook with a Chinese medicine angle with useful information about the energetics of foods.

The 30-Minute Cook. Nigel Slater. Penguin 0 14 023135 8

As the title suggests, quick but delicious recipes that will inspire even the most reluctant cook.

The Madhur Jaffrey Cookbook. Madhur Jaffrey. Tiger 1 85501 268 5

A classic compendium of Indian and international cuisine.

The Healing Cuisine of China. Zhuo Zhao and George Ellis. Healing Arts Press, 0 89281 778 X

Authentic traditional Chinese recipes with a focus on healing.

The Book of Jook. Bob Flaws. Blue Poppy Press, 0 936185 60 0

A book of Chinese medicinal porridges compiled from Chinese language sources.

Books about Food

Folk Remedies for Common Ailments. Anne McIntyre. Gaia 1 85675 086 8

A very accessible book on the medicinal uses of common foods.

Healing with Whole Foods. Paul Pitchford. North Atlantic Books
0 938190 64 4

An ambitious fusion of eastern and western nutritional theory, a book I tend to reach for when seeking information.

May All Be Fed. John Robbins. Morrow 0 688 11625 6

This book compassionately and wisely sets our cultural eating habits in the context of the whole planet's health and guides us towards an ecologically sustainable eating style. A vitally important book for the twenty-first century showing positive ways forward and, as a bonus, full of excellent recipes.

The Simple Path to Health. Kim Le. Rudra Press 0 915801 62 0

A guide to oriental nutrition and well-being for westerners, simply and elegantly presented. Includes recipes.

Food and Healing. Annemarie Colbin. Ballantine Books 0 345 30385 7

Something of a classic in the field, full of interesting insights into the link between nutrition and health from a largely energetic perspective.

Fruit as Medicine. Dai Yin-Fang and Liu Cheng-Jun. Rams Skull Press 0 909901 61 9

Vegetables As Medicine. Chang Chao-Liang, Cao Qing-Rong and Li Bao-Zhen. Rams Skull Press 0 909901 81 3

Available only in Australia so far as I know, two translations from the Chinese detailing the medicinal uses of common, and uncommon, fruits and vegetables. The best of its kind.

Genetic Engineering: Food and our Environment. Luke Anderson. Green Books 1 870 09878 1

Easy, informative and up-to-date information. A great introduction to the subject.

Books about Chinese Medicine

Principles of Chinese Medicine. Angela Hicks. Thorsons 0 7225 3215 6

A simple, concise and elegant introduction to Chinese medicine. One of the best around.

Five Laws for Healthy Living. Angela Hicks. Thorsons 0 7225 3500 7

Lifestyle advice from the viewpoint of Chinese medicine: accessible, simple and wise.

Principles of Chinese Herbal Medicine. John Hicks. Thorsons
0 7225 3341 1

A good place to start, very lucid and engaging.

Back to Balance. Dylana Accolla and Peter Yates. Kodansha
4 7700 1923 8

Focuses on self-help strategies from the viewpoint of traditional Chinese medicine including diet. A book to keep on the shelf to refer to.

Natural Medicine for Children. Julian Scott. Gaia 1 85675 082 5

Very accessible, includes nutritional advice and the approaches of Chinese medicine, homeopathy and flower remedies.

The Energetics of Western Herbs Volume I & II. Peter Holmes.
NatTrop Publishing 0 9623477 3 6/Snow Lotus Press 0 9623477 4 4

A treasure trove, very thorough and inspiring, and it takes up a lot of room on the shelf.

Reclaiming the Wisdom of the Body. Sandra Hill. Constable
0 09 477340 8

A personal interpretation of traditional Chinese medicine by a very experienced practitioner. Very wise and includes a good section on Qi Gong.

Between Heaven and Earth. Harriet Beinfeld and Efrem Korngold.
Ballantine Books 0 345 35942 7

Very articulately written book about Chinese medicine with a strong focus on Chinese herbs.

The Way of Energy. Lam Kam Chuen. Gaia 1 85675 020 5

An excellent book about Qi Gong, safe and easy to use.

Keeping Your Child Healthy with Chinese Medicine. Bob Flaws.
Blue Poppy Press 0 936185 71 6

A practical and readable book in which an experienced practitioner shares his wisdom.

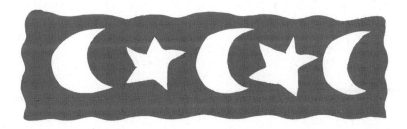

Useful Addresses

Organic and naturally grown food

UK

The Organic Directory (ISBN 1 900322 09 0), published by Green Earth Books, Foxhole, Dartington, Totnes TQ9 6EB tel: 01803 863260

A comprehensive compendium of retail outlets, home delivery schemes, organic farms, organic associations and so on. An immensely valuable directory that will guide you painlessly to your nearest source of organic produce.

USA

National Campaign for Sustainable Agriculture, PO Box 396, Pine Bush, NY 12556 tel: 914 744 8448

The Organic Trade Association, PO Box 1078, Greenfield, MA 01302 tel: 202 338 2900 www.ota.com

*Community Alliance for Family Farmer*s tel: 530 756 8518 e-mail: CAFF@caff.org. A good source for locating your nearest organic farmers. You could also try your local County Extension office or State Department of Agriculture for information. Alternatively, there are many CSA's (Community Supported Agriculture groups) through which it is possible to receive locally-produced food.

Qi Gong

UK

Zhixing Wang, Chinese Heritage, Katana House, Shillingford Bridge, Nr. Wallingford, Oxon OX10 8NA

Tse Qi Gong Centre, POBox 116, Manchester M20 3YN tel: 0161 929 4485

Lam Kam Chuen, The Lam Clinic, 70 Shaftesbury Avenue, London, W1V 7DF

BuQi College UK, 28 Withleigh Road, Knowle, Bristol BS4 2LQ tel: 0117 907 3380

USA

National Qi Gong Association, 571 Selby Avenue, St Paul MN 55102 tel: 888 218 7788

World Qi Gong Federation/American Qi Gong Association, 450 Sutter Street, Suite 2104, San Francisco, CA 94108 tel: 415 788 2227

Canada

World Natural Medical Foundation, 9904 106 Street, Edmonton, Alberta T5K IC4 tel: 403 426 2760 fax: 403 426 5650

Australia

Qi Gong Association of Australia, 458 White Horse Road, Surrey Hills, Victoria 3127 tel: 03 836 6961

Oriental Medicine

UK

British Acupuncture Council, Park House, 206 Latimer Road, London W10 6RE tel: 0181 964 0222

Register of Chinese Herbal Medicine, PO Box 400, Wembley, Middlesex HA9 9NZ tel: 0181 904 1357

The Shiatsu Society, Eastlands Court, St Peters Road, Rugby CV21 3QP tel: 01788 555051 www.shiatsu.org

USA

National Commission for Certified Acupuncturists and Oriental Medicine (NCCAOM), POBox 97075, Washington DC 97075 tel: (202) 232 1404

American Oriental Bodywork Association (AOBTA), 1000 Whitehouse Road, Suite 510, Voorhes NJ 08043 tel: (609) 782 1616

Australia

Australian Traditional Medicine Society, 120 Blaxland Road, Ryde, New South Wales 2112 tel: 809 6800

National Herbalists Association of Australia, POBox 61, Broadway, New South Wales 2007 tel: 02 211 6452

Environmental Organisations

UK

Friends of the Earth, 56-58 Alma Street, Luton, LU1 2PH tel: 01582 482297. A good source of information on a range of environmental issues with plenty of opportunity for you to get involved

Oxfam Trading, POBox 72, Bicester, Oxon, OX6 7LT. Oxfam Trading are a good source of fairtraded foods. They have a catalogue as well as many retail outlets throughout the country

Greenpeace, Canonbury Villas, London N1 2PN tel: 0171 865 8100 fax: 865 8200/1

USA

Greenpeace, 568 Howard Street, 3rd Floor, San Francisco, CA 94105

Genetic Engineering

UK

Genetic Engineering Network, PO Box 9656 London N4 4NL tel: 0181 374 9516 e-mail genetix@gn.apc.org

A good place to start to find local groups and information sources. They produce a free informative newsletter called Genetix Update.

Soil Association, Bristol House 40-56 Victoria Street, Bristol BS1 6B tel: 0117 9142449 The main accrediting body for organic produce

Gaia Foundation, 18 Well Walk, London NW3 1LD tel: 0171 4355000

USA

Campaign for Food Safety, 860 Highway 61, Little Marais, Minnesota 55614 tel: 218 226 4164 e-mail: http//www.purefood.org

The best place to start finding out about genetic engineering and other issues of food quality

Australia

Australian Gene Ethics Network, 340 Gore Street Fitzroy 3065 Victoria tel: 03 94 16 22 22 e-mail acsgcnet@teg.apc.org

Index of Foods and Recipes

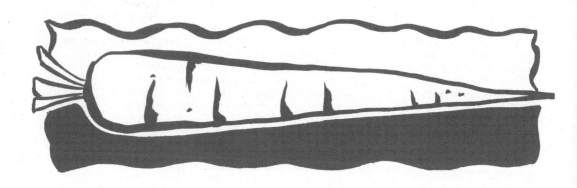

General Index

Other Publications by Meridian Press

Helping Ourselves: A Guide to Traditional Chinese Food Energetics by Daverick Leggett. Illustrations by Katheryn Trenshaw. ISBN 0 9524640 0 4

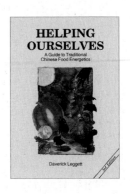

'There are other guides to Chinese dietary therapy on the market, but none that I have seen makes the subject so readily accessible.'
European Journal of Oriental Medicine

Helping Ourselves is a concise guide to traditional Chinese food energetics. The book contains charts detailing the energetic properties of about 300 common foods, and succinct explanations of the principles of Chinese medicine in an easy-to-read format. Highly acclaimed by the traditional Chinese medicine press, it has found its way into the homes of those with no previous knowledge of Chinese medicine as well as on to the recommended reading lists of many major schools of oriental medicine. As useful for the lay person as it is for the professional practitioner, it forms a trilogy with the *Energetics of Food wallchart* and *Recipes for Self-Healing*. Simple, accessible and brief, it is one of the most user-friendly guides on the market.

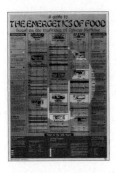

The Energetics of Food wallchart by Daverick Leggett. 45x64cm. Illustrations by Katheryn Trenshaw. ISBN 0 9524640 1 2

'A masterly condensation of information.' *Shiatsu Society News*

This full colour wallchart is the ideal companion to both *Recipes for Self-Healing* and *Helping Ourselves*. Attractively designed, fully laminated and easy to use, it enables you to find at a glance the energetic properties of about 300 common foods. For anyone wishing to apply the principles of food energetics in their own kitchen, *The Energetics of Food* is the perfect companion.

Prices and ordering

These publications can be ordered direct from Meridian Press.

Helping Ourselves £9.95 plus £1.50 p&p
The Energetics of Food £7.50 plus £1.50 p&p
Recipes for Self-Healing £16.95 plus £3 p&p

Discounted prices for combined purchases:

Recipes for Self-Healing plus *Helping Ourselves*
£24 plus £4.50 p&p
Recipes for Self-Healing plus *The Energetics of Food*
£21.50 plus £4.50 p&p
Helping Ourselves plus *The Energetics of Food*
£15 plus £3 p&p

All three titles £30 plus £6 p&p

European orders please add £1.50 per item and all other overseas orders add £3 per item. Please make cheques payable in pounds sterling.

Cheques should be made payable to **Meridian Press**. Please send payment with order to Meridian Press, PO Box 3, Totnes, Devon TQ9 5WJ, England.

For details of wholesale prices please contact Meridian Press.

Meridian Press publications are distributed in the USA by **Redwing Book Company**, 44 Linden Street, Brookline, MA 02445 tel: 1800 873 3946 fax: 617 738 4620 and in Australia by **China Books**, 234 Swanston Street, Melbourne, Victoria 3000 tel: 03 9663 8822 fax: 03 9663 8821

Meridian Press
PO Box 3, Totnes, Devon TQ9 5WJ, England
tel/fax: 01803 863552
e-mail: post@meridianpress.net
www.meridianpress.net

Notes

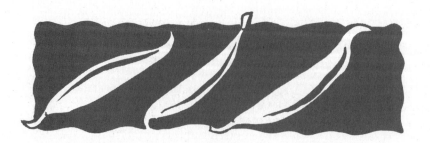

Notes

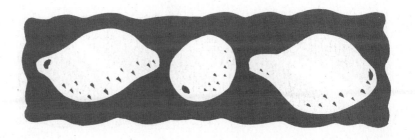

Notes

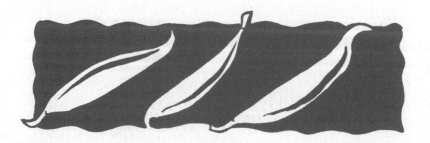

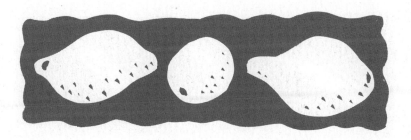

Notes

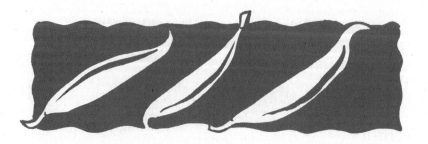

Notes

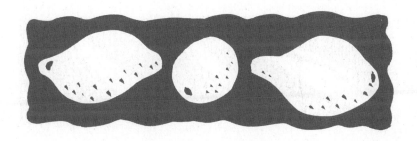

Notes

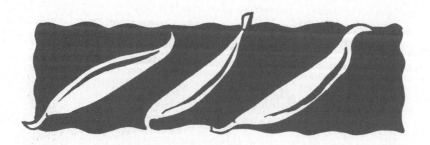

Notes

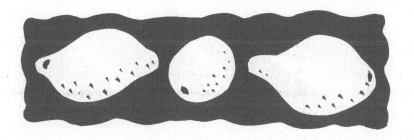

Notes

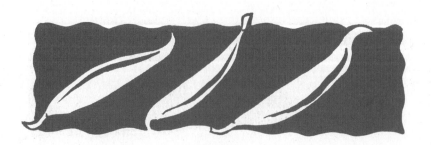

Notes

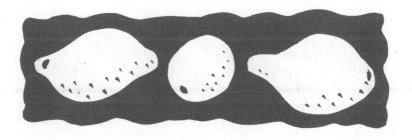

Notes

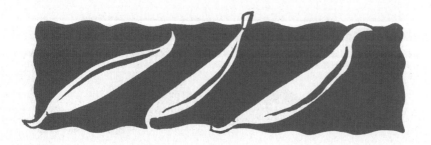

Notes

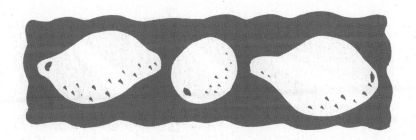

Notes

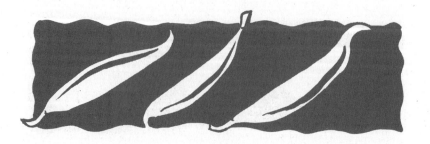

Notes

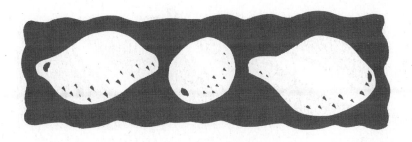

Notes

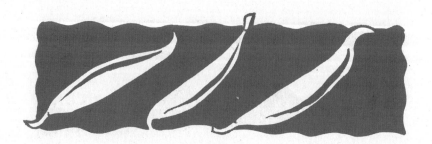

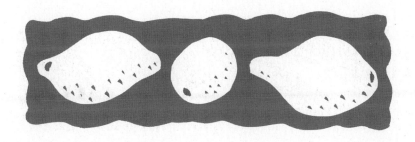